Radiology of the
Salivary Glands

Radiology of the Salivary Glands

Keith Rabinov, M.D.
Director of Radiology, Cardinal Cushing General Hospital
Brockton, Massachusetts
Assistant Clinical Professor of Radiology, Harvard Medical School
Lecturer in Radiology, Tufts Medical School
Boston, Massachusetts

Alfred L. Weber, M.D.
Chief of Radiology, Massachusetts Eye and Ear Infirmary
Radiologist, Massachusetts General Hospital
Associate Professor of Radiology, Harvard Medical School
Boston, Massachusetts

G. K. HALL MEDICAL PUBLISHERS • BOSTON

G. K. Hall Medical Publishers
70 Lincoln Street
Boston, Massachusetts 02111

85 86 87 88 / 4 3 2 1

Rabinov, Keith R.
  Radiology of the salivary glands.

  Includes index.
  1. Salivary glands—Radiography. 2. Diagnosis,
Radioscopic. I. Weber, Alfred L. II. Title.
RC815.5.R33 1984   616.3'1607572   84-19221
ISBN 0-8161-2111-7

Copyediting supervised by Michael Sims. Designed by
Carole Rollins. Set in 10½/13 ITC Garamond by R/tsi
Typografic Co., Inc.

The author and publisher have worked to ensure that all
information in this book concerning drug dosages,
schedules, and routes of administration is accurate at the
time of publication. As medical research and practice
advance, however, therapeutic standards may change. For
this reason, and because human and mechanical errors will
sometimes occur, we recommend that our readers consult
the *PDR* or a manufacturer's product information sheet
prior to prescribing or administering any drug discussed in
this volume.

Contents

Foreword

The growth and development of diagnostic radiology in its first 30 years or so was entirely in the hands of general diagnostic radiologists who developed an unusual ability to interpret radiographic and fluoroscopic findings and, to a certain extent, contributed to some of the technical advances in the specialty. As time went on, however, the increasing depth of required knowledge generated the need for special concentration of individuals in a specific organ system in order for them to be able to contribute to and advance the field. Nowhere is this more apparent than in this volume on the radiology of the salivary glands, written by two extremely experienced radiologists with special interest in this area. This book represents the cumulation of much of the professional experience of the two authors. Their case material illustrates nearly every disease entity and variation the radiologist is likely to encounter.

The discussion of how to examine the salivary glands radiologically is unusually thorough and complete, and the same is true of the chapters dealing with inflammatory and neoplastic conditions.

I am delighted to have been asked by the authors to write this foreword. The link between head and neck radiology and neuro-radiology continues to grow stronger with advances in the areas of computed tomography and magnetic resonance imaging. I believe that the ability of computed tomography to show calcifications and benign and malignant tumors, and to demonstrate the ductal system via radiopaque contrast material, will keep CT as the procedure of choice in the examination of the salivary glands.

I trust that this book will become a true classic in the evaluation of salivary gland diseases and that it will remain so for years to come.

Juan M. Taveras, M.D.
Radiologist-in-Chief
Massachusetts General Hospital
Professor of Radiology
Harvard Medical School

Preface

Pain, swelling, or palpable mass in the region of the salivary glands are common complaints. Diagnostic studies may be required to determine the nature and seriousness of such complaints and to demonstrate any underlying organic changes that may be present. This monograph concerns the radiologic examination of the salivary apparatus, with special attention to sialography and computed tomography (CT) of the parotid and submandibular glands.

Sialography, performed by opacifying the salivary ducts and glands with radiopaque contrast material, has been available for more than 50 years. Its lack of popularity in some centers may be related to past technical difficulties in performance, fear of complications, or doubt about its merits. Recent refinements in instrumentation and technique have augmented the speed, ease, and success of sialography, added to the accuracy of interpretation, and have sometimes been of therapeutic value.

CT is rapidly achieving a dominant role in the examination of masses in and about the salivary glands. Radionuclide scanning and ultrasonography may provide supplementary or complementary diagnostic information. The place of magnetic resonance imaging in the diagnosis of salivary gland disease is undetermined, but its multiplanar display and its enhanced ability to differentiate between various tissues suggest almost limitless imaging potential.

Based on courses that we conducted at the annual meetings of the Radiological Society of North America in 1978–1980, this book is intended to serve as a reference and didactic course in the radiology of the salivary glands.

Since the modern practice of sialography is constructed upon the past contributions of many and can best be appreciated in this light, the most important of these contributions are identified. Particular emphasis is placed upon those developments that have had a lasting impact and that we have found most useful and reliable in our practice.

We present detailed recommendations for the performance of sialography, with emphasis on understanding all aspects of normal sialography, including normal roentgen anatomy and a description of the events occurring within the salivary glands during sialography. Artifactual appearances, including a number of commonly seen but not necessarily widely recognized patterns of extravasation, are identified. The radiologic findings associated with local or systemic disease processes that affect the salivary glands are shown, with radiologic-pathologic correlations where possible. Pertinent embryologic, histologic, anatomic, physiologic, and pathologic information is integrated into the text where appropriate so that the radiologic findings may be more confidently understood.

The indications for the performance of sialography and CT, the practical clinical benefits that may be anticipated, and the pitfalls and limitations of these examinations are noted.

Although interventional procedures have had only limited application to diseases of the salivary glands and ducts, they can be quite effective in selected instances and the techniques and indications for their performance are described.

Needle biopsy is being used increasingly for histologic diagnosis, and its application and usefulness are discussed.

We would like to thank Dr. Kurt J. Bloch, Massachusetts General Hospital, for reviewing the chapter on Sjögren's syndrome. We would also like to thank Mrs. Nancy Richmond for her help in typing and preparation of the manuscript.

Chapter 1   The Technique of Sialography

Historical Background

Comprehensive historical accounts of the contributions of many early investigators have been published elsewhere (Thomas 1956; O'Hara 1973; Blair 1973; Micheli-Pellegrini and Polayes 1976) and cover production of models of anatomic specimens, early radiographs, and the first use and subsequent popularization of sialography.

Casts of anatomic specimens of salivary glands have been made after injection with plaster of paris or wax since the thirteenth century (Gioffre and DiPietro 1963). Study of such casts continues to be of value in the understanding of radiologic anatomy (Rubin et al. 1955; Winsten, Gould, and Ward 1956) (fig. 1.1).

The first radiographs of the ducts of the parotid gland were made in 1900 by Charpy following the injection of mercury into an isolated parotid gland. According to Redon (1955), Arcelin in 1902 was the first to conceive and accomplish sialography. Barraud (1931) cites a reference to the work of Arcelin (1913) who published a case report of a submandibular sialogram performed by injecting a bismuth solution into the submandibular duct prior to radiography. Unfortunately, despite extensive efforts, we have not been able to locate and confirm these references to the work of Arcelin, possibly because of the long interval of time since his work was reported.

Sialography was popularized as a clinical method by investigators reporting independently from different countries in 1925 (Barsony; Uslenghi) and 1926 (Carlsten; Wiskovsky; Jacobovici, Poplitza, and Albu). During the following three decades, technical refinements were made and radiologic-pathologic correlations were established; thorough reviews of the entire subject have been published periodically (Garusi 1964; O'Hara 1973).

Modern methods of sialography are based on techniques, equipment, materials, and concepts that have been progressively developed and highly refined over the past half-century, but especially in the past 25 to 30 years. Some of the most important refinements are:

1. Improvements in instruments such as probes, dilators, cannulas, and catheters.
2. The development of more suitable contrast materials.
3. Introduction of the "closed system" of injection.
4. Use of fluoroscopy, image intensification and television, and spot films.
5. Development of fine focal spot x-ray tubes.
6. Use of radiographic-photographic methods such as laminography, xerography, magnification, and subtraction.
7. Development of special methods of examination such as radioscintigraphy, ultrasound, and computed tomography (CT).
8. Description of the phases of sialography and events that occur during the injection of contrast material, especially demonstration of the radiologic-histologic correlation of events that occur during the acinar opacification phase.
9. Recognition of the patterns of extravasation of contrast material that occur as artifacts of injection in normal parenchyma and as a reflection of pathology in diseased glands.

The significance of each of these advances to the practice of clinical sialography will be discussed under the appropriate sections that follow. The historical background will be given first, followed by the current recommendations for technique.

Conventional sialography of only the parotid and submandibular glands is discussed in the text that follows. The sublingual gland can sometimes be examined by this method (Liliequist and Welander 1970), but such studies have not been shown to have much practical clinical value. Tumors of all the salivary glands, including those of the minor salivary glands can, of course, be demonstrated by CT.

Indications for Sialography

Although sialography can produce clinically useful information that may help to establish diagnosis and indicate appropriate therapy (Yune and Klatte 1972; Calcaterra et al. 1977), this examination is not universally applied to the diagnosis of salivary gland disease. Some use it rarely or only under limited circumstances (Quinn 1976). Others use it almost regularly, preferring to have as much information as possible before making a clinical decision and embarking upon a course of treatment (Yune and Klatte 1972). In a series of 100 patients reported by Adam and colleagues (1983), parotid sialography provided significant information in 54 patients, and in just under one third of patients it provided new or unexpected information. In 22% of patients the diagnosis was reached on sialographic appearances alone, or the sialographic findings altered the treatment. Some reasons (Gates 1977) for using sialography are: (1) clinical signs and symptoms of diseases of the salivary glands tend to be nonspecific, (2) concern on the part of the physician that a malignant tumor will be missed, (3) objective confirmation of pathology to the patient by a "test," and (4) help in determining whether treatment can be done on an outpatient basis.

The salivary glands, like many other organs, may react to diverse disease processes with a limited number of clinical manifestations, such as pain, enlargement, or diminished function, so that signs and symptoms tend to be nonspecific. Furthermore, there are situations where symptoms are present but without definite objective signs of disease; in such circumstances sialography can demonstrate normal salivary structures or indicate disease. The only alternative to the use of conventional sialography or one of the other radiologic examinations (such as CT) may be to rely upon the clinical impression alone or to perform exploratory surgery.

In addition to showing whether pathology is present, sialography may provide many kinds of specific information that may greatly influence clinical decisions. For example, it may demonstrate whether pathology arises from within or outside the salivary apparatus. It may show the exact site and extent of a disease process, and it may indicate whether the process is purely local or is a manifestation of a more generalized or even systemic disease. The findings are often diagnostic of a specific entity and, in most instances, will indicate an appropriate choice of treatment. Thus, sialography can provide important information that may have a direct influence on therapy.

The frequency with which sialography may change a clinical diagnosis and intended therapy has also been discussed by Yune and Klatte (1972). In their series, more than 50% of the patients with a clinical diagnosis of neoplasm of the salivary gland had their final diagnosis changed from neoplasm to inflammation or other nonneoplastic condition based upon the results of sialography. Calcaterra and colleagues (1977) pointed out the importance of distinguishing between intrinsic and extrinsic masses, since intrinsic masses in general require prompt surgical excision, while extrinsic masses, which may be due to adjacent infection, metastasis, or tumor of adjacent structures, might be better dealt with by other diagnostic or therapeutic measures such as treatment for infection or a search for an unknown primary tumor. These authors pointed out also that the demonstration of inflammatory changes in the duct system would indicate a workup for infectious disease, allowing time for treatment and resolution of a mass before considering surgery. Som and Biller (1980) and Stone and co-workers (1981) point out the further importance of determining the intrinsic versus the extrinsic origin of a tumor, since the surgical approaches to remove such masses may be technically entirely different according to their location and site of origin.

Some of the clinical situations in which we have found sialography or other radiologic studies of the salivary glands to be helpful are:

1. Sudden acute swelling of a salivary gland, especially during eating, commonly of a transitory nature and often recurrent; such swelling suggests obstruction of a salivary duct, most often caused by a calculus. It may also be caused by stricture, mucus impaction, or acute inflammation of a salivary gland.

2. Gradual progressive enlargement or chronic recurrent enlargement of one or several salivary glands lasting days, weeks, months, or years; such enlargement suggests chronic infection, sialosis (benign parotid hypertrophy), benign lymphoepithelial lesion, sarcoidosis, and occasionally, neoplasm. The submandibular salivary glands may normally become more prominent with increasing age, probably because the muscles and fascia supporting them weaken, allowing the glands to sag slightly.

3. A suspected or clinically palpable mass; this finding suggests a tumor, cyst, enlarged lymph node, or focal area of inflammation.

4. Recurrent sialadenitis.

5. Pain.

6. Dryness of the mouth; this may result from loss of function of the salivary gland such as occurs with benign lymphoepithelial disease, chronic infection, or other processes replacing the parenchyma or destroying its function. Radionuclide scanning can be very helpful in quantifying the functional capability of a salivary gland.

7. Postoperative or posttraumatic salivary fistula or soft fluctuant swelling suggesting sialocele.

8. Surgical considerations: to determine the amount of damage to a gland and its salvageability; to indicate an appropriate site for biopsy; to demonstrate whether a mass is intrinsic or extrinsic to the salivary glands, and if intrinsic, whether it is in the superficial or deep part of the gland; to demonstrate the likely relationship of a mass to the facial nerve and to adjacent structures. CT plays a dominant role not only in determining the presence or absence of a mass but also in demonstrating the pertinent anatomic details of the lesion.

9. The collection of saliva; measurement of the flow of saliva from a submandibular gland compared with that from the opposite gland may be used to determine the level of injury to the facial nerve in the presence of Bell's palsy, trauma, or tumor. By combining the information so obtained with data from other tests, the injury to the facial nerve can be determined to be above or below the temporal bone or at a specific location within the temporal bone (Schvey and Polayes 1976). For example, if a lesion involves the facial nerve above the separation of the chorda tympani, salivary flow from the affected submandibular gland will be diminished on that side accordingly. On the other hand, if the injury to the facial nerve is below the chorda tympani, salivary flow will not be disrupted and will be equal to that of the opposite side. Furthermore, prognostic value can be attached to the preservation of salivary gland function in the presence of Bell's palsy in that if 40% or more of normal salivary flow on stimulation is preserved, spontaneous remission of the paralysis is probable (Blatt 1962).

   Collection of saliva from the salivary glands for measurement of flow or qualitative or quantitative analysis may also help in the study of many other systemic conditions such as cystic fibrosis, Addison's disease, Cushing's disease, and hypertension (Wotman and Mandel 1976; Rice 1977).

10. Therapeutic reasons for performing cannulation and/or sialography include dilation of strictures of the salivary ducts and removal of calculi through the duct orifice.

Contraindications to Performing Sialography

There are conditions under which sialography should not be performed:

1. When there is acute infection in the salivary gland; the examination may aggravate symptoms.

2. Known sensitivity to iodine-containing compounds usually is considered to be a contraindication to performance of sialography. We have not experienced any cutaneous, pulmonary, cerebral, circulatory, or other systemic toxic or allergic reactions to contrast materials injected during sialography. One instance of a serious reaction has, however, been reported (Ansell 1968).

3. Anticipated thyroid function tests should be performed prior to sialography since retained iodine may interfere with these tests.

Instruments for Sialography

Probes and Dilators

Background

Various probes made of metal or other materials have been used to identify and dilate the salivary duct orifice, especially that of the submandibular gland. "Flexible" probes were used by Barsky and Silberman in 1932. Use of root canal probes was suggested by Drevattne and Stiris (1964), and whalebone bougies were suggested by Putney and Shapiro in 1950 and by Eisenbud and Cranin in 1963. Most authors have used lacrimal probes (Blady and Hocker 1938, 1939; Winsten, Gould, and Ward 1956; Ollerenshaw and Rose 1957; Rubin and Holt 1957; Gullmo and Book-Hederstrom 1958; Park and Mason 1966; Park and Bahn 1968; Reid 1969; Meine and Woloshin 1970; Yune and Klatte 1972; Blair 1973; Martin 1975; Lowman and Cheng 1976; Manashil 1976, 1978). Cook and Pollack (1966) used a fine polyethylene probe. A Teflon catheter with blunted stainless steel obturator was suggested by Hettwer (1969), and an obturator and plastic sheath from a spinal needle was suggested by Harwell (1978). Most of these instruments are rigid and their use entails some risk of perforation of the duct wall. Horsehairs or nylon suture material have been used to locate and dilate the duct orifice and to guide the catheter into the duct (Thomas 1956; Liverud 1959). Suzuki and Kawashima (1969) used a Seldinger wire as a guide for the catheter, but reported some failures in cannulating the submandibular duct. Use of flexible nylon eustachian bougies for sialography was reported by Marano, Smart, and Kolodny in 1971.

Recommended Technique

Preliminary use of a probe usually is not required for cannulation of the parotid duct but often is necessary for cannulation of the submandibular duct. We prefer to use the olive-tipped filiform nylon bougie recommended by Marano, Smart, and Kolodny (1971) as the initial instrument to identify and enter the duct (fig. 1.2). It is very flexible and safe to use and can be placed successfully in almost any salivary duct orifice. It is not an effective dilator, however, since it tapers over a relatively long distance (8 cm) and thus must be placed deeply into the duct in order to dilate the duct orifice to the full diameter of the shaft. Therefore, we have modified this probe into a second instrument by tapering it over a shorter distance (2.0 cm) so that it can function as a dilator and need not be advanced more than this distance into the duct in order to obtain full dilatation (fig. 1.2). Its distal portion is somewhat stiffer as a consequence, but it is still much more flexible than a metal probe. The diameter of these nylon probes and dilators is 0.020 inches at the olive tip and 0.038 inches at the shaft. A stainless steel dilator of similar measurements to the nylon dilator but tapering over 1.5 cm has also been made and has proved helpful in many instances (fig. 1.2).

Because the olive tip of each of these instruments is small enough to enter almost any duct orifice, even of most submandibular glands, and the shaft of the dilators is the diameter of the largest cannula used, it is not necessary to insert progressively larger probes in order to obtain a satisfactory orifice for cannulation. Several sets of such graduated probes are commercially available, however, and the smallest size of these may occasionally be helpful. Williams lacrimal probes are olive tipped and Bowman lacrimal probes are plain tipped. Great care must be used with any of these metal instruments to avoid perforation of the duct wall.

Cannulas and Catheters: The "Closed System"

Injection systems may be classified as open or closed, according to whether a column of contrast injectate is continuously maintained into the gland throughout the entire procedure (Rubin and Blatt 1955; Rubin et al. 1955). In the open system, injection is done through blunt needles or cannulas of various designs connected directly to the syringe and either disconnected or removed from the duct before films are obtained (Kimm, Spies, and Wolfe 1935; Eisenbud and Cranin 1963, Einstein 1966). This system has several disadvantages: the injection cannot be carried out under fluoroscopic monitoring because of radiation exposure to the operator's hand, although the injection could be done fractionally between fluoroscopic observations; the possibilities for moving the patient's head into optimal positions are limited for fear of dislodging the cannula; and the contrast material may leak out of the ducts and gland during exposure of the radiographs.

A number of blunt needles or cannulas for open sialography have been commercially available in the past. Many of these, including one recently designed by Lowman and Belleza (1976), can be connected either to a syringe or to an extension tubing, thereby creating a closed system (Gullmo and Book-Hederstrom 1958). In the closed system, a catheter is left in place in the duct so that evacuation of the contrast material from the duct and gland is prevented until the examination is completed. Although ureteral or other catheters had been used earlier (Carlsten 1926; Steinhardt 1942; Putney and Shapiro 1950), the widespread use of catheters for sialography had to await the development and ready availability of flexible plastic catheters. Their routine use in sialography was recommended by Rubin and associates (1955) and subsequently by others (Liverud 1959; Hettler and Lauth 1961; Drevattne and Stiris 1964; Park and Mason 1966; Potter 1973).

The use of flexible catheters allows the necessary time and mobility to perform a detailed examination with fluoroscopy and spot films, and special radiographic projections if necessary, and to observe and record the filling and evacuation phases. The rate of injection and the total amount of contrast material injected can be carefully adjusted under fluoroscopic monitoring. There is no danger of contrast material being lost from the gland prematurely. Injection of water-soluble contrast materials, which are absorbed through the gland, may be continued as necessary without interruption throughout the entire examination. Radiation exposure to the examiner's hands is avoided.

A number of investigators have drawn plastic catheters to a fine tip for easy insertion (Liverud 1959; Drevattne and Stiris 1964; Park and Mason 1966; Park and Bahn 1968; Suzuki and Kawashima 1969). Others have introduced the catheter over a metal stylet (Rubin and Blatt 1955), over a guide of horsehair or nylon thread (Liverud 1959; Drevattne and Stiris 1964), and over a Seldinger guidewire (Suzuki and Kawashima 1969).

In the past 10 years, flexible catheters with prepared metal cannulas attached have become available in various sizes (Rabinov and Joffe 1969; Manashil 1976; Rabinov 1981a,b). Manashil (1977) suggested modifying these cannulas by incorporating a metal coil into the distal part of the catheter. Som and Khilnani (1982) recommended a modified butterfly infusion set.

Recommended Technique

We prefer to use catheters with prepared metal cannulas attached. The array of cannulas already described (Rabinov and Joffe 1969; Rabinov 1981a) has been modified and expanded so that these are now available in four different diameters and two different lengths (Rabinov 1981b) (fig. 1.3). The largest, made from 18-gauge thin-walled metal tubing (0.049 inches overall diameter) has a blunt smooth closed tapering to an end 0.032 inches (21 gauge) in diameter. Its taper provides for wedging it into place to prevent loss of contrast material. The location of the port on the side of the cannula avoids blocking of flow, which sometimes can occur with end-port cannulas when the end of the cannula is against the duct wall (Gullmo and Book-Hederstrom 1958; Drevattne and Stiris 1964). If the duct diameter is very small or stenotic, however, an end-port cannula should be used, since the side port itself may be occluded by the tightly fitting duct wall. The other three cannulas have end ports and measure 0.022 inches (24 gauge), 0.016 inches (27 gauge), and 0.012 inches (30 gauge) in diameter.

The cannulas each come in a shorter length (approximately 1.5 cm for the side-port cannula and 0.8 cm for the end-port cannulas) and a longer length (approximately 4.5 cm).

The end-port cannulas are fitted with a tapered metal collar or plastic sheath for obturation of the duct orifice. This device is located approximately 8 mm proximal to the tip of the cannula. If the duct is unusually patulous, even the collar portion of the catheter may be placed into the orifice It is, however, ordinarily not necessary or desirable to extend a cannula deeply into the duct, since calculi may then be bypassed by the cannula.

These various cannulas, especially the largest one, provide an excellent method for the collection of saliva. The cannula may be placed into a duct orifice and the saliva allowed to drip into a receptacle.

Ethiodol may be injected through the three larger cannulas. Ethiodol will pass only slowly drop by drop through the 0.012-inch cannula even with considerable sustained hand pressure or by the hydrostatic delivery method. Water soluble contrast materials can be used with any of the cannulas.

Other helpful or necessary materials for sialography include cotton swabs, tongue blades, 2 × 2-inch gauze, lemon juice, stopcock, several small (5- to 10-ml) syringes, magnifying spectacles, contrast materials, and a shot pellet (BB) with tape to be affixed to the skin as a marker (fig. 1.4).

Contrast Materials

Background

The contrast materials used in sialography historically have developed in two general categories: those soluble or suspended in water and those soluble in fat (Lowman and Cheng 1976; Yune 1977). Arcelin is cited as having used a suspension of bismuth for the first sialogram (Redon 1955). In 1925, Barsony performed a sialogram with 20% potassium iodide, causing pain and a facial paralysis lasting one to two hours. Although Lipiodol was originally produced in 1901 and had been shown to be a suitable contrast material for several other radiologic examinations, it was first recommended for clinical use in sialography in 1925 (Uslenghi; Barsony) and in 1926 (Carlsten; Jacobovici, Poplitza, and Albu).

Since that time a large number of water-soluble iodinated organic compounds introduced for urologic studies or angiography have been used for sialography. A somewhat smaller number of fat-soluble contrast materials introduced since Lipiodol include Pantopaque, iodochlorol, and Ethiodol, which was recommended for sialography by Epsteen in 1956. Some investigators prefer to use water-soluble contrast materials while others prefer one of the fat-soluble contrast materials. An excellent review comparing the properties of the various contrast materials has been published by Lowman and Cheng (1976).

Recommended Technique

If an oily contrast material is to be used we believe Ethiodol (ethiodized poppy seed oil) to be the contrast medium of choice. It is the most fluid of the oily contrast materials (Lowman and Cheng 1976; Fischer 1977) and can be injected easily through any of the three larger cannulas described. It contains 37% iodine and has a high radiographic density so that it produces a very good ductogram and excellent acinar opacification. Other fat soluble contrast materials such as Lipiodol and Pantopaque are more viscid. Although foreign body inflammatory and granulomatous reactions can be seen in the tissues following extravasation of any of these oily contrast materials, such reactions do not appear to be clinically significant (Yune 1977). Nevertheless, if a situation exists in which retention of oily contrast material might be anticipated, a water-soluble contrast material may be preferable since such contrast materials are not retained in the duct or gland.

Any of the commercially available water-soluble iodinated organic compounds containing approximately 28% to 38% iodine can be used for conventional sialography. These water-soluble contrast materials do not produce images of the duct system as clear as those made with Ethiodol, nor are they nearly as reliable in producing dense opacification of the parenchyma; this is true even for those with equivalent iodine concentration (fig. 1.5). Indeed, Gullmo and Book-Hederstrom (1958) recommended the use of water-soluble contrast materials for this very reason. Nevertheless, quite dense acinar filling does occur with water-soluble contrast materials in some instances (fig. 1.37A,B).

The relatively pale parenchymal opacification produced by water-soluble contrast material may be explained by several mechanisms. First, the water-soluble contrast materials diffuse rapidly through the gland and are absorbed into the blood. The specific sites in the gland where such absorption occurs is not known, but because of this absorption it may be necessary to continue the injection of water-soluble contrast media during subsequent filming in order to maintain duct and acinar filling (Drevattne and Stiris 1964). Second, the water-soluble contrast materials are miscible with saliva and may become diluted by saliva. Furthermore, the water-soluble contrast materials are hypertonic and so may be diluted by additional fluid transferred into them by the osmotic effect.

In practice, if only duct opacification is needed, either the water-soluble or the oily contrast materials will be satisfactory. If the examination is being conducted to study a possible mass lesion, and the mass is large and contained within the gland, water-soluble contrast material ordinarily will provide adequate information. On the other hand, if a mass is small or located far peripherally in the gland or is suspected to be outside the gland, or its presence is questionable, Ethiodol is more likely to provide a definitive examination because of the dense parenchymal opacification and clear definition of the margin of the salivary gland with which it is associated (figs. 1.5B, 1.20A,B, 1.21B,C, 1.22). If sialography is to be performed in conjunction with CT scanning, water-soluble contrast materials are preferred since Ethiodol is denser than necessary, sometimes producing CT artifacts (fig. 1.39E), and may be retained if extravasated. The same water-soluble contrast material containing 28% iodine used in conventional sialography may be used, but less concentrated contrast material produces quite satisfactory opacification (fig. 1.34E). In practice, plain CT performed on modern equipment without any contrast material usually demonstrates the details of any mass within or outside the salivary gland quite satisfactorily (Bryan et al. 1982) (figs. 1.34A,B,C,D, 1.35A, 1.36A,C,D, 1.37D, 1.38A,B,C, 1.39B, 1.40B).

Preliminary Films

Plain films taken of the salivary region before injection of contrast material can be of great help in sialographic interpretation (figs. 1.6–1.10; see chapter 3). Calculi in the submandibular salivary ducts may be demonstrated by the standard views such as the oblique films of the mandibular area or by an intraoral film of the floor of the mouth or by panoramic radiography (Panella and Calenoff 1979), open mouth views (Heystek and Hildreth 1958), or anterior-oblique views with the chin tilted up (fig. 1.6A,B,C). Parotid stones may best be demonstrated by an anterior-posterior or axial tangential view (Hettler and Lauth 1961) (fig. 1.7), or with the cheek puffed out (fig. 2.18), or by a lateral view with a small film inside the cheek. Eighty percent of salivary calculi are opaque, although not all of these can be demonstrated on plain films. Preexisting calcification may be present in lymph nodes, tonsils, tumors, or phleboliths as well as in salivary calculi (figs. 1.8, 1.9). Awareness of the presence of such preexisting calcifications may prevent confusion when interpreting the subsequent sialogram. Pneumosialosis presents a characteristic appearance on plain films (O'Hara 1973; O'Hara and Keohane 1973) (fig. 3.32).

Preliminary films may also demonstrate pathology in structures other than salivary glands, such as the bones, rendering sialography unnecessary (fig. 1.10). Therefore, preliminary films are recommended in most instances.

Instructions to the Patient

Before beginning the examination, the patient's cooperation may be gained by explaining what is to be done, the information being sought, and how such information will be used to determine therapy. The patient is informed that as the examination progresses, the gland will feel full and distended, but not painful. If the examination is being performed to study a mass lesion so that acinar opacification is to be attained, the patient is notified that the gland may become considerably enlarged but that it may be expected to return to normal over the subsequent 24 to 48 hours. A prearranged hand signal or sound to indicate discomfort is established. The instruments are displayed, indicating that the nylon probes are quite flexible and that the cannulas are not sharp.

Premedication and Anesthesia

In the past, topical anesthetic (Rubin and Blatt 1955), nerve block (Eisenbud and Cranin 1963), intraductal anesthetic (Quinn 1971), or local anesthetic injected into the tissues (Gates 1977) have all been suggested for use with sialography. We have not found it necessary to use any premedication or local or general anesthesia for sialography, since neither the cannulation nor the injection of contrast material is painful if done carefully. Even young children will often tolerate the procedure without sedation or anesthetic if it is explained beforehand and reassurance is provided during its performance.

Cannulation

We perform the cannulation with the patient in the supine position on the x-ray table. Good illumination is essential.

Parotid Duct

The parotid duct orifice is located on the buccal mucosa opposite the second upper molar tooth (fig. 1.11A). It can sometimes be identified as a tiny dark spot on the raised mucosa. The tip of the papilla upon which it opens may overhang and obscure the duct orifice, from which a droplet of saliva often can be enticed by gentle massage. If the duct orifice cannot be identified, a sialogogue, such as lemon juice, can be given. In theory at least, it is probably preferable to cannulate without stimulation if possible, since the added salivary secretion, which may continue for a short while, can cause the gland to distend more than is necessary once the cannula is in place and contrast material is being injected. This may lead to patient discomfort and to dilution of the contrast material. Approximately 90% of the daily salivary flow of 1000 to 1500 ml comes from the parotid and submandibular glands in roughly equal volume (Wotman and Mandel 1976). According to these authors the flow rate of saliva from each major salivary gland at rest is less than 0.05 ml per minute. Ericson (1968) documented the variations in parotid gland flow rates among individuals in the resting and stimulated states. Mason and Chisholm (1975) present a detailed chart showing mean resting parotid flow rates in different age groups to vary from 0.06 ml per minute to 0.10 ml per minute. The rate of flow from the stimulated salivary gland may vary from 0.5 ml or greater per minute (Wotman and Mandel 1976) to as much as 3.0 to 4.0 ml per minute (Mason and Chisholm 1975). With these flow rates it is easy to see how a salivary gland with its duct obturated by a cannula could be become overdistended with saliva and contrast material, especially if cannulation is accomplished during stimulation. Rarely, the flow of saliva may become so copious as to render it difficult to maintain contrast material in the gland. Under such circumstances, atropine 0.5 mg administered intramuscularly can be helpful by diminishing salivary flow (Carter et al. 1981a).

Preliminary use of a probe may be required to dilate the duct orifice, or even to reestablish its patency if scarring has occurred, before the cannula can be successfully introduced (fig. 1.11B). Preliminary use of a probe generally is not necessary in the parotid gland, however. Usually the large closed-end cannula can be placed directly into the duct orifice. Occasionally, one of the smaller cannulas will be needed; rarely, the smallest one may be needed. When a cannula has been selected, a contrast-filled syringe and stopcock should be attached and the tubing and cannula filled with contrast material (fig. 1.4). The stopcock should then be closed to keep air from seeping back into the tubing.

Cannulation is facilitated by pulling the cheek forward (fig. 1.11A), thus straightening the right-angle bend in the parotid duct as it traverses the buccinator muscle (figs. 1.11B, 1.37C, 2.4A). If one of the shorter cannulas is selected, it should be grasped by the plastic tubing portion for insertion into the duct (fig. 1.12). This is preferable to grasping the metal cannula with a forceps because the assembly is then rigid, increasing the danger of perforation. The cannula ordinarily will seek its own direction into the duct. If one of the longer cannulas has been selected, cannulation attempts should be carried out gently to avoid perforation. The cannula should be wedged in place in the case of the tapered side-port cannula, or inserted up to the metal or plastic shoulder situated proximally along the shaft if an end-port cannula is used.

After the cannula has been inserted it should be packed firmly in place with 2×2-inch gauze and the mouth and lips firmly closed. There is no need to use sutures as suggested by Steinhardt (1942) or clips as suggested by Gullmo and Book-Hederstrom (1958) to prevent loss of contrast material from the duct or to fix the catheter in place either here or in the submandibular duct. If the cannula is inserted properly, it will rarely become displaced. The metal or plastic shoulder located along the shaft of the cannula prevents leakage of contrast material back into the mouth.

Cannulation almost always can be accomplished. The rare instances when it is not possible to identify and cannulate the parotid duct orifice usually are associated with inability of the gland to secrete saliva into the mouth. This may be due to loss of function of the gland such as may occur with previous radiation treatment (Wescott et al. 1978) or to other causes of destruction of the gland parenchyma such as inflammation or replacement by tumor. It also may be due to complete duct obstruction from scarring as a result of surgery, trauma, or chronic infection. A notable cause of parotid obstruction is trauma to the parotid papilla by ill-fitting dentures (Wakely 1948; Hutchinson 1954; Rubin and Blatt 1955), whereby the papilla repeatedly is caught between the denture plate and the alveolar ridge. The papilla is also particularly vulnerable to being traumatized by chewing during eruption of new teeth, following installation of new dental prostheses, or following dental extraction (Ollerenshaw and Rose 1957).

Submandibular Duct

The orifice of the submandibular duct is usually smaller than that of the parotid duct, and magnifying spectacles often are essential to identify it. The submandibular duct opens onto a papilla, the sublingual caruncle, on the floor of the mouth just lateral to the frenulum of the tongue (fig. 1.13). It may open on to the side of the papilla, however, and may be also covered by a fold and thus be obscured. Bartholin's duct (see chapter 2) may occasionally open on the papilla by a separate orifice, but when present it usually joins the main submandibular duct (fig. 1.30A). If initial injection demonstrates the cannula to have entered Bartholin's duct (fig. 1.14A,B), the cannula should be withdrawn and redirected until satisfactory placement in the main submandibular duct has been accomplished.

The papilla is exposed and steadied somewhat by having the patient place the tongue against the roof of the mouth. A piece of tongue blade, cotton swab, or forceps can be used gently to steady the papilla further if necessary. Administration of lemon juice into the mouth may be required before the submandibular duct orifice can be identified. The duct opening appears as a tiny black spot when it opens to deliver saliva. It is often possible, however, to enter the duct without stimulating the flow of saliva.

One of the probes or dilators may first be used to identify and dilate the submandibular duct orifice. It is not unusual to succeed in placing the cannula directly into the submandibular duct without preliminary probing, although this is possible less often than in exploration of the parotid duct.

In about one third of instances, the largest cannula can be used, but commonly a 24- or 27-gauge cannula is necessary, even after probing and dilation. Occasionally, the smallest cannula is the only instrument that can be inserted into the duct orifice. Cannulation should be accomplished as already described, allowing the cannula to seek its own way into the duct.

Drying the papilla with a cotton swab will often help to identify the duct orifice. If the probe or cannula will not enter the duct orifice readily or if the orifice is not easily identified, teasing the orifice with a twirling or to and fro motion of the probe or cannula will frequently be successful. If the cannula cannot be advanced beyond the duct orifice, swallowing motions or external massage of the floor of the mouth may force saliva forward, momentarily opening the orifice sufficiently for a cannula to slip into place. Leaving a probe in place in the duct for a short time will obstruct the flow of saliva sufficiently so that when it is removed, a copious flow of saliva results and a cannula may be easily exchanged for the probe. The submandibular duct angles posteriorly and downward (figs. 1.26A, 2.26) (Pernkopf 1963), and the cannula or probe should be inserted at the appropriate angle. Approximately 1 to 2 cm below its orifice the duct becomes more horizontal, and the direction of the probe should be altered accordingly at this point if deeper penetration is desired. The three smaller cannulas can be bent to facilitate insertion if necessary.

The cannula should be advanced fully until the orifice is obturated and then it is packed in place with gauze. The patient should be instructed to close the mouth and lips firmly about the catheter.

With gentle persistence, it usually is possible to identify and cannulate the duct. Occasionally a duct orifice may measure less than 0.010 inches in diameter. These tiny duct orifices tend to occur in patients who have obstructive symptoms, and we believe such restricted orifices are abnormal and stenotic. In such cases, the tip of a plastic toothpick or the tip of a blunted needle may be used (with great caution) to dilate the orifice enough to allow introduction of the nylon or metal probe.

Sonnabend (1968) cites a failure to cannulate the submandibular duct in 10% of patients. With the instruments currently in use, such failure is uncommon provided there is secretion of saliva from the gland into the mouth so that the duct orifice can be identified. While some causes for absent secretion have already been discussed, the most common cause of such deficiency in the submandibular gland is a prior surgical procedure resulting in scarring of the floor of the mouth so that the duct orifice has become occluded. If a sialogram is required but cannulation cannot be accomplished because the duct orifice is too tiny or cannot be identified at all, various minor surgical approaches have been suggested. For example, the duct orifice may be nicked or slit by the sharp point of a surgical blade (Schultze and Weisburger 1947; Eisenbud and Cranin 1963), or the caruncle may be removed surgically to expose the duct. Castigliano (1962), using a different approach, described a technique for producing a transverse incision halfway through the duct at a point 1 cm proximal to the duct orifice, with subsequent cannulation at the surgical opening. Fistulas from the submandibular duct to the floor of the mouth may result from prior surgery or, rarely, may be due to spontaneous passage of a calculus, or to trauma, infection, or tumor. In such instances, there may be no flow of saliva through the anatomic duct orifice, but sialography can be accomplished by cannulating the fistula directly (figs. 3.63A and B). If salivary flow occurs through both the anatomic orifice and the fistula, one or the other can be blocked by a probe or dilator while injection is done through the remaining orifice, or the cannula in the anatomic orifice may be advanced into the duct beyond the fistula (fig. 1.14C). Ranulas may be injected with contrast material directly using a small (23- to 25-gauge) needle (fig. 1.14D,E).

Method of Injection of Contrast Material

Hand Syringe Versus Hydrostatic Injection

Background

The earliest sialograms were performed by hand injection and syringe (Barsony 1925; Uslenghi 1925; Carlsten 1926), and this remains the most popular method (Rubin and Blatt 1955; Ollerenshaw and Rose 1957; Osmer and Pleasants 1966; Berg 1969; Suzuki and Kawashima 1969; Yune and Klatte 1972; Manashil 1976, 1978; Lowman and Cheng 1976; Gates 1977; Kushner and Weber 1978; Mancuso, Rice, and Hanafee 1979). The rate of flow of contrast material is determined by adjustment of manual pressures according to patient response and fluoroscopic observation.

In 1958, in order to control the rate of introduction of contrast material into the gland and to avoid parenchymatous filling of the gland, which they felt was harmful, Gullmo and Book-Hederstrom introduced the hydrostatic method of injection. A reservoir of contrast material was connected by tubing to a cannula in the salivary duct and elevated above the level of the patient so that contrast material flowed into the salivary duct by gravity at a pressure of 30 to 40 cm of water. Other authors recommending the hydrostatic method of injection are Drevattne and Stiris (1964), Park and Mason (1966), Park and Bahn (1968), Blair (1973), and Mason and Chisholm (1975). Most investigators employing this method have used water soluble contrast material, but personal experience has shown that Ethiodol will also flow quite briskly, drop by drop, through an adequate size cannula into the gland from an elevated reservoir.

The advantages of the hydrostatic method are that the pressure of injection can be standardized, measured by the height of the reservoir. The rate of flow and the amount of contrast material injected can be regulated easily by a stopcock, and continuous injection of contrast material during the entire examination is facilitated without the need for the person performing the study even to remain in the room.

Recommended Technique

For conventional sialography we prefer to inject the contrast material, either Ethiodol or water soluble, by syringe and constant gentle hand pressure. Sudden increases in pressure should be avoided since they may cause pain. We have measured injection pressures at the hub of the syringe and in the duct itself in five patients (fig. 1.15) (table 1.1). These patients were undergoing sialography to evaluate suspected masses or enlargement of the salivary glands. While it is certainly true that pressures at the syringe during hand injection measured 300 mm Hg or more, as shown by Ollerenshaw and Rose (1951), pressures measured in the duct at the same time ranged only from 33 to 75 mm

Table 1.1.
Salivary duct pressures during sialography

Case	Gland	Contrast	Acinar Filling	Resting Pressure in Duct (mmHg)	Range of Pressure in Duct During Injection (mmHg)
1	Submand	Ethiodol	Slight	10	53–65
2	Submand	Renografin 76	None	10	35–50
3	Submand	Renografin 76	Slight	—	52–75
4	Parotid	Ethiodol	Moderate	5	33–46
5	Parotid	Sinografin	Moderate	0	33–64

NOTE: Baseline initial resting pressures in the duct were measured before injection was initiated.

All pressures were measured during a steady state of hand injection pressure using a 10-ml syringe. Actual pressure measurements were obtained from direct digital readout during the injection.

The pressure at the hub of the syringe was greater than 280 mm Hg in all five instances.

In two patients (cases 1 and 3), masses were shown by sialography to be extrinsic to the salivary gland. Biopsy in these two cases showed lymphoma. One patient (case 2) had a calculus in a duct, with a tiny fistula to the floor of the mouth. The sialograms were normal in the other two patients (cases 4 and 5).

Hg. These pressures are only slightly higher than the secretory pressures of the parotid and submandibular glands, as measured by Mason and Chisholm (1975), which range from 40 to 54 mm Hg. They are similar to pressures measured externally by the method of Zijlstra and Ten Bosch (1975) but somewhat higher than those measured externally by the method of Ferguson, Evans, and Mason (1977). The reason for such a drop in pressure from the syringe to the duct may be related to the length of the tubing, to the narrow lumen of the cannulas, to the compliance of the tissues, or to other causes. At the pressures described, easily generated by hand pressure and syringe, Ethiodol can be injected without difficulty and in adequate amounts through any of the cannulas except the smallest.

The volume of contrast material injected is determined not only by the needs of a particular examination, such as whether duct filling only is needed or whether the examination must be carried to the acinar opacification phase, but also by the capacity of the duct system and by patient response.

If the examination is to be prolonged, as by laminography or CT, and water-soluble contrast is being used, it may be necessary to inject additional amounts of contrast material at frequent intervals. Injection by the hydrostatic method may be more convenient under such circumstances (Rabinov, Kell, and Gordon 1984) (figs. 1.34E,F). The reservoir containing contrast material should be raised to a level of approximately 50 to 70 cm above the gland (Drevattne and Stiris 1964; Park and Mason 1966; Blair 1973). Heights as great as 90 cm (Mason and Chisholm 1975, chapter 17) have not been found to be necessary and could contribute to extravasation of the contrast material.

The Phases of Sialography

According to Yune and Klatte (1972) there are three phases of sialography: duct filling, acinar filling, and postevacuation. In order to draw attention to the importance of observing the actual evacuation itself in evaluating obstruction, it is useful to distinguish an additional interim phase, that of active evacuation, thereby recognizing four phases of sialography. There are two filling phases, duct filling and acinar filling, and two emptying phases, evacuation and postevacuation (fig. 1.16).

The Filling Phases

Background

Early sialograms were performed primarily to demonstrate the ducts and their branches (Payne 1931). Since that time, some authors have continued to stress the radiologic appearances of the ducts in the filling and postevacuation phases (Rubin et al. 1955; Blatt et al. 1956; Rubin and Holt 1957; Blatt et al. 1959), describing in detail the appearances of the ducts in various kinds of intrinsic and extrinsic masses.

In 1935, Kimm, Spies, and Wolf defined sialography as the "roentgenographic demonstration of the ducts, ductules and parenchyma of the salivary glands by means of radiopaque substances introduced into the ducts." They recognized the value of the parenchymal opacification that occurred during sialography in distinguishing masses arising within the gland from those arising without. They stated, however, that the reason for such opacification was unknown.

In 1950, Samuel reported opacification of the salivary parenchyma in three patients undergoing sialography, calling this appearance "sialo-acinar reflux." He stated that this was caused at least partly by overfilling of the duct system and compared it with pyelotubular reflux in the kidney. He recognized this appearance to be due to regurgitation of contrast material into the acini, and differentiated it from rupture of the duct walls with resultant passage of the contrast material into the interstitial tissues of the gland. He noted that the entire gland showed a generalized increase in density and that the lobulated character of the gland was well shown, but he did not attribute any diagnostic value to this phenomenon.

An understanding of acinar filling as the mechanism that causes parenchymal opacification is most important to clinical sialography. In 1951 Ollerenshaw and Rose stated that parenchymal opacification was due to normal filling of the acini as a completed state of injection and called it simply "acinar filling." By injecting post-mortem salivary gland specimens with iodized oil containing particulate material, they showed that acini were beginning to fill toward the end of the injection, although the particulate matter that they included in the oil was too coarse to pass through the smaller intercalated ducts into the acini. They believed that normal acini could always be filled and that failure to opacify the acini was due either to their being already filled, obstructed, or destroyed, or to incomplete injection. They noted that the acini of the submandibular gland filled readily, while filling of the acini in the parotid gland required more pressure and volume of contrast material. They attributed this difference to anatomic differences in the intercalated ducts, which in the submandibular gland are short and wide, while those in the parotid gland are longer and narrower, thus offering much greater resistance to the passage of contrast material.

Ranger was able in 1957 to demonstrate and correlate in detail the radiologic and histologic events that occur during the injection of contrast material for sialography by injecting contrast material into 20 normal parotid gland specimens and 20 normal submandibular gland specimens. In all of the 20 normal parotid glands, duct filling was followed by patchy opacification of the parenchyma (fig. 1.17A). This irregular parenchymal opacification was shown to be due to filling of the acini in some areas (fig. 1.17B). In these and subsequent specimens, further injection of contrast material resulted in more acini being distended with contrast material. This caused the gland to become more opaque, and as a result the ducts became obscured.

The parotid specimens could be separated into two groups, depending on whether globular extravasations of contrast material occurred. In 7 of the 20 normal parotid glands, no such extravasations developed. In the other 13, a few small globular collections of contrast material appeared during the duct filling phase (fig. 1.17C), becoming larger and more numerous as the injection continued. These were shown to be due to extravasation of contrast material from the intralobular ducts. Such extravasations tended to appear before there was much acinar filling and occurred only in the parotid glands, never in the submandibular glands. Ranger, too, attributed their occurrence to the increased resistance to injection offered by the longer, narrower intralobular ducts in the parotid gland when compared with the shorter, wider intralobular ducts in the submandibular gland (fig. 2.3A). He stated further that the individual globular extravasations that occur in these normal parotid glands were of the same nature as the similar but much more numerous extravasations that can be seen in chronic parotitis where the widespread pathologic changes rendered the intralobular ducts more vulnerable to rupture (see fig. 1.49 and chapter 4).

In all normal submandibular gland specimens, duct filling and acinar filling occurred sequentially, as noted in the normal parotid gland specimens. Not only did globular extravasations not occur in the submandibular gland even with large volumes (5 ml) of contrast material, but acinar filling occurred earlier and more readily in the submandibular glands than in the parotid glands. Ranger attributed both of these findings to the short and wide intralobular ducts in the submandibular gland, which he felt offered less resistance to the passage of contrast material. He concluded that the parenchymal opacification observed during sialography in normal parotid and submandibular glands was due to normal filling of the acini with contrast material.

The appearances seen in normal clinical sialography of the parotid and submandibular glands during duct filling and parenchymal opacification are similar to those described in the injected specimens (figs. 1.18, 1.19).

Osmer and Pleasants (1966) recommended obtaining as complete acinar filling as possible by injecting as much contrast material as the gland would accept, calling this "distension sialography." The purpose of such maximum filling was to produce a marked difference between the radiolucency of a mass and the dense opacification of the normal surrounding parenchyma caused by such filling. The minimum amount injected into the submandibular gland was 2.5 ml, and in the parotid gland, 3 ml with amounts up to 4 to 5 ml in some cases. According to these authors, patient discomfort did not appear to increase significantly as the injection continued, and the discomfort diminished over the next four to eight hours; both discomfort and swelling usually disappeared by 24 to 36 hours after sialography.

Osmer and Pleasants (1966) further noted that, while no gross or microscopic inflammatory or obstructive changes secondary to distension sialography were demonstrated in tumor cases undergoing prompt surgery, there were some later histologic inflammatory changes that could be attributed to the procedure in some patients with benign salivary gland disease. These authors felt, however, that the significance of such changes was far outweighed by the more detailed diagnostic information produced by the distension sialogram and they recommended distension sialography for the diagnosis of suspected salivary gland masses.

Not all investigators agree that extensive acinar filling during sialography is desirable. Rubin and colleagues (1955) noted that the salivary glands may become enlarged to two to three times their normal size during filling of the acini. It was stated in this paper, and in a subsequent paper by Rubin and Holt (1957), that extensive acinar filling was undesirable and that only minimal delineation of the acini was preferred, with reliance placed almost entirely upon changes in the duct system during filling and evacuation to diagnose mass lesions. In both papers, the authors stated that overdistension caused rupture of acinar cells and obscured duct details. Gullmo and Book-Hederstrom (1958) felt that dense filling of the parenchyma with oily contrast medium caused pain and swelling of the gland by plugging of the small ducts and should be avoided. Liliequist and Welander (1969) stated that overfilling of the gland with contrast material was undesirable and should be avoided. Berg (1969) stated that he did not find such distension of the salivary glands helpful.

On the other hand, Ollerenshaw and Rose (1951, 1957) and Hettwer and Folsom (1968) felt that parenchymal opacification had diagnostic value. Drevattne and Stiris (1964) stated that parenchymal filling could demonstrate defects too small to affect the duct system, especially masses located peripherally in the gland. These authors injected water-soluble contrast material by the hydrostatic method but added that if a greater degree of parenchymal filling was required, additional contrast material could be injected by syringe. Park and Bahn (1968) stated that the presence or absence of acinar filling was critical to the interpretation of sialograms. They felt that its absence after injection of adequate amounts of contrast material meant that the gland was diseased and noted that space-occupying lesions were represented by "bare areas."

Reid (1969) stated that distension sialography could be very helpful in demonstrating some small masses that did not cause distortion of the duct system. In other cases, he felt that it obscured pathology and did not recommend its use when an inflammatory process or stricture was suspected. He suggested that when a mass is suspected, a two-stage examination should be performed, with filling of the ducts first and then repeating the radiographs after injecting enough additional contrast material to cause slight distension of the gland.

Yune and Klatte (1972) recommended injection under fluoroscopic control until filling of the acini could be recognized but did not advocate distension sialography as described by Osmer and Pleasants (1966). Yune and Klatte stated that the parenchymal phase was particularly useful in the presence of (1) subacute autoimmune sialosis where failure of acinar filling could be assumed to indicate diffuse parenchymal swelling and (2) peripheral mass lesions that could easily be missed by duct opacification alone.

Recommended Technique

It seems clear from the preceding studies that parenchymal opacification occurs normally if an adequate amount of contrast material is injected. It is seen with either oily or water-soluble contrast materials but, as noted, it is much denser and more reliably produced with the oily contrast material (fig. 1.5). Parenchymal opacification is extremely useful in outlining and defining masses within the salivary glands (fig. 1.20). Even very tiny masses can be demonstrated (fig. 1.20B). It is also necessary to obtain such parenchymal opacification in order to define the margin of the salivary glands so that clear distinction can be made between intrinsic and adjacent masses (figs. 1.5B, 1.8C, 1.21B). Failure of the acini to opacify is abnormal but nonspecific. Any process that causes marked swelling or edema of the gland or that fills the acinar lumens or causes destruction, infiltration, or replacement of the acini may prevent acinar opacification.

In clinical application of this information, it has been our practice and recommendation that the proper amount of contrast material to inject in any individual case is only that amount required to produce a diagnostic sialogram. The amount of contrast material, therefore, varies in each case and in different clinical situations, the examination being performed somewhat differently according to whether a mass lesion or a stone or obstruction is suspected. In any event, contrast material should be injected slowly with constant gentle pressure, in fractional amounts, under fluoroscopic monitoring.

In examination for a possible intrinsic or extrinsic mass lesion, the duct filling phase and especially the acinar filling phase should be performed (figs. 1.5B, 1.20, 2.13, 2.16B,C). Progressive acinar opacification should be accomplished until the gland parenchyma and the margins of the gland are clearly outlined (fig. 1.21A,B). On the other hand, when only stone, obstruction, or inflammation is suspected, it is sufficient to opacify only the ducts, and the acinar filling phase should be omitted. Injection of contrast material should continue only up to the point where a definite diagnosis can be made and therapy can be undertaken with confidence, or a definitely normal gland has been demonstrated and pathology has been excluded. We do not recommend the routine use of distension sialography as described by Osmer and Pleasants (1966) since it usually is not necessary to continue the injection to this degree. Furthermore, such injection practically always results in some extravasation of contrast material into the gland (figs. 1.43, 1.44). Nevertheless, distension sialography may be required in some instances to demonstrate conclusively whether a small mass is present (figs. 1.20B, 1.22, 2.13B) and to determine whether it is within the peripheral parts of the gland or adjacent to the gland, and we do not hesitate to perform distension sialography as needed. Laminography can be especially helpful in demonstrating the findings under these circumstances (figs. 1.27B, 1.32). The tail of the parotid gland usually is the most difficult part of the gland in which to obtain good acinar filling.

Distension sialography is accompanied by enlargement of the gland (fig. 2.15B). The enlargement, which presumably is related to the volume of injected contrast material, to secreted saliva, and to some edema and hyperemia, may seem to be of alarming proportions, but if the injection is performed slowly it is not painful. The increasing size of the gland, which causes it to bulge away from the adjacent bony structures, may even be helpful in identifying masses in or around the gland. Extensive acinar filling ultimately results in obscuration of the ducts, partly because they are compressed by the distended acini and swollen parenchyma, and also because the opacifying parenchyma obscures the outlines of the ducts. If the injection is continued beyond this point, it may result in extravasation of contrast material (fig. 1.23A) and ultimately in loss of definition of the gland margins (fig. 1.23B,C). When the injection has been finished, the stopcock should be closed until recording on film is completed to prevent return of contrast material into the syringe and to prevent any additional contrast material from entering the gland. Contrast material already in the ducts may continue to ooze slowly into the peripheral ducts and acini.

The filling phases should be completed as quickly as possible for several reasons. First, the appearance of the parenchymal opacification eventually deteriorates (fig. 1.23D), presumably owing to displacement of the contrast material by the continued secretion of saliva, to swelling of the gland tissue, and to mixture of the contrast material with saliva in the case of water-soluble contrast material. Areas of resulting deficient acinar filling may begin to simulate masses at this time. Second, extravasation of contrast material appears to be related not only to the volume of contrast material injected but also to the duration and pressure of the injection as well as to the length of time during which the contrast material remains in the gland. The increasing volume of saliva accumulating in the gland and a possible increase in permeability of the tissues of the duct wall may contribute to extravasation.

The Emptying Phases
Background

In 1955 Rubin with Blatt and with other associates, noting the value of evacuation films of other organs, studied the evacuation physiology of the salivary glands by observing their emptying under stimulation. They referred to such studies as "physiologic or secretory sialography." After filling of the ducts, the catheter was plugged with a toothpick and standard radiographs were taken. The catheter was then removed and the gland stimulated with lemon juice. Roentgenograms at five minutes showed the normal duct system to be empty in all cases. These authors stated that studies with rapid sequential films showed that all the glands emptied completely within the first minute(s) after stimulation. Even acinar filling was usually absent in one hour. In subsequent papers, Blatt and co-workers (1956), Rubin and Holt (1957), and Blatt and associates (1959) showed the value of the secretory phase in various pathologic conditions. In calculous disease, the ball-valve mechanism was illustrated. In chronic nonobstructive sialectasis, the residual secretory function of the gland could be evaluated by the rate of washout of contrast material. In the study of neoplasms, secretory sialography was suggested as an aid in differentiating between the various kinds of tumors within the salivary glands and distinguishing between intrinsic masses and those arising outside of the salivary glands. The appearances of the ducts in mass lesions were described in great detail by these authors, stressing in particular the value of secretory sialography. More recent recommendations for the use of the secretory phase of sialography in various conditions have been published by Park and Mason (1966), Yune and Klatte (1972), O'Hara (1973), Lowman and Cheng (1976), and Manashil (1978).

Recommended Technique

After recording of the filling phases has been completed, the cannula is tugged out of the duct, allowing the contrast material to spill into the gauze packing in the mouth. Ordinarily, even without stimulation, there is an immediate spill of much of the contrast material into the mouth (Berg 1969) (fig. 1.16C). This results from the elastic contraction of the tissues of the salivary ducts and gland, from active contraction of smooth muscle in the duct walls when such muscle fibers are present (Blount and Lachman 1953; Pick and Howden 1977), from pressure against the distended duct and gland by surrounding tissues, and from outflow of pent-up salivary secretions. Active secretion can be stimulated if desired by administration of lemon juice into the mouth, driving most of the remaining free contrast material from the ducts. Because the factors causing evacuation are all variable, and the amount and type of contrast material injected is quite variable, the actual rate of emptying and its completeness at any given moment in the normal gland as observed fluoroscopically and by film is variable. Also, since the main salivary duct, especially that of the submandibular gland, may be capacious, the ducts themselves may act as reservoirs for saliva (Rubin et al. 1955). We have observed that free contrast material may remain in such capacious normal ducts for many minutes before it is entirely removed by salivary flow. In general, however, we agree that most of the free contrast material has been evacuated even from capacious submandibular ducts and glands within five minutes, as described by Rubin and colleagues (1955) (fig. 1.16D). Any residual contrast material remaining in the normal gland after stimulated salivary flow may be either in the form of plugs in the smaller ducts or may be extravasated into the tissues.

In a similar fashion to the filling phases, the evacuation phases are also used differently according to whether the examination is being performed because of a suspected mass or because of suspected obstruction or inflammation. These phases are relatively unimportant in the study of mass lesions of the salivary glands, even though typical changes in the amount, distribution, and appearance of residual contrast material have been described in various kinds of intraglandular masses and in extrinsic masses (Blatt et al. 1956, 1959; Rubin and Holt 1957). The appearances of the filling phases, especially that of acinar opacification, usually are, more definitive. We have not found the evaluation of the amount and pattern of retained contrast material in postevacuation films to be of great additional diagnostic value in studying masses. Postevacuation films often are taken but are used primarily to record any extravasation of contrast material and to be certain that the gland has been emptied. Evacuation is not observed fluoroscopically in examination for mass lesions.

On the other hand, in the presence of inflammation or obstruction, the evacuation and postevacuation phases may be quite informative, and the findings should be recorded on spot films. We observe emptying in the active evacuation phase very carefully under fluoroscopy, looking particularly for any small calculi just beyond the duct orifice that may have been bypassed by the cannula, since such calculi (fig. 1.24) or those distal to a stricture may be detected only on evacuation films. The ball-valve mechanism of obstruction may also be clearly demonstrated at this time (figs. 1.24C, 1.25, 1.26B,E, 3.9A,B, 3.10A,B, 3.12E, 3.18B). One can also obtain an indication of the degree of obstruction to flow from strictures by observing the evacuation phase.

Delayed or incomplete evacuation of contrast material may also be associated with processes that cause parenchymal destruction, such as autoimmune sialosis, chronic infection, irradiation, or replacement by tumor. Such processes result not only in poor acinar filling, but also in decreased or absent secretion of saliva because of loss of acinar function. The amount of secretion, and therefore the functioning capacity of the gland, can be determined by observing the rate of clearance of contrast material during sialography, but this can be more easily measured directly by observing or collecting the salivary flow of a gland.

Examination for Mass Lesion versus Examination for Obstruction

The Tailored Sialogram

The sialographic examination should be tailored according to the clinical findings so that the required information will be produced with certainty and with the simplest procedure possible. Selection of a suitable contrast material, its injection in an optimal amount, and the appropriate use of the phases of sialography are especially important.

Examination for Mass Lesions

As noted, the phases of duct filling and especially acinar filling are the most important in the evaluation of the salivary glands for mass lesions.

At the beginning of the examination a BB, used as a marker, is taped on the skin directly over the palpable mass (figs. 1.20B, 1.22). This will be of great help subsequently in correlating the clinical and radiologic findings. Contrast material is injected slowly and fractionally under fluoroscopic monitoring with constant gentle pressure on the syringe. The rate of injection should be slowed if the patient signals the onset of pain. Filling of the major duct, interlobar, and intralobular ducts and acini is observed and recorded in anteroposterior, lateral, and various anterior-oblique and lateral-oblique projections. Particular and repeated attention is paid to the focus of suspected pathology indicated by the BB as the examination progresses.

Enough contrast material should be injected so that a moderate degree of parenchymal opacification occurs and the outline of any mass within the gland (fig. 1.20), and the outlines of the gland margins themselves, may be clearly seen and distinguished sharply from any adjacent masses (figs. 1.5B, 1.21). If the mass is suspected to be in the deep part of the gland, or is small or very peripherally located, it may be necessary to perform distension sialography as described by Osmer and Pleasants (1966) (fig. 1.22). Laminography is especially helpful in outlining masses clearly (Kushner and Weber 1978) (fig. 1.27B).

Serious errors of interpretation will be avoided by awareness that while it is possible to distinguish an encapsulated or circumscribed mass from an invasive one, these terms are not necessarily synonymous with benign and malignant (Blatt et al. 1956; Rubin and Holt 1957). Conventional sialography is often disappointing in its ability to distinguish between a benign and malignant mass (Yune and Klatte 1972) or even between an inflammatory and a neoplastic mass (Calcaterra et al. 1977) (see chapters 3 and 6). Malignant neoplasms may appear well circumscribed, while nonneoplastic processes may destroy the integrity of the duct walls, causing extravasation and puddling of contrast material that may be indistinguishable from that caused by an invasive tumor (Blatt et al. 1956). We agree with Rubin and Holt (1957) that no attempt should be made to diagnose the exact histologic type of a salivary gland tumor on the basis of the sialographic findings alone. Furthermore, the presence of inflammatory changes or sialectasis should not be interpreted as evidence that a mass is necessarily of an inflammatory nature, since tumors may also occur in such glands (figs. 1.27, 3.47).

When recording of the filling phases has been completed, the cannula is withdrawn and the contrast material is allowed to spill from the duct into the gauze packing used to keep the cannula in place. To complete the evacuation of contrast material from the duct, salivary flow should be stimulated with lemon juice. If a record of the degree of emptying is desired, a radiograph may be obtained at this time.

Examination for Suspected Stone, Obstruction, or Inflammation

The phases of duct filling, evacuation, and postevacuation are the most important. The acinar opacification phase should be omitted unless a mass is also suspected. Careful attention should be paid to filling of all branches of the duct as well as the main duct itself, since calculi or strictures may be present in the peripheral portions of the duct system.

Especially if obstruction or stone is suspected and none has been demonstrated, evacuation should be observed carefully under fluoroscopy and recorded by spot films during removal of the cannula since some calculi may best be brought to attention at this time (figs. 1.24–1.26). If necessary, salivary flow may be stimulated to encourage evacuation of contrast material. Postevacuation films are taken to record completeness of evacuation.

Since less contrast material is injected and acinar filling is minimal, little or no enlargement of the gland occurs during this type of study, and the patient need not be forewarned about swelling of the gland.

Several artifacts are known to occur. Air bubbles may be inadvertently injected with the contrast material. Such air bubbles can be distinguished from calculi because they may be dispersed into the small peripheral branches of the duct and disappear with continued injection; alternatively, they can be withdrawn back into the catheter (fig. 1.28). Calculi can be withdrawn, but only to the tip of the cannula (fig. 1.29).

Segments of oily contrast material within the duct may be separated from each other by saliva, giving the appearance of strictures, but these "strictures" can be seen to move back and forth in the duct and may disappear (fig. 1.30), while true strictures are fixed in position and unchanging.

Fluoroscopic Monitoring

Recommendations for the routine use of fluoroscopy with image intensification and television in sialography have been made by Hettler and Lauth (1961), Sonnabend (1968), Berg (1968), Rabinov and Joffe (1969), Yune and Klatte (1972), and Kushner and Weber (1978). For a number of reasons, it is very important to perform the examination under fluoroscopic monitoring. The ducts and gland structures and any pathologic changes can be projected into optimal profile and as free of interfering bony structures as possible. Position is helped by having the patient turn not just the head but the entire body into position under the fluoroscope and by having the assistant manipulate the patient's head into position with gloved hands. The radiologic findings are recorded on multiple spot films with a small focal-spot x-ray tube (0.3 to 0.6 mm).

The importance of fluoroscopic monitoring to identify and confirm any radiologic abnormalities and to ensure that just the appropriate amount of contrast material is injected cannot be overemphasized. Any leak back of contrast material into the mouth can be corrected, and extravasation of contrast material into the gland can be recognized early. It should be remembered that with the cannula wedged into a duct, a closed system exists and it is possible to cause extravasation of contrast material into the tissues of even normal glands if too much pressure or volume is used. Furthermore, pathologic processes in which retention of contrast material may be anticipated (e.g., autoimmune sialosis) can be identified promptly and the amount of oily contrast material injected limited or water-soluble contrast material selected. Occasionally, a cannula may be placed into a Bartholin's duct of the sublingual gland (fig. 1.14), or the major duct itself may be found to end blindly as a congenital anomaly. Timely awareness of these situations will lead to appropriate modifications of technique.

Radiographic Photographic Techniques

While fluoroscopic and spot film examination may be entirely diagnostic, it may be necessary or desirable under some circumstances to complete the study with additional radiographs. For example, it may be necessary to obtain views of a focal abnormality in two or three planes at right angles to each other before an abnormality has been demonstrated to the best advantage. The stopcock should remain closed and such additional studies performed as expeditiously as possible since the contrast material tends to be pushed out of the acini and peripheral radicals by salivary secretion (fig. 1.23D), and the appearance may sometimes begin to simulate masses within the gland. If water-soluble contrast material is being used, additional contrast material may have to be injected more or less continually because of its absorption through the gland.

The fine focal-spot tubes available in modern radiologic equipment are important to sialography because they produce not only greater resolution than was possible without them, but they also provide the capability for magnification if desired.

Xerosialography (Glassman, O'Hara, and Cregar 1974) (fig. 1.21C) may be especially helpful in demonstrating the extraglandular component of a lesion and in distinguishing between the extrinsic and intrinsic origin of a lesion. Panoramic radiography (Azouz 1978; Massouh and Dunscombe 1982) (figs. 1.6A, 1.10, 1.31A), magnification, subtraction (Liliequist and Welander 1970; Forman 1977) (fig. 1.18B and D), and stereoscopic films may be helpful in certain instances. Laminography is especially helpful in demonstrating masses within the salivary glands (Kushner and Weber 1978) (fig. 1.27B) and in showing the margin of the gland (fig. 1.32).

Special Methods of Examination

Computed Tomography

Background

For more than half a century, conventional sialography has been the standard method for radiologic examination of the salivary glands. For a number of reasons, however, the recent advent of CT has had a revolutionary impact upon the study of mass lesions in and around the salivary glands (Hanafee 1982a, 1982b).

When compared with conventional sialography alone, CT sialography (i.e., CT of the salivary glands following the injection of contrast material into the salivary duct and gland) has been reported to improve sensitivity in the detection of masses and in the determination of their intrinsic or extrinsic origin and their relationship to structures within and outside the salivary gland, as well as their benign or malignant nature (Som and Biller 1980; Stone et al. 1981). Conventional sialography alone is reported to be 75% (Yune and Klatte 1972) to 85% (Calcaterra et al. 1977) accurate in the detection of masses in or about the parotid salivary glands. Nevertheless, according to these latter authors and others (Som and Biller 1980; Stone et al. 1981), it is not always possible to distinguish by conventional sialography between extrinsic and intrinsic masses. This is especially true if the mass has arisen in a peripheral part of the gland. CT sialography often demonstrates tumors far more clearly and accurately than conventional sialography, indicating their site of origin and location more clearly and distinguishing more definitively between extrinsic and intrinsic masses.

Furthermore, according to Stone and associates (1981), the pattern of tumor growth as demonstrated by CT may be sufficiently characteristic to suggest the benign or malignant nature of a neoplasm. As noted, it often is not possible by conventional sialography alone to distinguish between benign and malignant neoplasms (Yune and Klatte 1972; Kushner and Weber 1978). It is true that typical malignant changes have been described (Blatt et al. 1956; Rubin and Holt 1957; Calcaterra et al. 1977), and that by paying careful attention to the details of the conventional sialogram it is possible in selected instances to make this distinction, such as when there is gross disruption of architecture, abrupt deformities and obstructions of ducts, and bizarre pooling of contrast materials known to occur in some infiltrating malignant tumors (fig. 1.35C). On the other hand, CT sialography, by demonstrating more or less characteristic appearances within the tumor itself, at its interface with the normal gland tissue, and in the surrounding structures, appears to increase the accuracy of differentiating benign from malignant tumors (Mancuso, Rice, and Hanafee 1979; Som and Biller 1980; Rice, Mancuso, and Hanafee 1980; Carter et al. 1981b). Nevertheless, as with conventional sialography, CT can distinguish between circumscribed and invasive tumors, but it often cannot distinguish between benign and malignant ones (Hanafee 1982a) since not all malignant tumors appear invasive (figs. 1.34D, E). Pathologic examination of the tissue must be done for accurate classification and grading of tumors, except in a few instances where CT is able to suggest the specific histologic nature of a mass (e.g., hemangioma, cyst, or lipoma) (Carter et al. and Panders 1981b) (Figs. 1.36A, D).

CT elegantly demonstrates the specific anatomic details of a tumor, its precise location with the gland, its relationship to landmarks within the gland such as the plane of the facial nerve (the nerves themselves cannot be seen), the vascular structures, and the ducts as well as to structures outside the gland such as the styloid process and the mastoid process. The axial display provided by CT is especially valuable to show the relationship of masses to other structures.

Carter and co-workers (1981a) correlated normal anatomy with normal CT sialography. These authors in a separate paper (1981b) also described the CT findings in 134 patients examined for pathology in and around the parotid and submandibular glands, stressing the value of CT sialography.

CT of the salivary glands has been performed either without contrast material (plain) or following opacification of the gland by injection of contrast material into the ducts (CT sialography).The use of intravenous contrast material combined with CT has not been necessary in the examination of most lesions within the salivary glands (Golding 1982), although it is helpful in occasional instances (Sone et al. 1982), particularly where there is a question of abnormal lymph nodes or vessel identification extrinsic to the gland (Bryan et al. 1982). It has also been shown to be useful in differentiating between various extrasalivary tumors (Som 1980).

According to Bryan and colleagues (1982), CT without intraductal contrast material can provide excellent definition of normal salivary glands. They showed that focal tumors are usually denser than the normal parotid gland and be easily differentiated on CT from diffuse enlargement such as may occur with inflammatory disease. These authors state also that it is often possible by plain CT to distinguish between intrinsic and extrinsic masses and that it is usually possible to differentiate between benign neoplasms and carcinoma. Golding (1982) similarly documented the accuracy of plain CT in demonstrating parotid gland tumors.

According to Som and Biller (1980), however, plain CT does not demonstrate the margins of the salivary glands or the lucent fat zone separating the gland from extrinsic masses as well as does CT following injection of contrast material into the ducts, nor can intraglandular detail be seen as well. Kassel (1982a, 1982b) recommended the routine use of intraductal contrast material in the CT examination of salivary gland mass lesions (CT sialography).

The parotid glands generally are somewhat lower in density than soft tissue since they tend to contain a varying amount of fat. According to Batsakis (1972), replacement of the acinar parenchyma of the major salivary glands by fibroadipose tissue is an age-related event, with approximately one quarter of the parenchymal cell volume normally being lost between childhood and old age. Thus the parotid gland usually provides a background of CT density that is relatively lower to a varying degree than the CT density of most tumors.

According to Sone and associates (1982), the normal density of parotid tissue extends over a wide range from patient to patient, varying between a slightly higher density than fat to a slightly lower density than muscle. Since tumors may also vary considerably in density, these investigators found it necessary to combine sialographic injection with CT in 9 of their 18 patients in order to demonstrate the parotid tumors clearly.

Recommended Technique

A thin smudge of barium paste is dabbed onto the skin overlying the clinically palpable mass and a BB is taped in place over this. These markers ensure that the mass is included in the imaging procedure and are useful subsequently for anatomic-radiologic correlation. The bolsters used to steady the patient's head are positioned craniad to the ears so that they will not deform or flatten the parotid glands. A digital radiograph (scout view or topogram) is exposed to aid in selecting optimal artifact-free projections as well as to provide a basis for a final summary of the anatomic planes that have been imaged (fig. 1.33). The BB is then removed (it might cause artifacts) and imaging planes are selected (Rabinov, Kell, and Gordon 1984).

Parotid Gland

If no dental amalgam is present, the straight axial projection may be used to image both the parotid and the submandibular gland (figs. 1.33A, 2.20). The imaging plane to be used, however, is most commonly dictated by the presence of dental amalgam since this may obscure the middle and lower portions of the parotid glands in the straight axial projection. The semiaxial projection with the head extended and the gantry angled 15 to 20 degrees craniad (figs. 1.33B, 2.21) is generally the most useful basic position and can be used to demonstrate in most patients practically the entire parotid gland as well as the submandibular gland, free of interfering metallic structures. The upper half or more of the parotid gland can also be well shown in the semiaxial projection with the head flexed (figs. 1.33C, 2.22). Care should be taken to position the head and gantry so that the lenses of the eyes are excluded from the planes of radiation insofar as possible. Use of the direct coronal view (figs. 1.33D, 2.23) is rarely needed to demonstrate the lesion itself, but it can provide additional anatomic data and may occasionally show the lesion to the best advantage. Some patients find this position uncomfortable.

Submandibular Glands

These are well imaged in the basic position just described (fig. 1.33B) or in a modified axial view with the chin tilted up slightly and the gantry angled slightly craniad (figs. 1.33E; 2.30). The submandibular glands may also be demonstrated in the direct coronal view, but this position is somewhat more uncomfortable than the others.

Patient Instructions

In order to minimize motion artifacts, the patient should be instructed with each exposure to stop breathing and not to swallow.

Contrast Material

Most intraparotid masses can be demonstrated by plain CT, which is conducted without the use of intraductal or intravenous contrast material (fig. 1.34) (Bryan et al. 1982; Golding 1982). This is possible because the parotid glands usually contain some fat and are relatively low in density, while masses are usually nearer the density of soft tissue. Masses differing in density from parotid tissue by even small amounts, such as 10 to 15 Hounsfield units, are usually demonstrable, especially if a capsule or pseudocapsule is present (figs. 1.34B, 1.36A,C). Injection of intraductal or intravenous contrast material may reveal additional anatomic and pathologic details (Kassel 1982b), but contrast material is rarely necessary to demonstrate the lesion itself and its location (fig. 1.34D,E). Indeed, intraductal contrast material may be associated with artifacts of incomplete filling if inadequate amounts are injected (Kassel 1982b) and may itself obscure anatomic and pathologic details. If the administration of intraductal contrast material is felt to be necessary, water-soluble contrast material containing 5% to 7% iodine is preferable. This may be easily obtained by diluting a small volume of standard water-soluble contrast material containing 28% iodine (e. g., Renografin-60 or Conray-60) with 3 or 4 volumes of normal saline (e. g., 10 ml contrast material and 30 to 40 ml of saline). Since water-soluble contrast materials are readily absorbed through the gland into the bloodstream, it may be necessary to inject additional contrast material with each one or two images (Stone et al. 1981). We prefer to administer these solutions continuously during imaging by hydrostatic drip from a reservoir placed at a height of 40 to 70 cm above the parotid gland (Gullmo and Book-Hederstrom 1958; Drevattne and Stiris 1964; Park and Mason 1966) (fig. 1.34F). The flow of this contrast material through the intraductal cannula can be regulated by a stopcock. Contrast materials containing 28% iodine, such as the undiluted water soluble ones already mentioned or Ethiodol (37% iodine), are unnecessarily dense and may create artifacts on the CT images. Furthermore, extravasated Ethiodol may remain in the gland for many months. If intravenous contrast material is selected, a 50-ml bolus of water-soluble contrast material containing approximately 28% iodine is suggested, to be followed by a continuous intravenous drip during the scanning procedure, the total amount of contrast material being 100 to 150 ml (fig. 1.35B).

With modern CT scanners and meticulous technique, the use of contrast material has become less and less necessary for diagnosis of parotid masses, and we rarely use it in such instances. Even very small lesions often can be identified in plain CT scans (fig. 1.38A).

In order to demonstrate masses within the submandibular gland it may be necessary to use intraductal contrast material more frequently than in the parotid gland, since the submandibular glands ordinarily contain little fat and thus are in the range of soft-tissue density (25 to 60 Hounsfield units) (Bryan et al. 1982). Thus a tumor that may be of nearly the same density may not be distinguishable. Fortunately, tumors occur less frequently in the submandibular glands than in the parotid glands.

Masses extrinsic to the salivary glands are usually well defined by plain CT. It must be noted, however, that additional anatomic detail, such as necrosis, often is more visible with intravenous contrast material because of enhancement of the viable tumor or of the surrounding structures (fig. 1.39A). Adjacent arteries and veins may be identified and differentiated from lymph nodes or other structures. Any compression, occlusion, or displacement of the vessels can be determined (fig. 1.35B). Also, the differential diagnosis of extrasalivary tumors such as carotid body tumors, glomus jugulare tumors, schwannomas, and minor salivary gland tumors may be aided, since these various lesions may enhance in different ways.

CT Parameters

Magnification of 2.5 to 4 times normal is helpful. Relatively narrow collimation, 4 mm for example, is recommended, with contiguous slices. A window width of 256 Hounsfield units (HU) is suitable in most instances, with the window center at approximately 35 HU. Because many variables may be present, including wide variation in density of parotid tissue as well as of tumor tissue, it is not wise to adhere rigidly to predetermined factors, and careful adjustment of display parameters will often result in images with superior diagnostic information. Thus, if the parotid gland is very low in density, e.g. 0 to −60 HU, a window center at 0 or lower that corresponds more closely to the density of the parotid gland may produce a more diagnostic image. If the density of the tumor and parotid gland are close, 10 to 20 HU apart for example, the lesion may become more clearly visible with the use of a very narrow window setting with the center line at the median density of the structures of interest.

CT Appearances of Various Lesions

Tumors Arising From Within the Salivary Gland

Tumors of intrinsic origin may be entirely, or almost entirely, surrounded by salivary tissue (figs. 1.34A,D,E, 2.23A), or they may extend beyond the gland and be only partly buried in the parotid tissue (fig. 1.34C). If such partly buried masses are benign, they are usually (fig. 1.34A), but not always (figs. 1.34B, 1.36A,C), separated from adjacent structures by a layer of fat. It should be noted, however, that often very little fat separates the parotid gland from the mandible, the masseter muscle, or the sternocleidomastoid muscle. The interface between the intraglandular portion of a mass and the salivary tissue is a direct one, without an intervening fat layer. A capsule or pseudocapsule of soft tissue density may be present (figs. 1.34B, 1.36A,C). Any extraglandular portion that abuts the adjacent parotid gland may be separated from it by an intervening fatty layer (fig. 1.34C) similar to that seen in the presence of entirely extrinsic masses. Either benign or malignant tumors may be sharply circumscribed (figs. 1.34A,D,E). Thus, it is not possible to know by CT alone whether a sharply circumscribed tumor is benign or malignant. Similarly, either benign or malignant tumors may be lobulated (figs. 1.34C,D,E). On the other hand, invasive malignant tumors may have indistinct margins at their interface with the parotid tissue, or they may infiltrate outside the gland into the surrounding fat (fig. 1.35). According to Kassel (1982b), three morphologic patterns of salivary gland tumors may be described:

1. Round, smoothly outlined masses correlating well with benign, seldom recurrent tumors (fig. 1.34A)

2. Lobulated but still sharply outlined masses tending to be slightly more aggressive, with a higher likelihood of recurrence (figs. 1.34D,E)

3. Infiltrating masses with poorly defined margins (figs. 1.35A,B).

Hounsfield numbers of tumors are variable and except for specific cases, such as cyst or lipoma (figs. 1.36A,D), it is not possible in the usual case to know the histology of a tumor from its density. Cysts may have Hounsfield numbers varying from near that of water to as high as that of some soft tissue tumors depending on the amount of mucus or other contents within the cyst (figs. 1.36A,C).

When a mass occupies a position in the parotid gland along the anatomic course of the facial nerve (figs. 1.34A,B,C,D,E, 1.36A), the nerve structures may be displaced (Sone et al. 1982; (Bryan et al. 1982). Depending upon the particular location of the mass, the nerves may be displaced in a superficial or a deep direction or in a craniad or a caudad direction by the mass, or the nerve structures may be enveloped or invaded by the mass (figs. 1.35A,B). It is theoretically possible to predict the direction of displacement of the nerves, but most commonly it is not possible to do so with certainty (fig. 1.36A,C) since the nerve trunks themselves are not identified on CT images.

General Enlargement of a Salivary Gland or Glands; Inflammation; Calculi

Many disease processes are known to cause enlargement of one or several salivary glands. These include sialosis; Sjögren's syndrome; recurrent parotitis in children or adults; acute, chronic, or recurrent purulent infections; tuberculosis; sarcoid; lymphoma; and bilateral tumors such as Warthin's tumors. Varying degrees of inflammation may be present clinically in some of these entities.

If the enlargement of the parotid glands is relatively bland and the parotid glands are relatively low in density on CT, indicating a high fat content, the findings may be considered to be diagnostic of sialosis in the presence of appropriate clinical findings (figs. 5.6E, 5.7B, 5.8A, 5.9, 5.10A). If the parotid glands are in the soft tissue range, however (fig. 5.4C) the CT findings alone are not specific. A needle biopsy can be recommended here as in other instances when the radiologic and clinical findings alone are not diagnostic.

CT examination of inflammatory processes in the salivary glands may demonstrate enlargement and diffuse increase in density of the gland, sometimes with irregular areas of mixed density (Bryan et al. 1982) (fig. 1.37C,D). Focal inflammatory masses of soft tissue density are often present within such glands. The CT densities of these masses may be similar to those of tumors so that it is not possible to distinguish between inflammatory masses and benign or malignant neoplastic masses by CT alone. Multiple masses within the salivary glands (figs. 1.38A,B,C) often are lymph nodes that may be enlarged by inflammatory processes or tumor. The lobular pattern is usually preserved elsewhere in the gland, and the soft tissue septa surrounding the lower density parotid lobules may be somewhat thickened (fig. 1.37D). Inflammatory processes may extend into tissues adjacent to the salivary gland, in similar fashion to malignant tumors (fig. 1.37D). CT of the parotid glands in Sjögren's syndrome has shown enlargement of the salivary glands, particularly of the parotid glands, which tend to be of soft tissue density because of replacement of fat. Such parotid glands may contain irregular, small to moderate-sized areas of low density (Bryan et al. 1982) (see chapter 4). Calculi, even small ones, are well visualized on CT (fig. 1.26C), perhaps even more reliably than on plain film since CT is more sensitive to the demonstration of calcifications that are small or relatively faint.

Masses Arising from Outside the Salivary Glands

The apparent location of the mass outside the salivary gland or the presence of some intervening structures between the salivary gland and the mass will often indicate an extrasalivary origin (fig. 1.39A). Often, though not invariably (fig. 1.39B), a thin fat layer separates the mass from the gland (figs. 1.39A, 1.40A). Extrinsic masses may deform and/or displace the adjacent salivary gland which is, however, otherwise normal (fig. 1.39B). As with intrinsic masses, it may not be possible by CT appearances alone to distinguish between benign and malignant processes or between inflammatory and neoplastic masses.

The most common extrinsic masses adjacent to the salivary glands are either abscesses or lymph nodes enlarged by metastases, lymphoma, or infection (figs. 1.39A,D,E, 1.40A). Branchial cleft cysts may also occur in this location (figs. 1.39B,C). Arteriovenous malformations (figs. 1.40B–D) glomus vagale tumors, carotid body tumors, minor salivary gland tumors, and schwannomas may also present as masses that may be indistinguishable on clinical grounds alone from primary tumors in the major salivary glands.

Hypertrophy of the masticatory muscles (see chapter 7) may also present clinically as a mass in the parotid region on one or both sides. CT examination is able to identify such masses as consisting of masseter or masseter and temporalis muscles and thus to identify this condition without further examination.

The Role of CT

CT is the method of choice for the radiologic examination of masses in or about the salivary glands as well as for the study of diffuse noninflammatory enlargement of one or several salivary glands. CT is less invasive than conventional sialography since it can usually be performed without contrast material. Furthermore, it is more sensitive in determining the presence or absence of a mass and more accurate in demonstrating the extent and intrinsic or extrinsic nature of a mass. CT provides exquisite anatomic detail, showing the precise location of a mass within the parotid gland from which the probability of displacement of the facial nerve may be inferred, information that is useful to the surgeon and is especially well displayed in the axial projection. CT demonstrates whether a mass is circumscribed or invasive and can even demonstrate the precise histologic nature of some pathologic processes, such as lipoma, cyst, sialosis, or masseter muscle hypertrophy. The appearances in sialosis are often diagnostic (see chapter 5).

On the other hand, some caveats are in order. It should be remembered that with these few exceptions, CT is not a reliable histologic method (Martinez et al. 1983) and cannot differentiate with certainty between a benign tumor and a malignant one unless there is obvious infiltration into the gland at the margin of the tumor or invasion of surrounding structures. Nor is CT able to distinguish with certainty between an inflammatory and a neoplastic mass. Nevertheless, sensitivity in the detection of salivary gland lesions may approach 100% (Bryan et al. 1982). According to these authors, specificity of the CT findings alone in distinguishing between benign and malignant neoplasms and inflammation is only about 75%, although it may reach 90% when the radiologic findings are integrated with clinical and laboratory data.

The role of CT in the examination for calculi, obstruction, sialectasis, and inflammation is still controversial, and no consensus has yet been reached on the place of CT in these disorders (Golding 1982; Martinez et al. 1983). CT is able accurately to demonstrate the presence of salivary calculi (fig. 1.26C) as well as of diffuse or focal abnormalities such as can be caused by inflammatory processes in the salivary gland. It may be less reliable than conventional sialography for the demonstration of sialectasis or obstruction (Bryan et al. 1982), although it is possible to demonstrate duct dilatation, as seen in fig. 1.26C. Our current practice is to perform conventional sialography for the evaluation of calculi, obstruction, or sialectasis. If signs and symptoms of acute infection are present and acute parotitis is suspected, antibiotic treatment is administered. If the gland remains enlarged, plain CT is performed.

Sjögren's syndrome is diagnosed preferably on clinical and serological grounds, with biopsy of minor salivary glands of the lip for confirmation if necessary. Nevertheless, because of the presence of enlarged salivary glands with or without inflammation or a mass, radiological examination may be requested and changes consistent with Sjögren's syndrome involving the salivary glands may be demonstrated (see chapter 4).

Ultrasound

Ultrasound examination may be useful in differentiating between intrinsic and extrinsic masses and between solid and cystic masses (figs. 1.21D, 1.36B, 1.41E, 1.42C, 1.43B) and may even demonstrate calculi (Gooding 1980).

Nuclear Medicine

Radioisotope scans with ^{99m}Tc–pertechnetate are not as accurate as contrast sialography in demonstrating focal abnormalities of the salivary glands (Schmitt et al. 1976). This technique can confirm the presence of an occult mass in the gland but is more particularly of value in establishing the diagnosis of Warthin's tumor and oncocytomas, since these are the only tumors that regularly show an increased uptake of the isotope (Sorsdahl, Williams, and Bruno 1969; Schall and DiChiro 1972; Pogrel 1981; Cogan and Gill 1981). Furthermore, since it can assess salivary gland function, it also provides insight into the pathophysiology and course of Sjögren's syndrome (Alarcon-Segovia et al. 1971; Daniels et al. 1979), and aids in distinguishing between benign parotid hypertrophy (sialosis) and benign lymphoepithelial lesions (Sjögren's syndrome) (Hausler et al. 1977) (fig. 5.11), and in identifying subclinical involvement of the salivary gland by such systemic disease as sarcoidosis and various collagen diseases (Mishkin 1981). The application of radioisotopic studies to various diseases of the salivary glands is further discussed by de Rossi (1978), Parret and Peyrin (1979), Tainmont, Dubois, and Hennebert (1979), Schall, Smith, and Barsocchini (1981), Pretorius and Taylor (1982), Ohrt and Shafer (1982), and Sucupira et al. (1983).

Angiography

Although some masses in the salivary glands and their arterial supply and venous drainage can be demonstrated by arteriography

(Lowman and Cheng 1976), this procedure does not ordinarily provide additional information considered to be necessary for the clinical care of the patient and is not widely applied to the study of intrinsic diseases of the salivary gland. Nevertheless, arteriography or venography can be useful in the diagnosis and, in some instances, in the treatment of extrasalivary tumors of the neck (figs. 1.40B,C,D).

Pneumoradiography of the submandibular gland (Granone and Juliani 1968) has been reported but has never been widely practiced. In any event, much the same information can now be obtained with CT.

Biopsy

Needle biopsy (Godwin 1952; Eneroth and Hamberger 1974) is being used increasingly to obtain histologic diagnosis of masses in and around the salivary glands.

Pathologic examination of aspiration biopsy specimens of masses in and around the salivary glands can be used to diagnose the specific type of tumor present as well as to demonstrate the presence of infection and obtain specific bacteriologic data. A high degree of accuracy has been obtained (Kline, Merriam, and Shapshay 1981). Such biopsies are recommended wherever clinically indicated since the results often will help to determine the most appropriate therapy. Indeed, it has been suggested that aspiration biopsy may be the only workup needed in selected instances (Hanafee 1982b).

In a series of 51 fine-needle (22-gauge) biopsies performed on 44 patients with major salivary gland masses, 96% of the benign lesions and 85% of the malignant lesions were identified correctly (Sismanis et al. 1981). The exact histologic diagnosis of benign lesions was made in 87% and of malignant tumors in 60% of patients so examined. The overall concurrence rate between cystologic and histologic findings was 91%.

CT-guided aspiration biopsy using a 22-gauge needle (fig. 1.40A) can be performed under local anesthesia, with premedication if desired (Gatenby, Mulhern, and Strawitz 1983). Direct lateral, retromandibular, or inferior approaches may be used.

Care after Sialography

The patient is instructed to report any increase in pain or swelling after the examination. The gland enlargement that accompanies acinar filling ordinarily diminishes and disappears over the next 24 to 48 hours. Although patients rarely complain of much discomfort after the examination, pain and swelling may occasionally require symptomatic treatment. Normal eating habits may be resumed without any restrictions related to the performance of sialography.

Complications of Sialography

Perforation of Salivary Ducts

Mandel and Baurmash (1962) reported the appearance of a painless granulomatous mass in the cheek of a patient following Lipiodol extravasation through an accidental perforation of the parotid duct during sialography performed elsewhere five years previously. In a national survey, Ansell (1968) noted a patient with extravasation of Endografin through a false passage during submandibular sialography, with resulting sterile induration of the floor of the mouth lasting two weeks.

Perforation occasionally occurs with the use of the metal probe, although it rarely occurs with the nylon probes. Overdilatation may cause minor tearing of the tissues near the duct orifice and injection should be observed carefully with fluoroscopic monitoring under these circumstances to be certain that significant extravasation is not occurring.

Infection

Rarely, infection in the salivary gland may occur following sialography, or a previously existing infection may be exacerbated. Stasis or obstruction resulting from stone or stricture predisposes to the development of infection. An appropriate antibiotic may be required.

Clinical Reactions to Contrast Material

Very few untoward reactions to contrast material injected into salivary ducts have been reported (Sonnabend 1968). Ansell (1968) reviewed several cases. The most severe reaction was the development of edema of the glottis after injection of only a drop or two of viscous Neohydriol. Another patient developed painful swelling of the parotid gland following the injection of 1 ml of 76% Urografin, with the swelling subsiding after three days. Cook and Pollack (1966) state that allergic reactions are rare but mention one case in which a severe reaction occurred. According to Trester (1968), allergic reactions to water-soluble contrast materials injected at sialography had not been reported up to that time.

According to Yune (1977), the parotid gland may become edematous and painful as a result of coming in contact with a high concentration of iodine such as may occur either with elevated iodine levels in the blood or from direct injection of iodine-containing substances into the salivary ducts. While such "iodine parotitis" (Kohri et al. 1977) is a theoretical complication of sialography, to our knowledge no cases have been reported as such following sialography. Most instances of iodine parotitis have followed intravenous injection of iodinated contrast materials, especially in the presence of severe kidney or liver disease; even under these circumstances the condition is rare (Talner et al. 1971). The swelling and tenderness, which may appear in the parotid and/or submandibular glands within minutes

(Navani et al. 1972) to a few days (Talner et al. 1971) after the intravenous injection of contrast material, is of benign nature and disappears within hours or days. Presumably this reaction is related to the excretion into the saliva of a high concentration of iodine that may be toxic to the acinar cells. References to isolated instances of iodine parotitis following administration of bronchographic and cholecysto-graphic agents are quoted by Talner and co-workers (1971).

Extravasation of Contrast Material into the Salivary Glands

Radiologic Appearances

Overzealous injection may cause actual rupture of the gland with gross extravasation of contrast material (Cook and Pollack 1966). Even with carefully controlled injection, however, varying degrees of focal or widespread interstitial extravasation of contrast material within the gland may occur in salivary glands that are normal or normal except for the presence of a focal mass (figs. 1.23A,B,C,D, 1.31B, 1.43C, 1.44, 1.45), especially if injection is made too rapidly, at too high a pressure, in too great a volume, or over too prolonged a period (figs. 1.50, 1.51) (Ranger 1957). Various patterns of interstitial extravasation may be identified radiologically according to the distribution and location of the extravasated contrast material in the tissues. Extravasation may occur in normal or mass-containing submandibular glands also, although it is seen less commonly than in parotid glands (figs. 1.31B, 1.43C).

Extravasation is a common occurrence in diseased salivary glands (figs. 1.46–1.49, 3.53, 5.3C,D,E; see also chapter 4). Some contrast material may thus remain in the gland following sialography, even after stimulated salivary flow has removed the free contrast material from the ducts. Such residual oily contrast material may remain either as plugs in the smaller ductules or as actual extravasate into the tissues (Rubin et al. 1955; Rubin and Holt 1957; Ranger 1957; Gullmo and Book-Hederstrom 1958). Some of this may disappear over the ensuing few days (fig. 1.50), but much may remain in the tissues for many months. Thus, follow-up in a randomized series of our patients during the months following the examination have shown gradual disappearance of the residual contrast material extravasated interstitially at the time of the injection, with most of it having disappeared within six months to one year (fig. 1.51). Clinical signs or symptoms associated with the retention and gradual disappearance of this contrast material are not apparent. Our own observations and CT studies by Golding (1982) have shown retention and subsequent gradual disappearance of oily contrast material in the parotid gland following sialography.

Water-soluble contrast materials used for sialography presumably extravasate in a fashion similar to the oily contrast materials, but they are quickly absorbed into the blood and disappear.

Although the precise site or sites at which extravasation occurs have not been extensively studied, the small punctate extravasations that can be produced in normal parotid glands (Ranger 1957) and inflamed parotid glands (Patey and Thackray 1955) have been shown to occur from the intralobular ducts. Presumably, extravasation occurs at the weakest sites exposed to the injected contrast material. Intercellular spaces have been demonstrated between the adjacent serous acinar cells (intercellular canaliculi or intercellular territories) (Provenza 1964; Young and Van Lennep 1978) (fig. 2.3B,C). It is conjectural whether extravasation might occur through these intercellular intervals or through the intercellular spaces between the cells lining the ducts. Rubin and colleagues (1955) suggested that even the acinar cells themselves may be ruptured by overinjection.

Histologic Appearances

Previous authors have reported varying degrees of chronic inflammatory changes following the injection of Lipiodol, Dionosil, iodochlorol, or other fat soluble contrast materials into the salivary ducts and glands of humans or dogs (Epsteen and Bendix 1954; Thackray 1955; Rubin et al. 1955; Trester 1968; Lilly, Cutcher, and Steiner 1968). According to Thackray (1955), this granulomatous and fibrotic reaction may make dissection of salivary glands more difficult and may make the difference between resolution and persistence of an inflammatory process.

Epsteen (1956), who introduced Ethiodol for sialography, reported that it did not cause foreign body reaction in the salivary glands in three dogs studied for as long as eight weeks. Trester (1968) noted that while such early reports indicated that Ethiodol did not cause any acute or chronic reaction when injected into the salivary glands, more recent reports showed that it could cause a granulomatous reaction. Lilly, Cutcher, and Steiner (1968) showed that while no acute reaction occurred in salivary glands injected with Ethiodol or Lipiodol, chronic granulomatous reactions did occur when this contrast material was injected interstitially into the subcutaneous tissues of nipples of dogs. These authors suggested that because contrast material may be extravasated during sialography, this reaction compromises the use of Ethiodol and Lipiodol for sialography. Fischer (1977) reported temporary histologic inflammatory changes with giant cells, lasting several months, in lymph nodes that contained Ethiodol, apparently not clinically significant. Chronic tissue reaction to extravasated Ethiodol has been shown by Patey and Thackray (1955) and Thackray (1955).

Water-soluble contrast materials have also been studied. Epsteen and Bendix (1954) reported only a moderate tissue reaction to methiodal. Lilly, Cutcher, and Steiner (1968) reported that aqueous Dionosil produced sialadenitis and marked proliferation of ductal epithelium in dogs. No granulomatous reactions in the salivary glands have been reported from the injection of the water soluble contrast materials in current use such as the salts of diatrizoate, iodipamide, or iothalamate: Hypaque, Renografin, Sinografin, and Conray (Lilly, Cutcher, and Steiner 1968; Trester 1968; Lowman and Cheng 1976).

CASES

Parotid duct system

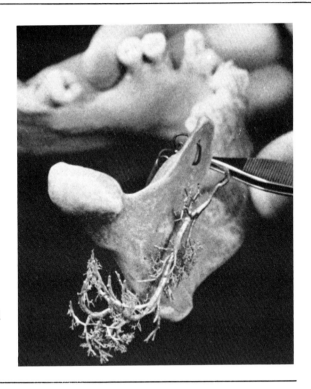

Figure 1.1

Lateral oblique view of a metal cast of the right parotid duct system as viewed from above, behind, and lateral to the mandibular condyle. There is a single main duct with many branches. Those to the deep part of the gland swing medially behind the ramus of the mandible at a right angle, while those to the superficial part continue in a general dorsal direction. The parotid gland is thus a single-lobed gland with deep and superficial portions. (Winsten, Gould, and Ward 1956. Reprinted by permission.)

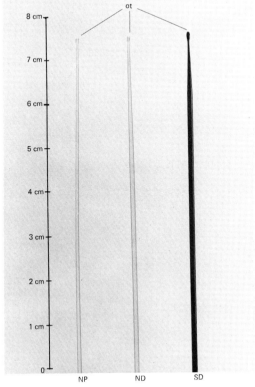

Probes and dilators for sialography

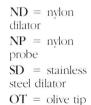

ND = nylon dilator
NP = nylon probe
SD = stainless steel dilator
OT = olive tip

Figure 1.2

Each probe is approximately 15 cm in total length. Nylon probe (Marano, Smart, and Kolodny 1971) tapers over a distance of 8 cm; nylon dilator tapers over a distance of 2 cm (both are available from U.S. Catheter and Instrument Corp., Billerica, Mass.). The stainless steel dilator tapers over a distance of 1.5 cm (E.M. Parker, Inc., Brookline, Mass.). (Rabinov 1981b. Reprinted with permission.)

Cannulas for sialography

CS = closed
smooth end
EP = end port
PS = plastic or
metal shoulder
SP = side port

Figure 1.3

These are manufactured in four diameters, each in a longer and shorter model. The attached plastic catheter is 30 cm long in each instance: 21-gauge long (4.5 cm) tapered side-port cannula, closed end (*21LT*); 21-gauge short (1.5 cm) tapered side-port cannula, closed end (*21ST*); 24-gauge long (4.5 cm) end-port cannula (*24L*); 24-gauge short (0.8 cm) end-port cannula (*24S*).

The end-port cannulas are available also in 27-gauge and 30-gauge sizes, long and short lengths as above (all may be ordered from Cook, Inc., Bloomington, Ind. and E.M. Parker Co., Brookline, Mass.).

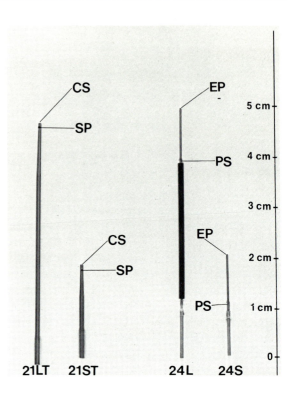

Equipment for sialography

Figure 1.4

Metal and nylon probes and dilators, 10-ml syringe with contrast material and attached stopcock and cannula, additional vials of contrast material, 10-ml syringe containing lemon juice, tongue blade, cotton swabs, 2″ × 2″ gauze, BB (used as marker) attached to tape; magnifying spectacles are not shown.

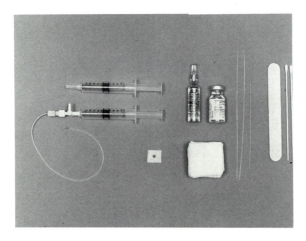

Water-soluble versus oily contrast material

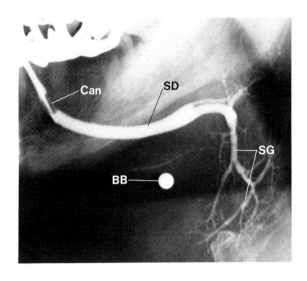

BB = marker taped to the skin overlying the palpable mass anterior to the submandibular gland
Can = cannula
M = mass anterior to the submandibular gland
MG = margin of the submandibular gland
SD = submandibular duct
SG = submandibular gland
U = uncinate process of the submandibular gland

Figure 1.5A

Submandibular sialogram, lateral view, performed with Renografin 76. The ducts are adequately demonstrated but the parenchyma could not be well opacified, even at pressures in the duct measured to range between 52 and 75 mm Hg (see Case 3, table 1.1). The BB is taped to the skin overlying the palpable mass anterior to the submandibular gland.

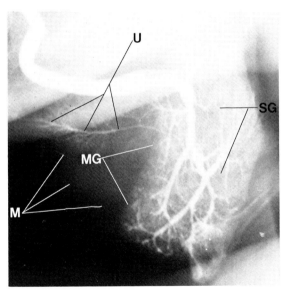

Figure 1.5B

Same patient, submandibular sialogram, lateral view, performed a few minutes later with Ethiodol. The parenchyma is well opacified, and the margin of the gland against the mass anterior to it is sharply delineated and intact. The findings indicate a mass outside the salivary gland. At surgery, the mass was found to be markedly enlarged lymph nodes. Biopsy of the mass revealed Hodgkin's disease.

Preliminary films

C   = calculus
CSP = cervical spine
MA = mandible
MP = mastoid process

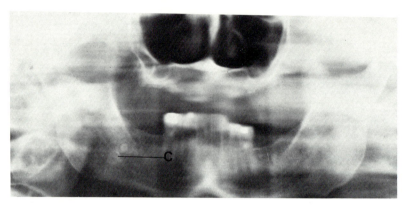

Figure 1.6A

Orthopantomogram.

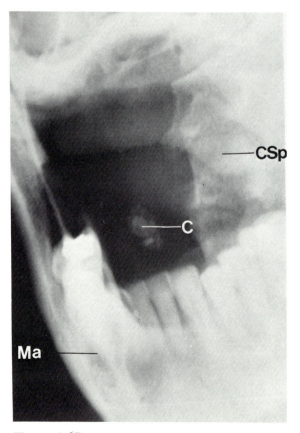

Figure 1.6B

Open mouth view; see Figure 2.17A for the radiographic position. Same patient as shown in Figures 1.6A, 2.27C, 2.28.

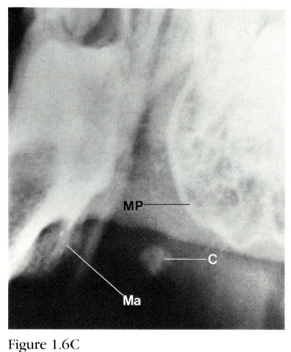

Figure 1.6C

Anterior-oblique view with the chin tilted up. The calculus is visualized beneath the mandible; from a different case. See figure 2.27A for radiographic positioning.

Parotid gland

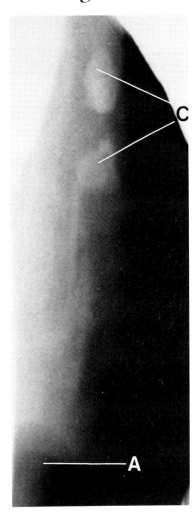

A = air in the cavum conchae
BB = marks location of palpable calculi
C = calculi in the parotid duct

Figure 1.7A

Preliminary axial-tangential view of the parotid gland; several calculi are visible. See figure 2.16A for the actual position in which this film was taken.

Figure 1.7B

Same patient, lateral view of the parotid duct, after injection of the contrast material, showing the calculi in the parotid duct.

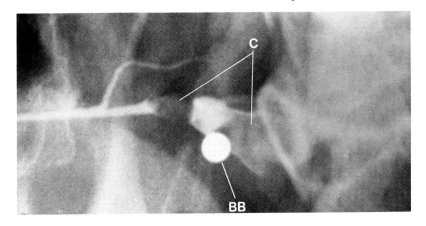

Panoramic radiography

T = metastatic tumor causing destruction of the ramus of the mandible

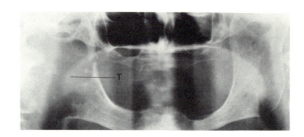

A palpable mass was thought possibly to be in the parotid gland, but this preliminary study showed the mass to be due to a destructive lesion in the mandible, and sialography was not performed. Biopsy subsequently showed metastasis to the mandible from a primary breast carcinoma.

Figure 1.10

Orthopantomogram obtained before sialography.

Parotid sialography

BB = marker
Can = cannula
Ma = mandible
O = orifice of the parotid duct
P = probe
PD = parotid duct
PG = parotid gland

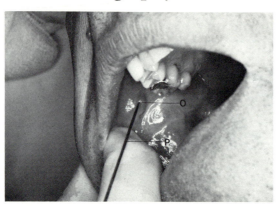

Figure 1.11A

Probe in the parotid duct orifice, located on the buccal mucosa opposite the second upper molar tooth. The cheek is pulled forward to facilitate advancement of the instrument into the duct.

The patient was a 75-year-old woman with a mass present in the left cheek for five months. The sialogram demonstrates moderately severe sialectasis. A fluctuant mass was present in the posterior portion of the gland beneath the BB, presumably an abscess. The gland returned to normal size and the mass disappeared following this dilation and drainage and antibiotic therapy. Because of recurrent symptoms, the duct orifice was redilated approximately 14 months later, with good results. It is possible that the stricture at the duct orifice may have been due to trauma from the patient's denture.

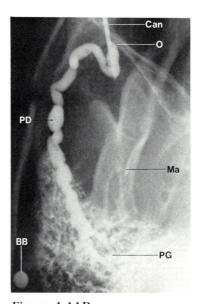

Figure 1.11B

Axial view; contrast material is Ethiodol. Stricture at the duct orifice, dilated by a probe; initially there was no secretion visible from the duct but a probe was eventually maneuvered into the orifice and satisfactory dilation was accomplished. The duct was filled with purulent material. This is the same patient shown in figure 3.66.

Cannula insertion

For insertion into the duct, the cannula should be grasped by the plastic portion so that the flexibility of the plastic can provide safety from perforation.

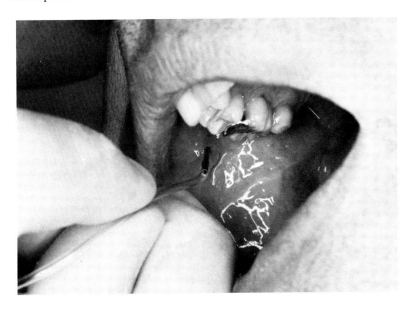

Figure 1.12

The cheek has been pulled forward and the cannula has been wedged into the parotid duct orifice.

Cannula insertion

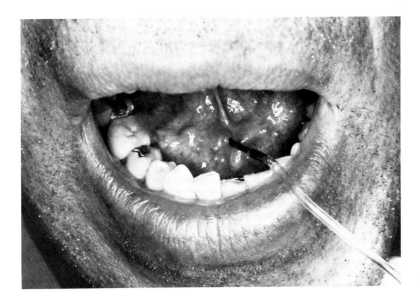

Figure 1.13

A side-port cannula in the orifice of the right submandibular duct, located on the sublingual caruncle. The cannula is wedged into place.

Cannula insertion and ranula injection

B   = Bartholin's duct
C   = calculus
Can   = cannula
Ma   = mandible
SD   = submandibular duct
SG   = submandibular gland
R   = ranula
N   = needle

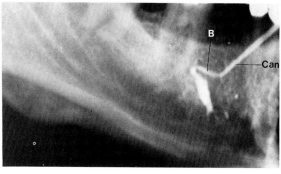

Figure 1.14A

Lateral view of the submandibular region. Fluoroscopy and spot films showed that the cannula had entered Bartholin's duct, which has been opacified by injection of Sinografin.

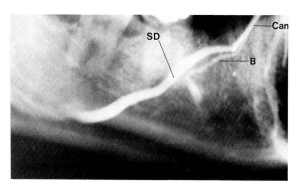

Figure 1.14B

The cannula has been withdrawn slightly and redirected into the main submandibular duct. Both the main submandibular duct and Bartholin's duct are now opacified with Sinografin.

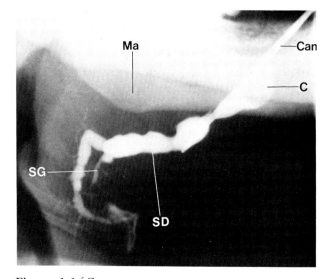

Figure 1.14C

Submandibular sialogram performed in the presence of a surgical fistula from the submandibular duct to the floor of the mouth. The long cannula has been placed in the anatomic duct orifice and passed easily into the duct, beyond the fistula site so that the fistula is not visualized. There is evidence of moderate sialectasis, and a stone is present in the anterior portion of the submandibular duct.

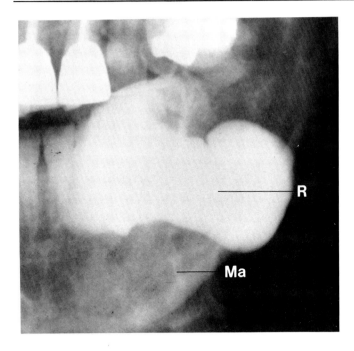

Figure 1.14D

AP view after ranula injection with water-soluble contrast material by direct puncture with a 23-gauge needle.

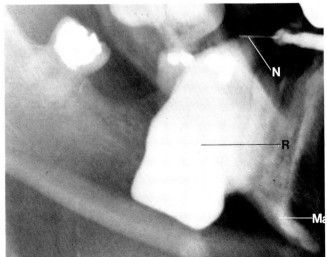

Figure 1.14E

Lateral oblique view of the floor of the mouth. The inferior margin of the ranula is flattened, probably at its interface with the mylohyoid muscle. Fifteen ml of slightly bloody watery fluid was removed prior to the injection of contrast material into this cavity, and the contrast material was subsequently aspirated from the ranula following this examination.

The patient in figures 1.14D and E was a 34-year old woman with a soft mass in the floor of the mouth. It had been explored and considerable bleeding had occurred; the mass was thought possibly to be an arteriovenous malformation. Carotid angiography did not demonstrate any vascular mass, however, and this injection into the cystic space was carried out to confirm that the mass was a ranula and to demonstrate its extent. The cystic mass was removed and pathologic analysis showed changes consistent with a ranula.

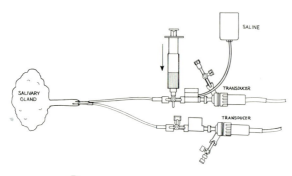

Figure 1.15A

Diagram of the arrangement used for the measurement of pressures at the hub of the syringe and in the duct during sialography. See figure 1.15B.

Gould transducers were used, with fluid-filled pressure monitoring systems. The flushing system (Sorenson Research) was clamped off after the system was filled, so that no fluid except contrast material would enter the duct. Digital pressure display was provided on blood pressure monitoring equipment (American Optical Company). MFE two-channel recorder was used to record simultaneous pressure tracings at the syringe hub and within the duct.

After recording of baseline pressures, contrast materials were injected by hand through either the short 27-gauge thin-wall cannula (0.016 inches overall diameter) or the short 30-gauge thin-wall cannula (0.012 inches overall diameter) end port, shown in figure 1.3. The tip of this cannula was just within the duct orifice. The pressures of injection at the syringe hub were measured through a four-way stopcock open to the duct as well as to the transducer and to the syringe.

Pressures within the duct were measured simultaneously through the short side-port cannula, 18-gauge thin-wall metal tubing (0.048 inches OD) drawn at the tip to 21-gauge (0.032 inches OD), shown in figure 1.3. The tip of this cannula was inserted at least a few millimeters beyond the tip of the injecting cannula. The upper limit of accuracy of the recording device was 280 mm Hg.

Measurement of pressures within the salivary ducts

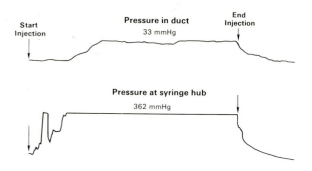

Figure 1.15B

Simultaneous tracing of pressures at the hub of the syringe (*bottom tracing*) and in the salivary duct (*top tracing*) during sialography, using the arrangement shown in figure 1.15A. These tracings are from case 4 in table 1.1. The examination was performed without any stimulation of salivary flow with lemon juice, at a steady state of hand injection pressure. The sialogram was normal. Note that the pressure at the hub of the syringe rose above 280 mm Hg, the upper limit of accuracy of the recording device used. The pressure within the duct at the same time was measured to range from 33 to 46 mm Hg. The specific numbers recorded above the tracings were obtained from direct digital readout during the injection. In this instance, as in all others, there was a uniform tendency for the pressure at the hub of the syringe to rise quickly at the beginning of the injection and to fall quickly at the end of the injection, while the pressure in the duct rose somewhat more slowly at the beginning of the injection and fell slightly more gradually toward the base at the end of the injection.

The four phases of sialography, illustrated by submandibular sialography using Ethiodol, lateral views

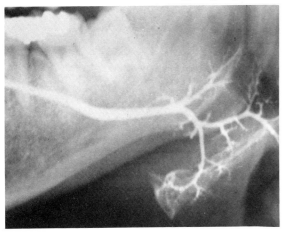

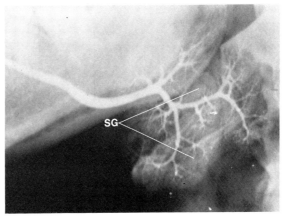

CM = evacuated contrast material on the floor of the patient's mouth

O = orifice of submandibular duct

SG = submandibular salivary gland

Figure 1.16A

The duct filling phase; a few branches have not yet filled completely.

Figure 1.16B

The acinar filling phase; the parenchyma has become opacified.

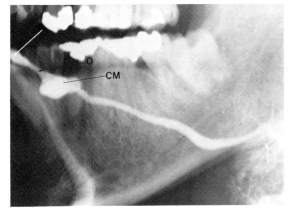

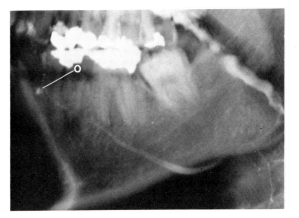

Figure 1.16C

The evacuation phase; the main submandibular duct can be seen all the way from the gland to the orifice of the duct, with spill of contrast material out of the duct (*arrow*) and onto the floor of the mouth immediately following removal of the cannula.

Figure 1.16D

The postevacuation phase taken several minutes after withdrawal of the cannula. Most of the contrast material has been evacuated from the duct spontaneously.

Radiographs of normal parotid gland specimens during injection of neo-hydriol

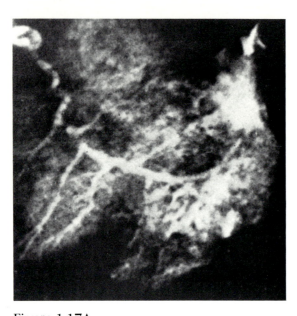

Figure 1.17A

Radiograph of a normal parotid gland specimen injected with 2 ml of neo-hydriol. The parenchyma shows mottled opacification. All 20 glands had this appearance.

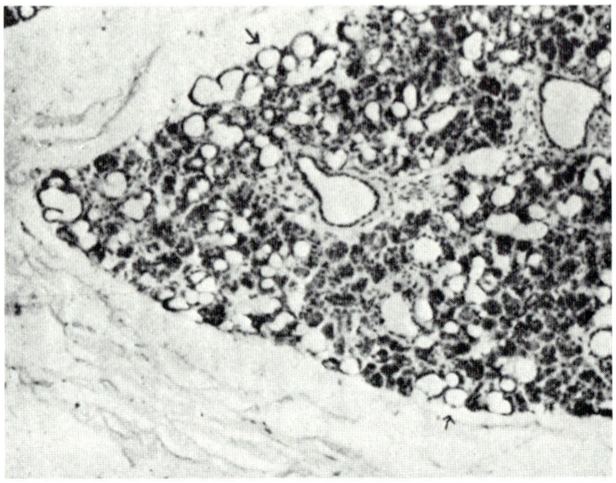

Figure 1.17B

Histologic section corresponding with figure 1.17A. Some of the ducts and acini are distended with contrast material that has been removed in processing. The mottled parenchymal opacification shown in figure 1.17A is due to patchy acinar filling.

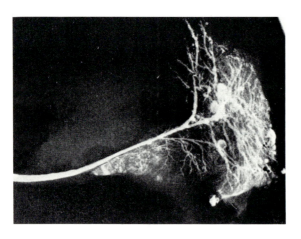

Figure 1.17C

Radiograph of a normal parotid gland specimen showing globules of contrast material adjacent to some of the ducts, in addition to the mottled parenchymal opacification. These globules became more numerous and larger as the examination progressed. Thirteen of 20 specimens showed this pattern. (Ranger 1957. Reprinted with permission.)

Parotid sialography showing the duct opacification and parenchymal opacification phases, lateral views

The contrast material is Ethiodol. The gland is normal except for deformity caused by an extrinsic mass inferiorly. Note the lobular character of the opacified parotid gland. A broad shallow deformity and irregular margin along the posterior inferior margin of the parotid gland was caused by a mass of adjacent lymph nodes (*arrows*) that were enlarged by metastases.

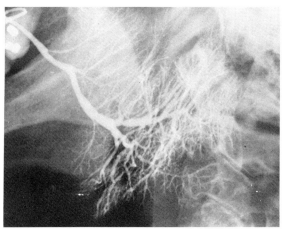

Figure 1.18A

Parotid sialogram, duct opacification phase.

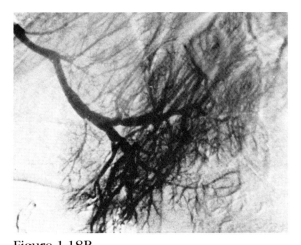

Figure 1.18B

Parotid sialogram, duct opacification, subtraction technique.

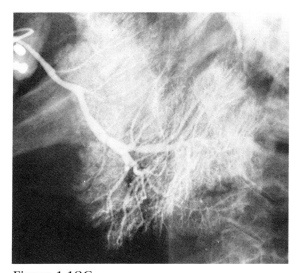

Figure 1.18C

Parotid sialogram, acinar opacification phase.

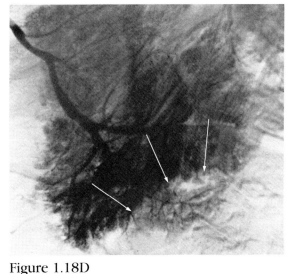

Figure 1.18D

Parotid sialogram, acinar opacification phase, subtraction technique.

Submandibular sialography showing the duct opacification and acinar opacification phases, lateral views

The contrast material is Ethiodol; the lobular character of the submandibular gland is well shown. The gland is normal.

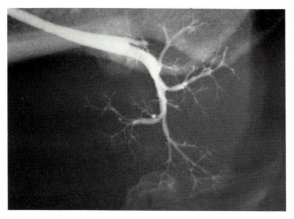

Figure 1.19A

Submandibular sialogram, duct opacification phase.

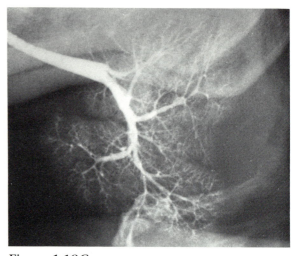

Figure 1.19C

Submandibular sialogram, acinar opacification phase.

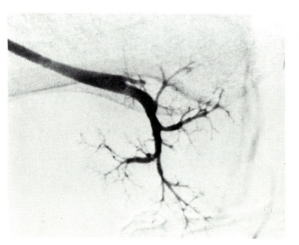

Figure 1.19B

Submandibular sialogram, duct opacification phase, subtraction technique.

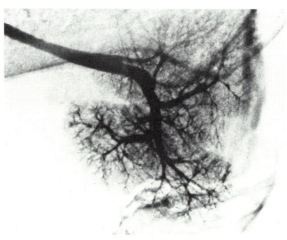

Figure 1.19D

Submandibular sialogram, acinar opacification phase, subtraction technique.

Sialography, acinar opacification phase, showing intrinsic masses

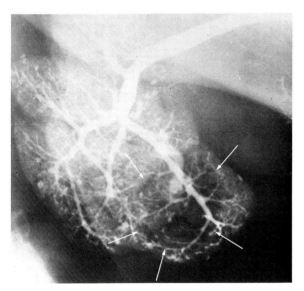

Figure 1.20A

A mass is seen in the anterior portion of the body of the submandibular gland (*arrows*). The pathologic examination showed a mixed tumor; same patient as in figure 1.31. Submandibular sialogram, lateral view, acinar opacification phase performed with Ethiodol.

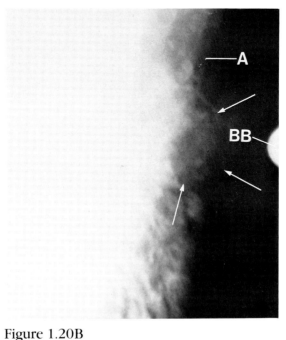

A = air in cavum conchae
BB = marker

Figure 1.20B

Parotid sialography, AP view, distention sialography, late acinar opacification phase with Ethiodol, showing a small mass (*arrows*) in the superficial part of the parotid gland covered by a very thin layer of parenchyma. The overlying BB, used for clinical-radiologic correlation, indicates the tiny size of the mass that has been demonstrated. Pathologic interpretation was a tiny benign mixed tumor. The radiolucency above the mass is air in the cavum conchae.

Submandibular sialography showing progressive acinar opacification; the contrast material is Ethiodol

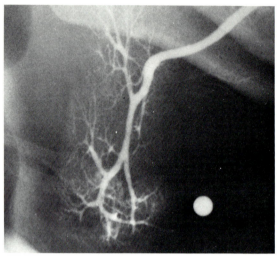

Figure 1.21A

Duct opacification phase, lateral view; the gland shows very early acinar opacification, but the gland margin is not distinctly outlined. The BB indicates the location of a palpable mass anterior to the submandibular gland.

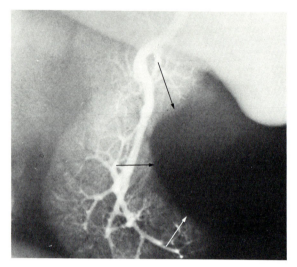

Figure 1.21B

Acinar opacification phase, lateral oblique view, same patient; the margin of the gland adjacent to the mass is now sharply delineated and the mass (*arrows*) can be seen to be extrinsic to the gland.

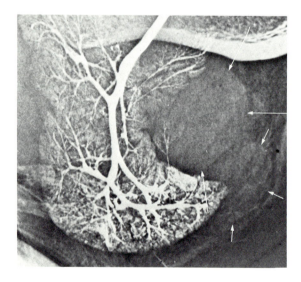

Figure 1.21C

Xeroradiography, lateral view, same patient; the enlarged lymph nodes themselves are now demonstrated (*arrows*) in the soft tissues just anterior to the gland.

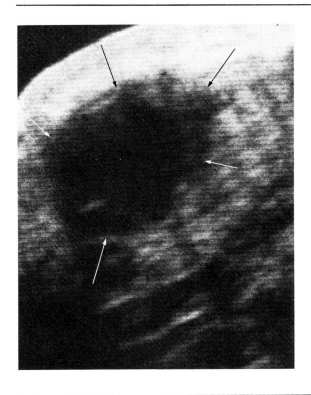

Figure 1.21D

Ultrasound examination, same patient, showing that the mass (*arrows*) anterior to the submandibular salivary gland is relatively sonolucent, although a few internal echoes are seen. The sound waves are not transmitted as well as might be expected with a fluid filled structure, however, nor is the posterior wall as well defined as would be expected, suggesting that the mass may be solid.

    Exploration revealed enlarged lymph nodes in the anterior part of the submaxillary triangle. Pathologic examination revealed lymphoma.

Distension sialography performed with Ethiodol

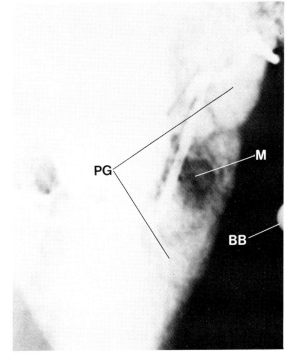

BB = marker
M = mass
PG = parotid gland

Figure 1.22

AP view of the parotid gland, with extensive filling of the acini, so-called distension sialography, to demonstrate a small mass within the parotid gland. The margin of the gland is intact. The gland is distended with contrast material and enlarged, and is densely opacified. Distension sialography may be necessary to demonstrate such small masses definitively. The mass was a tiny mixed tumor.

Extravasation of contrast material

BB = marker

CM = focal collections of extravasates contrast material

SG = submandibular gland

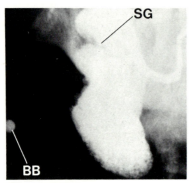 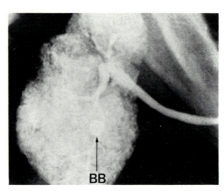

Figure 1.23A

Submandibular sialogram performed with Ethiodol; *left*, AP view; *right*, lateral view. An excessive amount of contrast material has been injected, resulting in interstitial extravasation throughout the gland. A large mass between the BB and the gland, with some extension between the lobules of the gland, was due to an extrinsic abscess.

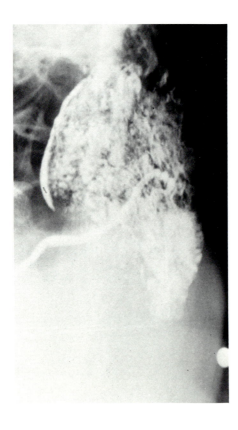

Figure 1.23B

Parotid sialogram in another patient, performed with Ethiodol, AP view.

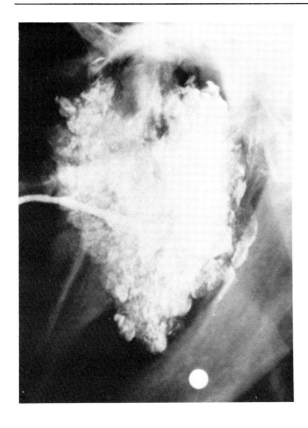

Figure 1.23C

Lateral view, same patient as in figure 1.23B; excessive injection has resulted in extravasation of contrast material interstitially in a lobular pattern and also beneath the parotid capsule. As a consequence, the definition of the margin of the gland has been lost. The large extrinsic mass underlying the BB was metastatic carcinoma.

Figure 1.23D

Parotid sialogram, another patient, lateral view, prolonged examination with Ethiodol. The appearance of the sialogram has deteriorated; the ducts and parenchyma are no longer clearly demonstrated. The irregular clearing of the contrast material under such circumstances may simulate masses within the gland. Most of the tiny collections of contrast material, as well as the larger ones, are outside of the visualized ducts and represent contrast material that has been extravasated into the interstitial tissues. The parotid sialogram was performed because of a clinically suspected mass. None could be demonstrated during the filling phases and the sialogram was reported as normal. The parotid glands were slightly to moderately larger than normal and the ducts were slightly spread apart, suggesting the possibility of sialosis, cause undetermined; same patient as in figure 1.50.

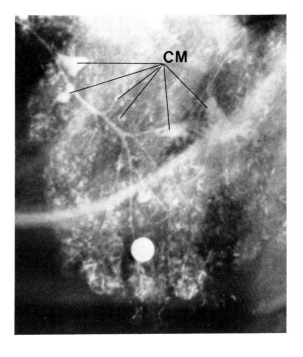

Calculi bypassed by cannula; detected on evacuation film

Submandibular sialography in an eight-year-old boy who complained of intermittent swelling and pain in the submandibular region for several months. The swelling would come suddenly, remain for an hour or less, and then disappear. Upon direct inspection, the small calculi could be seen through the duct orifice and through the mucosa; the duct orifice was slightly enlarged by a small surgical slit under local anesthesia, and the calculi were then easily teased out, followed immediately by ready evacuation of the contrast material.

C   = calculi
Can = cannula
Di = diverticulum

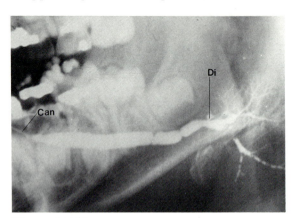

Figure 1.24A

Lateral view.

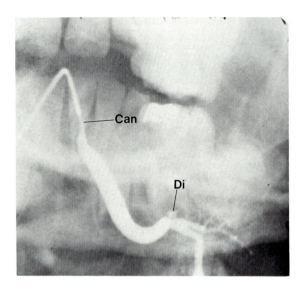

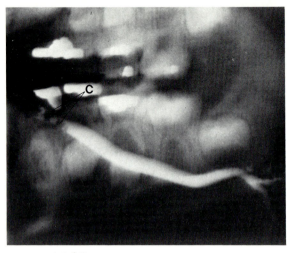

Figure 1.24C

The cannula was reinserted and additional study done. Several small calculi can now be seen near the duct orifice in this lateral view. These had been previously bypassed by the cannula.

Figure 1.24B

AP view. No calculi could be seen in either of these views, but it was noted that when the cannula was removed, there was practically no evacuation of the contrast material over the next ten minutes. A small diverticulum could be seen in the posterior part of the main duct near the hilum of the gland.

Submandibular sialogram, lateral views, to illustrate the ball-valve mechanism of obstruction

C   = calculus
Can = cannula

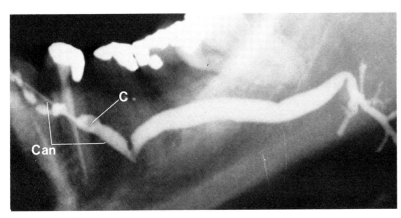

Figure 1.25A

During the injection of Ethiodol note that the cannula has bypassed this calculus also, although the calculus is visible.

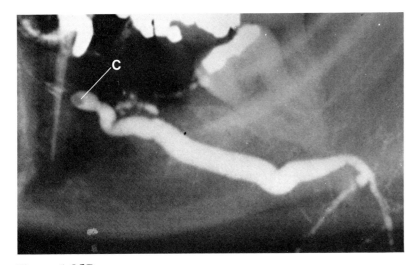

Figure 1.25B

The evacuation phase; the calculus has moved slightly forward and is now obstructing the sub-mandibular duct.

Submandibular sialography, lateral-oblique views

These images demonstrate the ball-valve action of a stone in the duct at the hilum of the gland.

C = calculus
Can = cannula
PD = dilated parotid main duct
PG = parotid gland

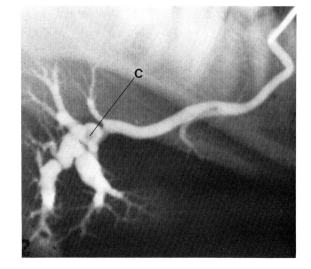

Figure 1.26A

Sialography demonstrates a calculus (*c*) as a relatively radiolucent filling defect in the duct within the gland. A moderate degree of sialectasia is present in the intraglandular branches.

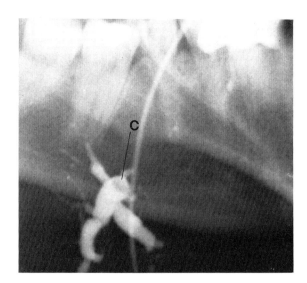

Figure 1.26B

The evacuation phase shows the obstruction caused by the calculus.

Small calculus in the parotid duct. Another case

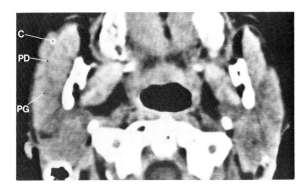

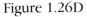

Figure 1.26C

CT performed without contrast material. A small calcification is seen in the anterior part of the parotid duct which can be seen to be moderately dilated. This calculus could not be seen on plain films.

Figure 1.26D

Parotid sialogram lateral view during injection of Sinografin. The main parotid duct is moderately dilated. Irregular sialectasis and stricture formation is present in the intraglandular ducts. The calculus appears as a triangular radiolucent filling defect in the anterior part of the duct.

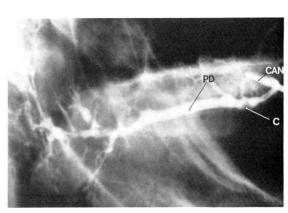

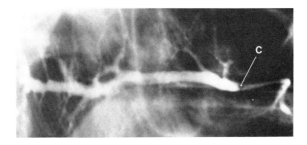

Figure 1.26E

Lateral view during evacuation. The calculus has moved anteriorly and now obstructs the duct.

The patient was a 74-year-old woman with recurrent episodes of swelling of the right parotid gland. A mass was palpable in the posterior part of the parotid gland, presumably inflammatory as it decreased in size with antibiotic therapy.

Inflammatory changes and tumor occurring in the same gland

BB = marker
Can = cannula
PD = parotid duct showing advanced sialectasis
S   = stricture
SMP = stylo-mandibular process

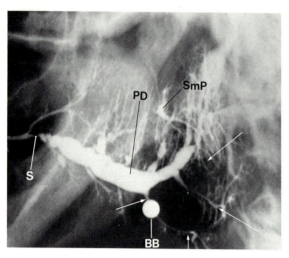

Figure 1.27A

Parotid sialogram, lateral view, performed with Ethiodol; duct-filling phase. The BB indicates the clinical location of the mass. The branches underlying the BB are distorted and the smaller ducts are poorly filled. The parotid duct is moderately sialectatic.

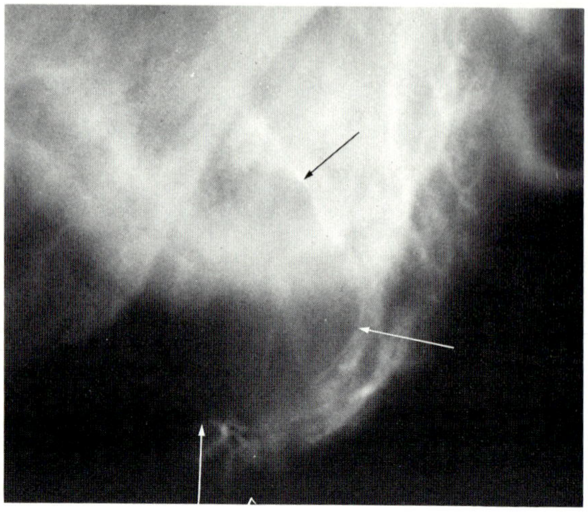

Figure 1.27B

Same patient, laminogram, lateral view, early acinar opacification phase; the mass (*arrows*) can now be seen to be much more clearly outlined, smoothly lobular in character.

At surgery, a tumor was resected from the deep portion of the gland. The inferior division facial nerve structures were in fact found to be displaced laterally and to be splayed over the mass. Pathologic interpretation was mixed tumor. This case demonstrates the presence of advanced sialectasis and inflammatory changes, and a tumor, in the same gland. Parenthetically, note that the anterior-most portion of the parotid duct, which is anatomically in a coronal plane, has been straightened during cannulation and is now held in almost a sagittal plane by the cannula.

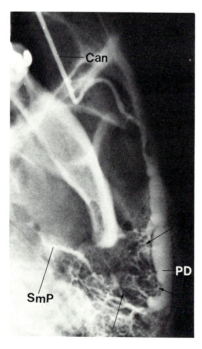

Figure 1.27C

Same patient, axial view; the mass (*arrows*) has arisen in the deep portion of the parotid gland and is situated along the course of the facial nerve. Since it has displaced the duct laterally, it would be expected to displace the nerves laterally also.

Submandibular sialogram, lateral views, showing air bubbles in the duct

A   = air bubble
Can = cannula

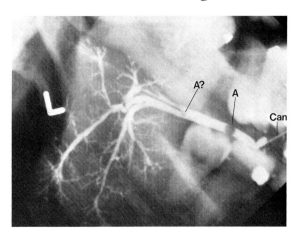

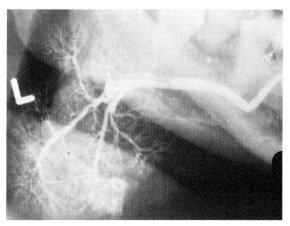

Figure 1.28A

A large oval filling defect is present in the anterior part of the duct, and there is possibly a second smaller one more posteriorly near the site of branching of the duct. The appearance could be due either to calculi or air bubbles. These filling defects were easily aspirated back through the cannula into the tubing, together with some contrast material, indicating that they were air bubbles.

Figure 1.28B

Reinjection demonstrates a normal appearance.

Submandibular sialogram showing a calculus in the submandibular duct

C   = calculus
Can = cannula

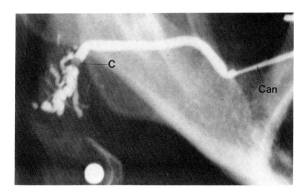

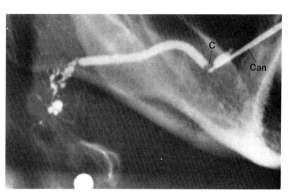

Figure 1.29A

Submandibular sialogram, lateral view, during the injection of Ethiodol, showing a small filling defect in the posterior portion of the submandibular duct, with sialectasia behind it.

Figure 1.29B

Lateral view during withdrawal of contrast material, showing the filling defect at the tip of the cannula; it could not be aspirated into the cannula, indicating that it was a calculus rather than an air bubble.

Submandibular sialogram, lateral views, sialectasia and stricture

B = Bartholin's duct
S = strictures
SD = submandibular duct
Seg = segmentation
SG = submandibular gland

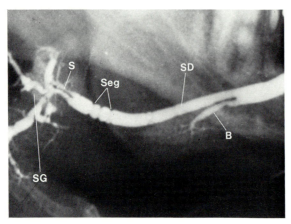

Figure 1.30A

Segmentation of the column of Ethiodol in the submandibular duct; the indentations could be seen to move during the injection.

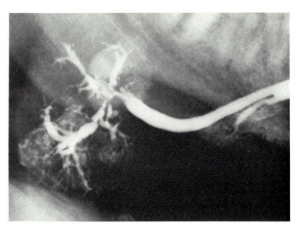

Figure 1.30B

The segmentations ultimately disappeared with continued injection.

Sialectasis and inflammatory changes are present in the intraglandular ducts. There are strictures of the ducts at the hilum of the gland.

Radiographic techniques

Submandibular sialogram, lateral views; the contrast material is Ethiodol.

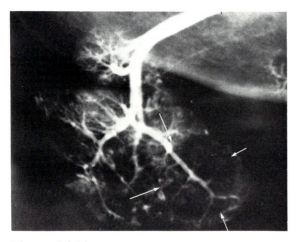

Figure 1.31A

Orthopantomogram; same patient as in figure 1.20A. The mass is outlined by the arrows.

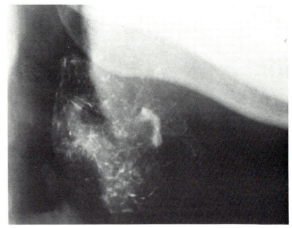

Figure 1.31B

Six days later a film shows residual contrast material outlining the gland. This contrast material is presumably extravasated into the interstitial tissues of the submandibular gland.

Parotid sialogram performed
with Ethiodol, late acinar
phase with moderate
distension of the gland by
contrast material; laminogram
(polytome)

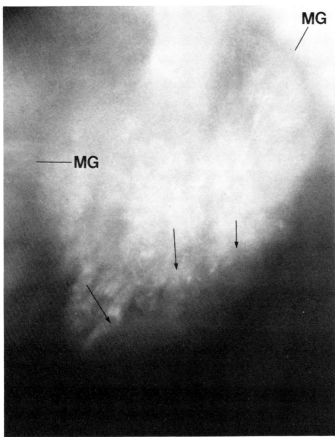

MG = margin of
the normal part of
the parotid gland

Figure 1.32

Lateral view; the portions of the gland that are in
the plane of section are sharply outlined except
for the posterior-inferior portion of the gland,
where the margin is indistinct. The arrows point
to the defect in the margin and superficial part of
the parotid gland, caused by the enlarged hyperplastic intraparotid lymph node.

The patient is a 32-year-old man with a
gradually increasing mass in the tail of the
parotid gland, thought to be a tumor. Pathologic
examination of the surgical specimen, however,
revealed the mass to be a large intraparotid
lymph node with reactive hyperplasia.

CT examination

Digital radiographs ("topograms" or "scout views") taken at the initial stage of CT examination provide a basis for selection of optimal planes for imaging as well as a basis for summarizing the anatomic planes that have been imaged. The BB indicates the clinically palpable mass in each instance.

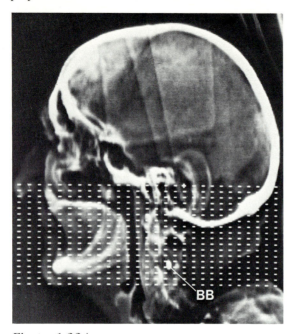

Figure 1.33A

Straight axial projection; if no metallic structures are present, both the parotid and the submandibular glands may be well shown in this projection; same patient as in figure 1.36C.

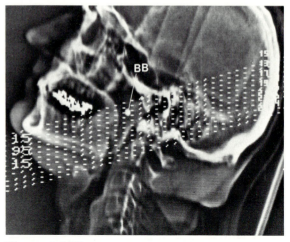

Figure 1.33B

The semiaxial view with the chin extended and the gantry angled 15 to 20 degrees craniad. This basic view may be used for imaging the entire parotid and submandibular glands in most patients; same patient as in figure 2.21A.

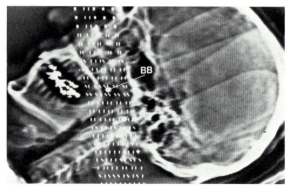

Figure 1.33C

The semiaxial view with the head flexed and the gantry straight or angled slightly can be used to image the upper half of the parotid gland; same patient as in figure 2.22A and B.

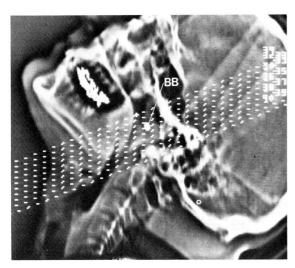

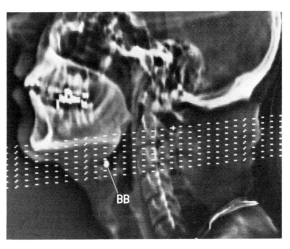

BB = marker indicating the clinically palpable mass

Figure 1.33D

The coronal view can be used to examine the parotid or submandibular glands. This view cannot be sustained by all patients; same patient as in figure 2.23A, B, and C.

Figure 1.33E

The near axial view with the chin slightly extended and the gantry angled slightly craniad can be used to examine the submandibular glands. (Rabinov, Kell, and Gordon, 1984. With permission.)

CT of intraparotid tumors

C = calcification of unidentified nature

CA = common or internal carotid artery

CM = contrast material in opacified part of parotid gland

F = fat layer separating the extraparotid lobule of tumor from the adjacent parotid gland

IJV = internal jugular vein

MA = mandible

MM = masseter muscle

MPM = medial pterygoid muscle

PBD = posterior belly of the digastric muscle

PG = parotid gland

PP = posterior process of parotid gland

SCM = sterno-cleidomastoid muscle

SG = sub-mandibular gland

ST = calcified stylohyoid ligament

T = tumor

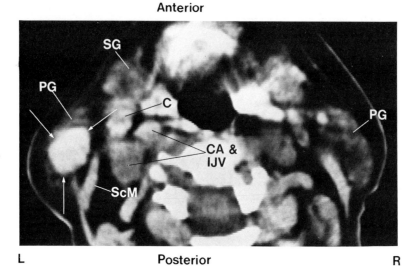

Figure 1.34A

Plain CT of the parotid glands performed in the position illustrated in figure 1.33B. The tumor (*arrows*) is surrounded on three sides by parotid tissue, which it abuts directly. A normal layer of fat is present medial to the tumor.

The patient in figure 1.34A is a 66-year-old woman with a seven-month history of a hard movable nodule in the left side of the neck, growing slowly larger. Pathologic examination revealed Warthin's tumor.

The patient in figure 1.34B is a 23-year-old woman with a palpable left parotid mass. At surgery the mass was deep to the facial nerve branches, which it splayed widely apart, displacing them superiorly and inferiorly. Superficial and deep parotidectomies were performed. The tumor was adherent to the mandible and masseter muscle. Examination of the specimen showed benign mixed tumor, but there were extensions of the tumor into the adjacent fat and skeletal muscle. In such instances, where large tumors are present in the deep portions of the gland, it is well to forewarn the surgeon that the facial nerve

structures may be displaced from their usual location and may sometimes be encountered in very superficial positions.

The patient in figure 1.34C is a 68-year-old man with a palpable mass in the left parotid region. Surgery revealed a Warthin's tumor occupying both the deep and superficial portions of the parotid gland, the larger extrinsic component extending downward along the medial aspect of the tail of the parotid gland.

Warthin's tumors tend to have multiple lobules and may originate from relatively small intraglandular components connected with larger extraglandular lobules. At different sites, this lesion illustrates the characteristics of both intrinsic and extrinsic lesions.

The tumor in figures 1.34D and E occupies both the deep and superficial portions of the parotid gland and is located in the plane of the facial nerve. Its outline against the adjacent parotid tissue is quite sharp. The mass is not completely separable from the masseter muscle (*arrow*). The anterior contour of the mass shows a fine lobulation at its interface with the normal parotid tissue, an appearance suggests

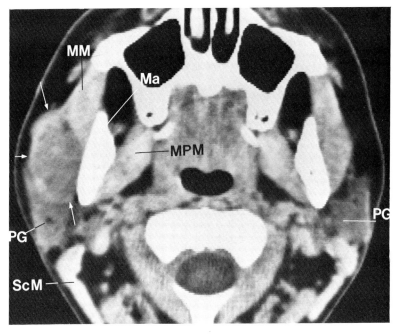

Figure 1.34B

Axial CT in another patient, also performed without contrast material; the tumor (*arrows*) is located in the deep anterior portion of the parotid gland. It measures 22 to 33 Hounsfield units, while the parotid tissue measures 15 to 23 Hounsfield units. A capsule or pseudocapsule of soft tissue density surrounds the tumor. The mass is inseparable from the masseter muscle.

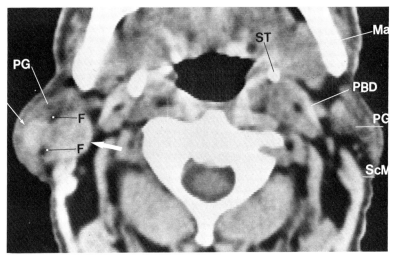

Figure 1.34C

Axial CT with the head flexed; a smaller intra-parotid lobule of the tumor abuts the parotid tissue directly (*small arrow*), while a larger extraparotid component (*larger arrow*) extends down along the parotid gland, from which it is separated by a low-density fat layer indicating its extraparotid location.

an increased level of aggressiveness. A calcified cyst (not shown) was also present within the gland. Aspiration biopsy revealed benign mixed tumor, but at surgery the mass was found to involve the facial nerve and a radical paroti-dectomy was done. Pathologic examination of the specimen revealed benign mixed tumor and also acinic cell carcinoma. The patient was a 64-year-old woman in whom a small lump had been present posteriorly in the parotid gland on the right side for many years, but there had been increase in size of the mass recently.

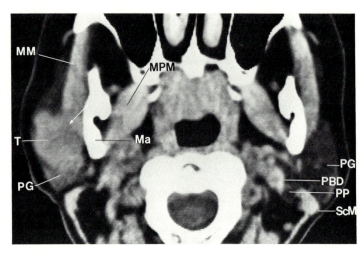

Figure 1.34D

Axial CT performed plain.

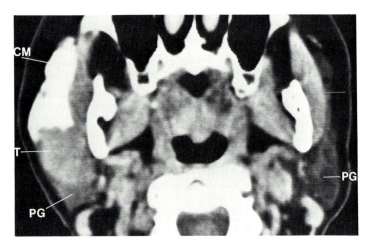

Figure 1.34E

Axial CT performed during infusion of 20% Renografin into the duct by the hydrostatic method.

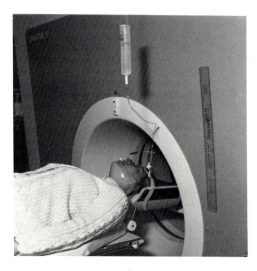

Figure 1.34F

Photograph of a patient undergoing CT sialography. A cannula placed in a salivary duct is connected to a reservoir elevated approximately 50 cm above the patient. Flow is regulated by a stopcock. (Rabinov, Kell, and Gordon 1984. With permission.)

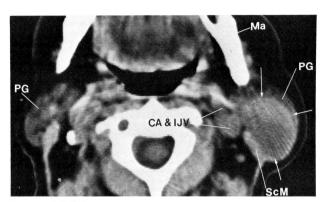

Figure 1.36C

Straight axial CT of the parotid glands in another patient. A large mass (*arrows*) is present in the right parotid gland, surrounded by a thin mantle of remaining parotid tissue. The mass is separated from the parotid tissue by a capsule or pseudo-capsule of soft tissue density. The mass itself measures 30 Hounsfield units. No contrast material has been used.

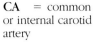

CA = common or internal carotid artery
IJV = internal jugular vein
Li = lipoma
Ma = mandible
PBD = posterior belly of the digastric muscle
PG = parotid gland
SCF = superficial cervical fascia, external layer
SCM = sterno-cleidomastoid muscle
SG = sub-mandibular gland

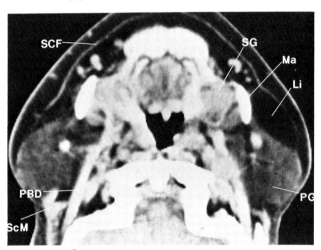

Figure 1.36D

Semiaxial CT of the parotid glands, in a different patient, with the chin extended and the gantry angled 20 degrees craniad. The parotid glands are moderately enlarged and are low in density (−28 to −50 Hounsfield units), consistent with sialosis. In addition, there is a biconvex lipoma (−117 Hounsfield units) located within the parotid capsule anteriorly, somewhat compressing the parotid tissue behind it. No contrast material has been used.

Infection in the parotid gland

CAB = corpus adiposum buccae
CM = residual contrast material
D = areas of deficient acinar opacification
LPM = lateral pterygoid muscle
LPP = lateral pterygoid plate
M = masses
Ma = mandible
MM = masseter muscle
MPM = medial pterygoid muscle
MPP = medial pterygoid plate
PD = parotid ducts
PG = parotid gland
Ph = pharynx
PPh = parapharyngeal space
Se = prominent septa within the parotid gland

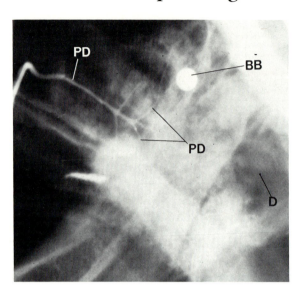

Figure 1.37A

Lateral view of conventional left parotid sialogram performed with Sinografin. The parotid gland is enlarged with irregular large areas of deficient acinar filling. The intraglandular duct branches are compressed. The BB corresponds to one area of particular enlargement, palpable clinically.

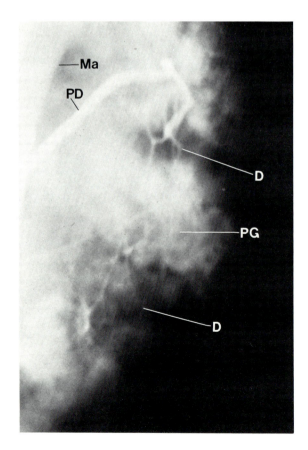

Figure 1.37B

AP view, same patient.

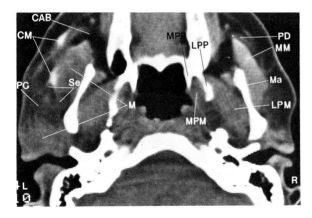

Figure 1.37C

CT examination, in the same patient, carried out following the conventional sialogram. There are still small amounts of residual water-soluble contrast material within the parotid gland. The left parotid gland is moderately enlarged, somewhat increased in density, with thickening of the septa within the gland. Several soft-tissue masses with ill-defined borders are present within the gland.

The patient in figures 1.37A–C was a 34-year-old woman with increasing soreness and swelling in the left parotid region of one week's duration. Incision and drainage were carried out with evacuation of 5 ml of pus from an abscess in the left parotid region. Culture grew *Staphylococcus epidermidis*, coagulase negative.

The patient in figure 1.37D is an 81-year-old woman with clinical signs and symptoms of acute parotitis following a dental extraction. Antibiotics and incision and drainage had been carried out but pain, swelling, and dysphagia persisted. The patient eventually recovered with further therapy.

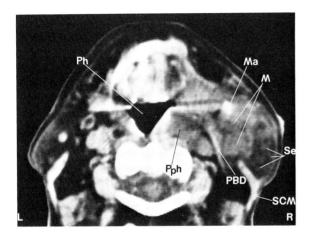

Figure 1.37D

Acute parotitis, another patient, plain axial CT with the head extended and the gantry angled 14 degrees craniad; the right parotid gland is enlarged and increased in density. The septa within the gland are thickened. Several soft-tissue masses are present within the gland. The infection extends medially into the parapharyngeal space, where the fat planes are obliterated. (Rabinov, Kell, and Gordon 1984. With permission.)

Infection in the parotid gland

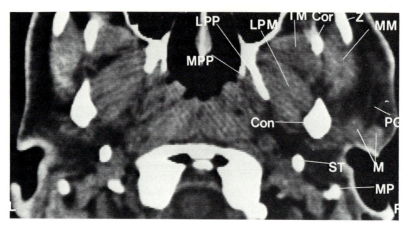

Figure 1.38A

Axial CT section, with the head slightly flexed and
the gantry vertical, through the upper part of the
gland. Each of the two small masses in the
posterior part of the parotid gland measure 6 × 9
mm.

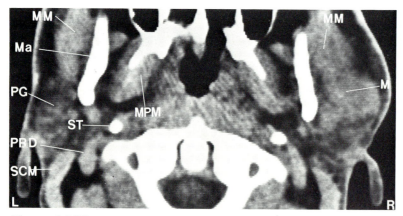

Figure 1.38B

Section through the mid-part of the parotid gland.

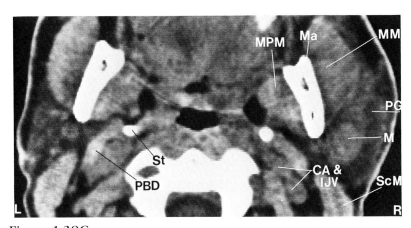

Figure 1.38C

Section through the lower part of the parotid gland. (Rabinov, Kell, and Gordon 1984. With permission.)

CA = internal or common carotid artery
Con = condyloid process of mandible
Cor = coronoid process of mandible
IJV = internal jugular vein
LPM = lateral pterygoid muscle
LPP = lateral pterygoid plate
M = mass
Ma = mandible
MM = masseter muscle
MP = mastoid process tip
MPM = medial pterygoid muscle
MPP = medial pterygoid plate
PBD = posterior belly of the digastric muscle
PG = parotid gland
SCM = sternocleidomastoid muscle
St = styloid process
TM = temporalis muscle
Z = zygomatic process of frontal bone

This 34-year-old male truck driver had noted onset of a nontender mass in the right parotid region of approximately three weeks' duration. The smaller oval masses in the parotid gland are most likely enlarged lymph nodes. The larger mass in the anterior portion of the gland shown in figure 1.38B could be a markedly enlarged lymph node or possibly a focal parenchymal inflammatory process. It is inseparable from the adjacent masseter muscle. The right parotid gland is moderately enlarged but only slightly increased in overall density from the normal gland on the other side. A ruptured gangrenous appendix had been removed 10 weeks previously. Aspiration biopsy of the mass in the parotid gland shown in figure 1.38B was performed. Pathologic examination revealed evidence of infection with large numbers of polymorphonuclear leukocytes, scattered histiocytes, many lymphocytes, and no granulomas. No specific organisms grew from the cultures. The mass disappeared on antibiotic therapy. No surgery was performed.

Masses extrinsic to the salivary glands

Art = artifact
F = fat layer between the submandibular gland and the mass
H = hyoid bone
M = mass
Ma = mandible
PG = lower tip of the parotid gland
SCM = sterno-cleidomastoid muscle
SG = sub-mandibular gland

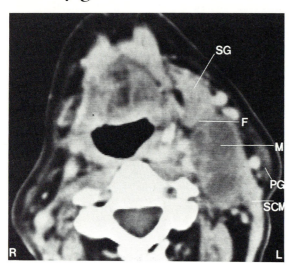

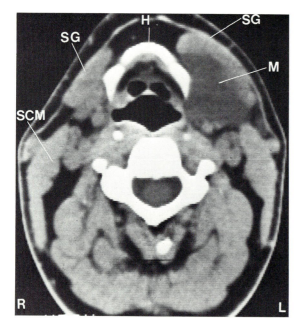

Figure 1.39A

Axial CT with the head flexed and bolus intravenous contrast material. A large oval mass is present behind the left submandibular gland from which it is separated by a low density fat layer. The center of the mass is low density, presumably necrotic metastatic lymph nodes. The opposite submandibular gland was removed at prior surgery. The mass is separated from the lower tip of the parotid gland by the sternocleidomastoid muscle.

The patient in figure 1.39A is a 77-year-old woman with a history of carcinoma of the larynx and metastatic lymph nodes on the opposite side, removed at prior surgery.

The patient in figures 1.39B and C was a 33-year-old man with a vague ill-defined gradually increasing mass in the region of the angle of the mandible for several months. The mass was removed surgically; it was immediately beneath the submandibular gland but was separable from it, and the submandibular gland was not removed. Pathologic analysis revealed a branchial cleft cyst, without infection.

The patient in figures 1.39D and E was a 60-year-old woman with a history of pain, soreness, and swelling of one month's duration in the right side of the upper neck. At surgery, an abscess was removed with the adjacent right submandibular salivary gland, which showed considerable inflammatory changes.

Figure 1.39B

Plain CT, axial view, another patient. A low density mass displaces the left submandibular gland anteriorly. In this instance no fat layer can be seen between the mass and the submandibular gland. The mass measured 17 Hounsfield units.

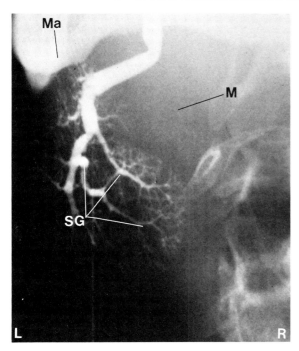

Figure 1.39C

Conventional left submandibular sialogram in the same patient as in figure 1.39B; the contrast material is Ethiodol. The chin has been extended and rotated toward the side of the lesion. (See figure 2.27A for position.) The submandibular gland is displaced downward and laterally by the mass, which did not alter the margin of the gland either on this duct-filling phase or on the subsequent acinar-filling phase.

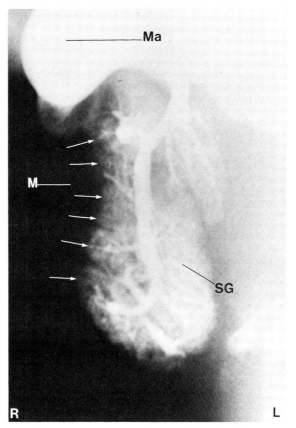

Figure 1.39D

Conventional sialogram performed in another patient. The contrast material is Ethiodol. The chin is extended and turned toward the side of the lesion. A mass has deformed the lateral margin of the submandibular gland in this acinar opacification phase. The lobular anatomy of the gland is well shown. The margin of the gland (*arrows*) including the lobular architecture, is intact, indicating the extrinsic location of the mass.

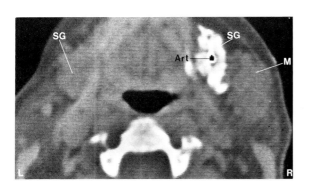

Figure 1.39E

Axial CT of the submandibular glands, same patient as in figure 1.39D, performed the same day as the conventional sialogram. The right submandibular gland is opacified with Ethiodol and can be compared with the unopacified submandibular gland on the opposite side. A moderate sized irregular mass is located posterolateral to the opacified submandibular gland.

Masses extrinsic to the salivary glands

AV = arteriovenous malformation
CA = internal or common carotid artery
CP = capsule or pseudocapsule
F = fat
IJV = internal jugular vein
M = mass
Ma = mandible
MM = masseter muscle
MPM = medial pterygoid muscle
PBD = posterior belly of the digastric muscle
PD = parotid duct
PG = parotid gland
SCM = sternocleidomastoid muscle
SG = submandibular gland
St = styloid process

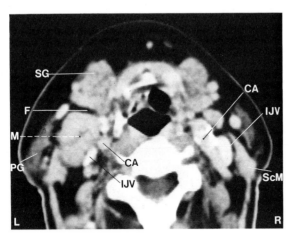

Figure 1.40A

Axial CT with bolus of intravenous contrast material, venous phase; a large extrinsic soft tissue mass is present behind the left submandibular gland, clearly separated from it by a layer of fat. The course traversed by the biopsy needle is indicated by the dotted line.

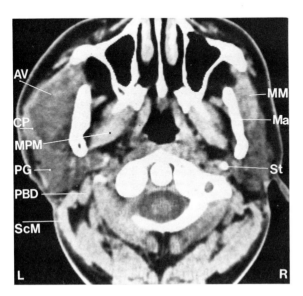

The patient in figure 1.40A was an 84-year-old woman with a two-month history of a mass in the left side of the neck. Percutaneous needle biopsy of the mass was performed from the direct lateral approach, revealing poorly differentiated carcinoma, with the same histology as was shown in a small tumor of the palate that was previously removed. Presumably the mass represents metastasis in lymph node(s).

Figures 1.40B, C, and D demonstrate an arteriovenous malformation of the masseter muscle.

Figure 1.40B

Plain axial CT showing a large relatively low density (25 Hounsfield units) mass replacing the left masseter muscle and displacing the parotid tissue laterally. The mass is separated from the normal parotid tissue lateral to it and behind it by a capsule or pseudocapsule of soft-tissue density.

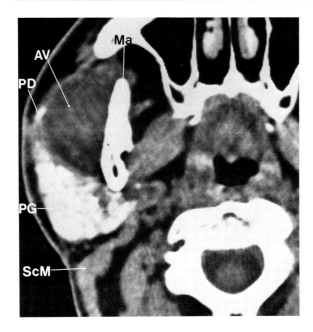

Figure 1.40C

CT sialography with the head flexed and the gantry vertical; 15% Renografin, containing approximately 7% iodine, was injected into the parotid duct by the hydrostatic method with the reservoir at a height of 50 cm above the parotid gland. The parotid tissue and the parotid duct are displaced posteriorly and laterally by the mass.

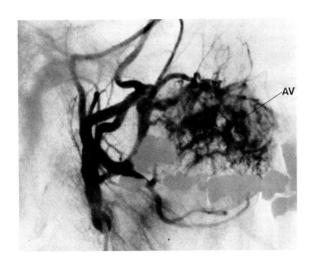

Figure 1.40D

Left external carotid arteriogram showing opacification of the arteriovenous malformation in the masseter muscle; embolization of the vessels leading to the mass was carried out with good results. (Photograph courtesy of Dr. Jerry Beers, Boston University Medical School.)

Tumor in the parotid gland

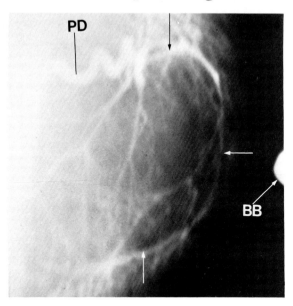

Figure 1.41A

Parotid sialogram, anterior-posterior view. The contrast material is Ethiodol. Arrows indicate tumor boundaries.

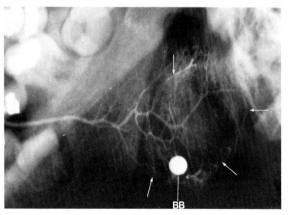

Figure 1.41B

Same patient, lateral view. Arrows indicate tumor boundaries; BB is taped over clinically apparent mass.

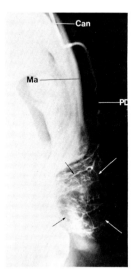

Figure 1.41C

Same patient, axial tangential view, positioned as shown in figure 2.16A. The mass (*arrows*) is primarily in the superficial portion of the gland but extends to the region of the plane of the facial nerve. At surgery the mass was found to be extending down to and just between several divisions of the facial nerve.

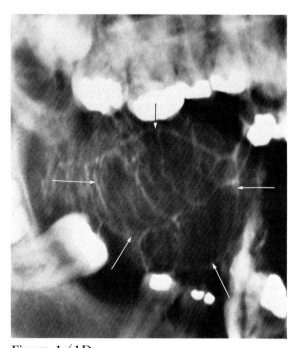

Figure 1.41D

Same patient, open-mouth view, positioned as shown in figure 2.17A. Arrows indicate the mass.

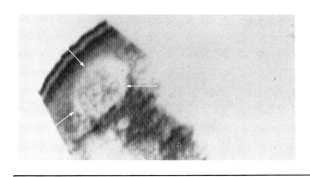

Figure 1.41E

Ultrasound examination in the same patient showing the mass (*arrows*) to have characteristics of a solid structure. Echoes are present within the lesion and the transmission of sound through the lesion is poor. Pathologic examination showed a mixed tumor of the parotid gland.

BB = marker
Can= cannula
Ma = mandible
PD = parotid duct

Abscess in the parotid gland

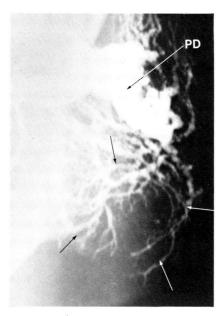

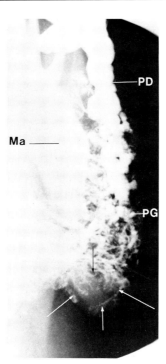

Ma = mandible
PD = parotid duct
PG = parotid gland

Figure 1.42A

Parotid sialography, AP view; contrast material is Ethiodol. Moderate sialectasia is evident, in addition to a mass (*arrows*) in the inferior portion of the parotid gland.

Figure 1.42B

Axial tangential view, as shown in figure 2.16A. A mass (*arrows*) is visible posteriorly in the superficial part of the parotid gland.

Total parotidectomy was performed. An abscess was found in the posterior portion of the gland; the pathologic report suggested possible actinomycosis.

Figure 1.42C

Ultrasound examination shows the mass (*arrows*) to be sonolucent, with good transmission; the posterior wall is fairly sharply outlined. There is some echogenic material in the posterior portion of the sonolucent mass.

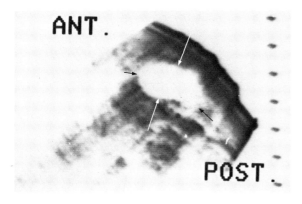

Retained contrast material; cystic structure between the parotid gland and the submandibular gland

CM = retained contrast material
Ma = mandible
PG = parotid gland
SG = submandibular gland

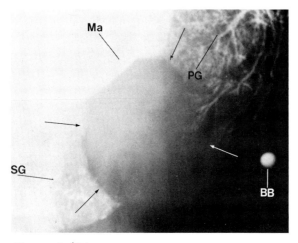

Figure 1.43A

Anterior view; the submandibular gland has been filled and allowed to evacuate and the parotid ducts are being filled with Ethiodol. A spherical mass separates the submandibular gland from the parotid gland. Note the residual contrast material in the submandibular gland.

The patient did not return subsequently for surgery and the nature of the cystic mass is unknown. Contrast material is Ethiodol.

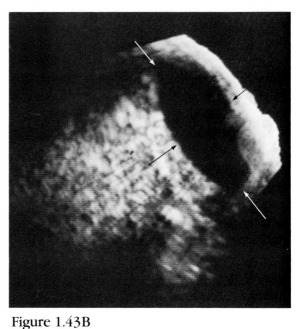

Figure 1.43B

Ultrasound shows an oval sonolucent mass (*arrows*) with good transmission and sharp posterior wall, consistent with a cystic mass.

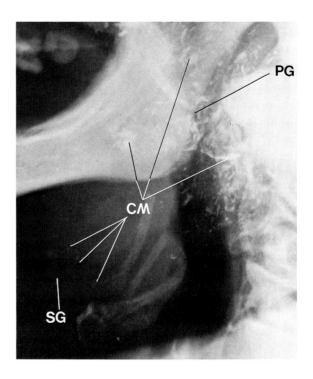

Figure 1.43C

Lateral view five days after sialography shows considerable retained contrast material in the parotid gland and a few tiny droplets of contrast material in the submandibular gland, presumably all extravasated into the interstitial tissues.

Retained contrast material; mass in the parotid gland

Parotid sialogram with Ethiodol. A mass is present in the upper portion of the gland. Considerable retained Ethiodol is present in the gland following evacuation, presumably extravasated into the interstitial tissues. Pathologic examination showed the mass to be a muco-epidermoid carcinoma.

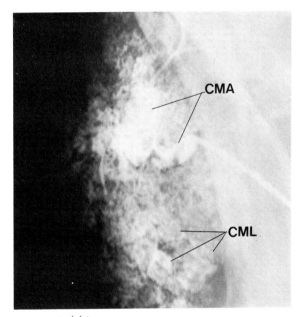

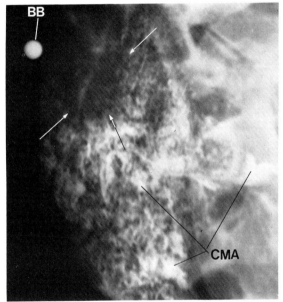

CMa = amorphous collections of extravasated contrast material
CMl = lobular pattern of extravasated contrast material

Figure 1.44A

AP view at the end of the injection; the large amorphous collections of contrast material in the upper part of the gland and the perilobular pattern of contrast material seen elsewhere in the gland parenchyma are consistent with an extraductal location of the contrast material. The mass in the upper lateral part of the gland is not well seen.

Figure 1.44B

Anterior oblique view, same patient, head turned toward the left, after evacuation. Most of the retained contrast material presumably is extravasated. The mass (*arrows*) is better visualized in this projection.

Mass in the parotid gland; retained contrast material

CMSC = contrast material extravasated in a subcapsular pattern

CM = contrast material extravasated into the gland parenchyma

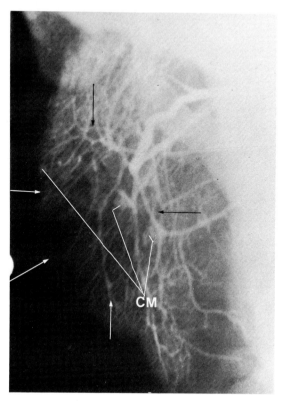

Figure 1.45A

Parotid sialogram, anterior oblique view with the head turned toward the left. A mass (*arrows*) is present in the inferolateral portion of the parotid gland. Some extravasated contrast material is already visible.

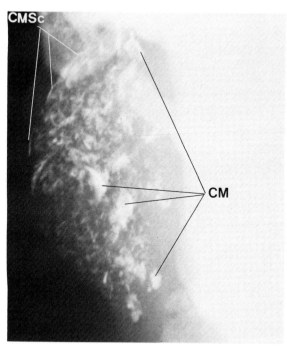

Figure 1.45B

Same position, as in figure 1.45A, immediately after evacuation. Retained interstitial contrast material is evident throughout the gland as well as beneath the capsule of the upper part of the gland.

Parotid sialograms show retained Ethiodol in the gland following evacuation. The mass subsequently disappeared upon treatment with antibiotics. Enlarged lymph nodes were palpable in the neck, and the intraparotid mass presumably represented an inflammatory process, most likely in an enlarged lymph node. The patient was a 19-year-old man who had previously been treated for pulmonary tuberculosis with antituberculous medication.

Retained contrast material following sialography

The patient was a 19-year-old woman who complained of intermittent swelling in the parotid region over the past one and a half years. The lower pole of the gland showed slight firmness. It was not possible during sialography to obtain good acinar filling, but the cause for this was undetermined. Failure of acinar filling to occur is consistent with parenchymal abnormality of undetermined nature.

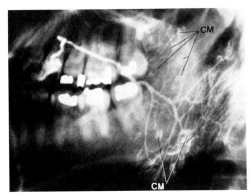

Figure 1.46A

Parotid sialogram, lateral view, at the end of the injection. The ducts are well filled but there is poor acinar opacification. Some extravasation of contrast material is already visible.

CM = extravasated retained contrast material

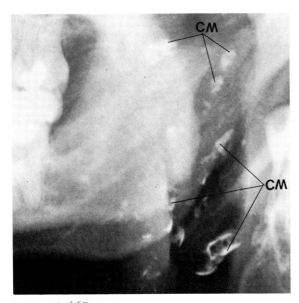

Figure 1.46B

Lateral view of the parotid gland at completion of evacuation, approximately 10 minutes after the end of the examination, and following repeated administrations of lemon juice. The pattern of retained contrast material is consistent with interstitial extravasation.

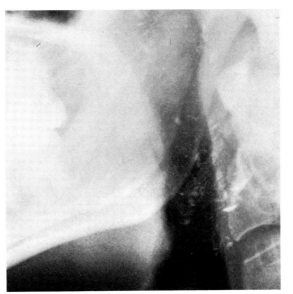

Figure 1.46C

Lateral film of the parotid gland 10 days following the sialogram, showing a moderate amount of retained contrast material in the gland. Prolonged sialography in an attempt to obtain acinar filling has resulted in some extravasation of contrast material.

Retained contrast material following sialography

C = calculus in parotid duct
CM = contrast material extravasated into the interstitial tissues of the lower part of the parotid gland
PD = parotid duct

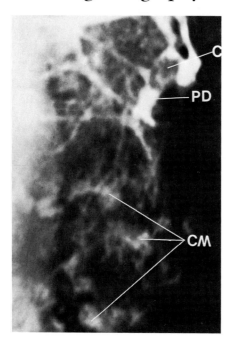

Figure 1.47

Parotid sialogram, antero-posterior view showing a stone in the posterior part of the main parotid duct. There is extravasation of Ethiodol into the interstitial tissues of the lower half of the parotid gland. This contrast remained in the gland after evacuation, together with a lesser amount in the upper portion of the gland.

Retained contrast material following sialography

Submandibular sialogram performed with Ethiodol; note was made that during injection very little pressure was used since the contrast material easily bypassed the obstruction caused by the stone. Most of the contrast material visible in this evacuation film has been extravasated into the tissues of the gland, including some beneath the capsule in the region of the lower portion of the gland, and remained following final evacuation film taken that day.

C = calculus
CM = contrast material extravasated into the tissues of the submandibular gland
CMSC = contrast material in subcapsular configuration
SD = sub-mandibular duct showing sialectasia

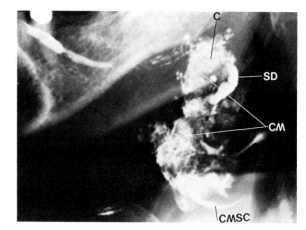

Figure 1.48

Evacuation phase, lateral view. A large calculus, obscured by the contrast material here, partly obstructs the posterior-most portion of the main submandibular duct; sialectasia is visible within the intraglandular portion of the duct.

Retained contrast material following sialography

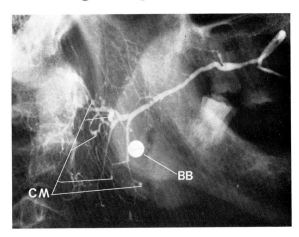

Parotid sialogram performed with Ethiodol. It was not possible to obtain good acinar filling. The patient was a poor historian but the clinical findings were thought to be consistent with chronic inflammation of the parotid gland (see also fig. 1.17C).

Figure 1.49A

Lateral view, duct filling phase. Tiny globules of contrast material are present adjacent to many of the intraglandular duct branches. A small lump palpable in the anterior lower parotid region is marked with a BB. No specific mass could be demonstrated by sialography.

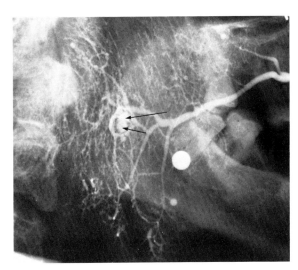

Figure 1.49B

Lateral view, later in the injection, showing good filling of the ducts. Acinar filling, however, could not be obtained, probably indicating abnormality in the gland parenchyma. Some of the small globules near the ducts have increased in size, especially the large collections in the central portion of the gland (*arrows*) and a few additional small globular collections are now visible. The gland itself is also considerably enlarged.

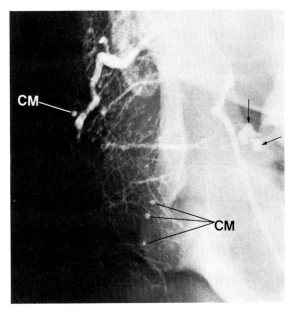

CM = contrast material existing as small globules adjacent to the ducts. This is believed to be extravasated into the tissues adjacent to the ducts.

Figure 1.49C

Antero-posterior view; the small globules can be seen to exist both in the superficial and deep portions of the gland. The large globules seen in the central part of the gland on the lateral view can now be seen to lie in the deep part of the gland (*arrow*).

Retained contrast material following sialography

Parotid sialogram performed with Ethiodol; same patient as in figures 1.23D and 2.14A.

CM = contrast material retained in the gland following sialography, presumably extravasated interstitially into the tissues of the parotid gland

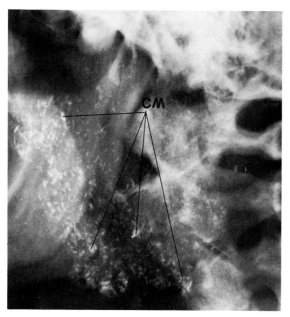

Figure 1.50A

Lateral view of the parotid region 20 minutes after the final evacuation film of the sialogram. Prolonged examination. A myriad of small flecks of residual interstitial contrast material can be seen distributed throughout the gland.

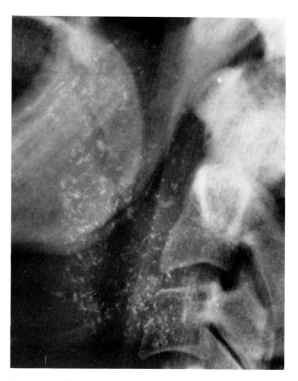

Figure 1.50B

Lateral view of the parotid area four days after the sialogram. There has been slight reduction in the amount of contrast material, but much remains.

Retained contrast material following sialography

Parotid sialogram, lateral views, performed with Ethiodol; same patient as in figure 1.18.

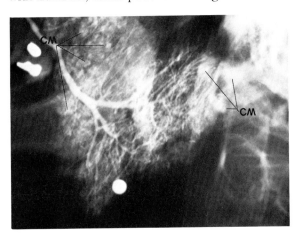

CM = contrast material extravasated outside the duct system into the interstitial tissues

Figure 1.51A

Lateral view of the parotid sialogram, late acinar opacification stage. There is already some interstitial contrast material visible in the gland. This was a moderately prolonged examination since the changes in the inferior-posterior portion of the gland caused by the adjacent enlarged metastatic nodes were difficult to demonstrate.

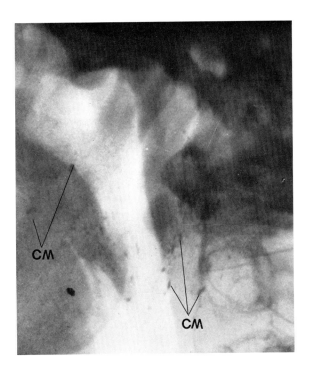

Figure 1.51B

Lateral view six months later still shows some flecks of residual Ethiodol. There were interim films that showed slow disappearance of the contrast material. The patient had no signs or symptoms related to this retained contrast material. The tones of the film have been reversed so that the small flecks of contrast material are dark. The very black spot in the anterior-inferior corner of the photograph is an artifact.

References

Adam, E. J., et al. The value of parotid sialography. *Br. J. Surg.* 70:108–110, 1983.

Alarcón-Segovia, D., et al. Radioisotopic evaluation of salivary gland dysfunction in Sjögren's syndrome. *Am. J. Roentgenol.* 112:373–379, 1971.

Ansell, G. A national survey of radiological complications: interim report. *Clin. Radiol.* 19:175–191, 1968.

Arcelin. *Revue pratique d'electrologie et de radiologie medicales,* no. 3, May 1913.

Azouz, E. M. The panoramic view in sialography. *Rdiology* 127:267–268, 1978.

Barsky, A. J., and Silberman, H. Roentgen visualization of the parotid gland by means of Lipiodol injection. *Ann. Surg.* 95:46–51, 1932.

Barraud, A. Méthod moderne d'exploration des canaux et des glandes salivaires. *Revue de Laryngologie, D'otologie et de Rhinologie* 52:453–457, 1931.

Barsony, T. Idiopathische stenongang-dilatation. *Klin. Wochenschr.* 4:2500–2501, 1925.

Batsakis, J. G. *Tumors of the head and neck. Clinical and pathological considerations.* Baltimore: Williams & Wilkins, 1972, pp. 112–114.

Berg, R. A. Sialography by image-intensified fluoroscopy. *Radiology* 93:1200–1201, 1969.

Blady, J. V., and Hocker, A. F. Sialography, its technique and application in the roentgen study of neoplasms of the parotid gland. *Surg. Gynecol. Obstet.* 67:777–787, 1938.

Blady, J. V., and Hocker, A. F. The application of sialography in non-neoplastic diseases of the parotid gland. *Radiology* 32:131–141, 1939.

Blair, G. S. Hydrostatic sialography: an analysis of a technique. *Oral Surg.* 36:116–130, 1973.

Blatt, I. M. Submaxillary salivary flow: a test of chorda tympani nerve function as a basis for surgical intervention in Bell's palsy: a study of 61 patients. *Transactions American Academy of Ophthalmology and Otolaryngology* 66:723–735, 1962.

Blatt, I. M., et al. Secretory sialography in diseases of the major salivary glands. *Ann. Otol. Rhinol. Laryngol.* 65:295–317, 1956.

Blatt, I. M., et al. Secretory sialography in diseases external to the major salivary glands. *Ann. Otol. Rhinol. Laryngol.* 68:175–186, 1959.

Blount, R. F., and Lachman, E. The digestive system. In *Morris' human anatomy,* 11th edition, ed. J. P. Schaeffer. New York: Blackiston, 1953, pp. 1308–1309.

Bryan, R. N., et al. Computerized tomography of the major salivary glands. *AJR* 139:547–554, September 1982.

Calcaterra, T. C., et al. The value of sialography in the diagnosis of parotid tumors. *Arch. Otolaryngol.* 103:727–729, 1977.

Carlsten, D. B. Lipiodolinjektion in den ausfuhrungs-gang der speicheldrusen. *Acta Radiol.* 6:221–223, 1926.

Carter, B. L., et al. CT and sialography: 1. Normal anatomy. *J. Comput. Assist. Tomogr.* 5:42–45, 1981a.

Carter, B. L., et al. Sialography and computed tomography: 2. Pathology. *J. Comput. Assist. Tomogr.* 5:46–53, 1981b.

Castigliano, S. G. Sialography of the submaxillary salivary gland: a new technique. *Am. J. Roentgenol.* 87:385–386, 1962.

Charpy, A. In *Traite d'anatomie humaine,* vol. 4, by P. Poirer and A. Charpy. Paris: Masson et Cie, 1900, p. 669, fig. 345.

Cogan, M. I., and Gill, P. S. Value of sialography and scintigraphy in diagnosis of salivary gland disorders. *Int. J. Oral Surg.* 10(suppl. 1):216–222, 1981.

Cook, T. J., and Pollack, J. Sialography: pathologic-radiologic correlation. *Oral Surg.* 21:559–573, 1966.

Daniels, T. E. et al. An evaluation of salivary scintigraphy in Sjögren's syndrome. *Arthritis Rheum.* 22:809–814, 1979.

de Rossi, G. The diagnostic value of radioisotopes and thermography in salivary gland diseases. *Radiol. Diagn. (Berl.)* 19:505–511, 1978.

Drevattne, T., and Stiris, G. Sialography by means of a polyethylene catheter and water soluble contrast medium (Isopaque 75%). *Br. J. Radiol.* 37:317–321, 1964.

Einstein, R. A. J. Sialography in the differential diagnosis of parotid masses. *Surg. Gynecol. Obstet.* 123:1079–1083, 1966.

Eisenbud, L., and Cranin, N. The role of sialography in the diagnosis and therapy of chronic obstructive sialadenitis. *Oral Surg.* 16:1181–1199, 1963.

Eneroth, C. M., and Hamberger, C. A. Principals of treatment of different types of parotid tumors. *Laryngoscope* 84:1732–1740, 1974.

Epsteen, C. M. Sialography: a non-irritating medium. *Am. J. Surg.* 92:603–605, 1956.

Epsteen, C. M., and Bendix, R. Effect of non-volatile substances on salivary glands in sialography. *Plast. Reconstr. Surg.* 13:299–306, 1954.

Ericson, S. The parotid gland in subjects with and without rheumatoid arthritis. *Acta Radiol. (Suppl.) (Stockh.)* 275:53–66, 1968.

Ferguson, M. M.; Evans, A.; and Mason, W. N. Continuous infusion pressure-monitored sialography. *Int. J. Oral Surg.* 6:84–89, 1977.

Fischer, H. W. Lymphographic contrast agents. In *Radiographic contrast agents*, ed. R. E. Miller and J. Skucas. Baltimore: University Park Press, 1977, pp. 463–475.

Forman, W. H. Subtraction sialography. *Radiology* 122:533, 1977.

Garusi, G. F. The salivary glands in radiological diagnosis. *Bibl. Radiol.* 4:1–125, 1964.

Gatenby, R. A.; Mulhern, C. B.; and Strawitz, J. CT-guided percutaneous biopsies of head and neck masses. *Radiology* 146:717–719, 1983.

Gates, G. A. Sialography and scanning of the salivary glands. *Otolaryngol. Clin. North Am.* 10:379–390, 1977.

Gioffre, L., and DiPietro, P. La storia della scialografia. *Otorinolaringologie* 32:349–354, 1963.

Glassman, L. M.; O'Hara, A. E.; and Cregar, D. Xerosialography. *Arch. Otolaryngol.* 100:341–343, 1974.

Godwin, J. T. Benign lymphoepithelial lesion of the parotid gland. Adenolymphoma, chronic inflammation, lymphoepithelioma, lymphocytic tumor, Mikulicz disease. Report of eleven cases. *Cancer* 5:1089–1103, 1952.

Golding, S. Computed tomography in the diagnosis of parotid gland tumors. *Br. J. Radiol.* 55:182–188, 1982.

Gooding, G. A. Gray scale ultrasound of the parotid gland. *AJR* 134:469–472, 1980.

Granone, F. G., and Juliani, G. Submaxillary sialography in combination with pneumoradiography and tomography. *Am. J. Roentgenol.* 104:692–696, 1968.

Gray's anatomy. Ed. T. P. Pick and R. Howden. New York: Bounty Books, 1977, p. 886.

Gullmo, A., and Book-Hederstrom, G. A method of sialography. *Acta Radiol. (Diagn.) (Stockh.)* 49:17–24, 1958.

Hanafee, W. N. Sialography. In *Radiology of the ear, nose and throat*, ed. G. E. Valvassori, et al. Philadelphia: W. B. Saunders, 1982a, pp. 312–332.

Hanafee, W. N. Notes and impressions from meetings. The Ninth International Congress of Radiology in Otolaryngology and the American Society of Head and Neck Radiology. Abbaye de Fontevraud, France, June 6–9, 1982. *Comput. Assist. Tomogr.* 6:1219, 1982b.

Harwell, E. L. Sialography made easier. *Radiology* 127:545, 1978.

Hausler, R. J., et al. Differential diagnosis of xerostomia by quantitative salivary gland scintigraphy. *Ann. Otol. Rhinol. Laryngol.* 86:333–341, 1977.

Hettler, M., and Lauth, G. Die gezielte sialographie. *Fortschr. Rontgenstr.* 95:493–505, 1961.

Hettwer, K. J. Simplified duct cannulation in sialography. *Oral Surg.* 28:639–640, 1969.

Hettwer, K. J., and Folsom, T. C. The normal sialogram. *Oral Surg.* 26:790–799, 1968.

Heystek, H. D., and Hildreth, R. C. Radiography of calcified submandibular calculi. *Med. Radiogr. Photogr.* 34:20–22, 1958.

Hutchinson, A. C. W. *Dental and oral x-ray diagnosis.* London: E. & S. Livingstone, 1954, pp. 309.

Jacobovici, J.; Poplitza, W.; and Albu, L. La sialographie. *Presse Med.* 34:1188, 1926.

Kassel, E. E. CT sialography, part I: introduction, technique, anatomy, and normal variants. *J. Otolaryngol.* 11, suppl. 12, 1982, pp. 1–10.

Kassel, E. E. CT sialography, part II: parotid masses. *J. Otolaryngol.* 11, suppl. 12, 1982b, pp. 11–24.

Kimm, H. T.; Spies, J. W.; and Wolfe, J. J. Sialography: with particular reference to neoplastic diseases. *Am. J. Roentgenol.* 34:289–296, 1935.

Kline, T. S.; Merriam, J. M.; and Shapshay, S. M. Aspiration biopsy cytology of the salivary gland. *Am. J. Clin. Pathol.* 76:263–269, 1981.

Kohri, K., et al. Bilateral parotid enlargement ("iodide mumps") following excretory urography. *Radiology* 122:654, 1977.

Kushner, D. C., and Weber, A. L. Sialography of salivary gland tumors with fluoroscopy and tomography. *AJR* 130:941–944, 1978.

Liliequist, B., and Welander, U. Sialography: new application of the subtraction technique. *Acta Radiol. (Diagn.) (Stockh.)* 8:228–234, 1969.

Liliequist, B., and Welander, U. Sialography of the sublingual gland: a modified technique enabling subtraction. *Acta Radiol. (Diagn.) (Stockh.)* 10:187–192, 1970.

Lilly, G. E.; Cutcher, J. L.; and Steiner, M. Radiopaque contrast mediums: effect on dog salivary gland and subcutaneous tissues. *J. Oral Surg.* 26:94–98, 1968.

Liverud, K. Sialographic technique with a polyethylene catheter. *Br. J. Radiol.* 32:627–628, 1959.

Lowman, R. M., and Belleza, N. A. An aid in sialographic studies: a newly devised curved sialographic obturator cannula. *Radiology* 121:747–748, 1976.

Lowman, R. M., and Cheng, G. K. Diagnostic roentgenology. In *Diseases of the salivary glands,* ed. R. M. Rankow and I. M. Polayes. Philadelphia: W. B. Saunders, 1976, pp. 54–98.

Manashil, G. B. Sialography—a simple procedure. *Med. Radiogr. Photogr.* 52:34–42, 1976.

Manashil, G. B. A new catheter for sialography. *AJR* 128:518, 1977.

Manashil, G. B. *Clinical sialography.* Springfield, Ill.: Charles C Thomas, 1978.

Mancuso, A; Rice, D.; and Hanafee, W. Computed tomography of the parotid gland during contrast sialography. *Radiology* 132:211–213, 1979.

Mandel, L., and Baurmash, H. Pathologic changes from sialographic media: report of case. *Journal of Oral Surgery, Anesthesia, and Hospital Dental Service* 20:341–344, 1962.

Marano, P. D.; Smart, E. A.; and Kolodny, S. C. Chronic obstructive sialadenitis. *Oral Surg.* 31:316–319, 1971.

Martin, B. H. Instrumentation for salivary duct cannulation. *Radiology* 115:213, 1975.

Martinez, C. B., et al. Computed tomography of the neck. *Radiographics* 3:9–40, 1983.

Mason, D. K., and Chisholm, D. M. Salivary glands in health and disease. Philadelphia: W. B. Saunders, 1975.

Massouh, H., and Dunscombe, P. B. Panoramic sialography: an alternative technique. *Br. J. Radiol.* 55:735–739, 1982.

Meine, F. J., and Woloshin, H. J. Radiologic diagnosis of salivary gland tumors. *Radiol. Clin. North Am.* 8:475–485, 1970.

Micheli-Pellegrini, V., and Polayes, I. M. Historical background. In *Diseases of the salivary glands,* ed. R. M. Rankow and I. M. Polayes. Philadelphia: W. B. Saunders, 1976, pp. 1–16.

Mishkin, F. S. Radionuclide salivary gland imaging. *Semin. Nucl. Med.* 11:258–265, 1981.

Navani, S., et al.. Evanescent enlargement of salivary glands following tri-iodinated contrast media. *Br. J. Radiol.* 45:19–20, 1972.

O'Hara, A. E. Sialography: past, present, and future. *CRC Crit Rev Radiol. Sci.* 4:87–139, 1973.

O'Hara, A. E., and Keohane, R. B. Sialography in an unusual case of subcutaneous emphysema of the neck. *Arch. Otolaryngol.* 98:354–355, 1973.

Ohrt, H. J., and Shafer, R. B. An atlas of salivary gland disorders. *Clin. Nucl. Med.* 7:370–376, 1982.

Ollerenshaw, R., and Rose, S. Radiological diagnosis of salivary gland disease. *Br. J. Radiol.* 24:538–548, 1951.

Ollerenshaw, R., and Rose, S. Sialography: a valuable diagnostic method. *Med. Radiogr. Photogr.* 33:93–102, 1957.

Osmer, J. C., and Pleasants, J. E. Distention sialography. *Radiology* 87:116–118, 1966.

Panella, J. S., and Calenoff, L. Medical uses of the orthopantomogram. *JAMA* 242:1295–1296, 1979.

Park, W. M., and Bahn, S. L. Sialography simplified. *Oral Surg.* 26:728–735, 1968.

Park, W. M., and Mason, D. K. Hydrostatic sialography. *Radiology* 86:116–121, 1966.

Parret, J., and Peyrin, J. O. Radioisotopic investigations in salivary pathology. *Clin. Nucl. Med.* 4:250–261, 1979.

Patey, D. H., and Thackray, A. C. Chronic 'sialectatic' parotitis in the light of pathological studies on parotidectomy material. *Br. J. Surg.* 43:43–50, 1955.

Payne, R. T. Sialography: its technique and applications. *Br. J. Surg.* 19:142–148, 1931.

Pernkopf, E. *Head and neck.* In *Atlas of topographical and applied human anatomy,* vol. I, ed. H. Ferner. Philadelphia: W. B. Saunders, 1963, fig. 145.

Pogrel, M. A. Some applications of salivary gland scintigraphy. *Int. J. Oral Surg.* 10 (suppl. 1):212–215, 1981.

Potter, G. D. Sialography and the salivary glands. *Otolaryngol. Clin. North Am.* 6:509–522, 1973.

Pretorius, D., and Taylor, A. The role of nuclear scanning in head and neck surgery. *Head Neck Surg.* 4:427–432, 1982.

Provenza, D. V. Oral histology—inheritance and development. Philadelphia: J. B. Lippincott, 1964, pp. 420.

Putney, F. J., and Shapiro, M. J. Sialography. *Arch. Otolaryngol.* 51:526–534, 1950.

Quinn, H. J. Diagnosis of parotid gland swelling. *Laryngoscope* 86:22–24, 1976.

Quinn, J. H. Intraductal anesthesia of salivary glands. *J. Oral Surg.* 29:230–231, 1971.

Rabinov, K. Sialography. *Contemporary Diagnostic Radiology* 4:1–5, 1981a.

Rabinov, K. Improved instruments for sialography. *Radiology* 141:245–246, 1981b.

Rabinov, K., and Joffe, N. A blunt-tip side-injecting cannula for sialography. *Radiology* 92:1438, 1969.

Rabinov, K.; Kell, T.; and Gordon, P. CT of the salivary glands. *Radiol. Clin. North Am.* 22:145–159, 1984.

Ranger, I. An experimental study of sialography, and its correlation with histological appearances, in normal parotid and submandibular glands. *Br. J. Surg.* 44:415–418, 1957.

Redon, H. *Chirurgie des glandes salivaires.* Paris: Masson et Cie, 1955, pp. 56–57.

Reid, J. M. Sialography. *Australas. Radiol.* 13:148–160, 1969.

Rice, D. H. Salivary gland physiology. *Otolaryngol. Clin. North Am.* 10:273–285, 1977.

Rice, D. H.; Mancuso, A. A.; and Hanafee, W. N. Computerized tomography with simultaneous sialography in evaluating parotid tumors. *Arch. Otolaryngol.* 106:472–473, 1980.

Rubin, P., et al. Physiological or secretory sialography. *Ann. Otol. Rhinol. Laryngol.* 64:667–688, 1955.

Rubin, P., and Blatt, I. A modification of sialography (preliminary report). *Univ. Mich. Med. Bull.* 21:57–63, 1955.

Rubin, P., and Holt, J. F. Secretory sialography in diseases of the major salivary glands. *Am. J. Roentgenol.* 77:575–598, 1957.

Samuel, E. Sialo-acinar reflux in sialography. *Br. J. Radiol.* 23:157–161, 1950.

Schall, G. L., and DiChiro, G. Clinical usefulness of salivary gland scanning. *Semin. Nucl. Med.* 2:270–277, 1972.

Schall, G. L.; Smith, R. R.; and Barsocchini, L. M. Radionuclide salivary imaging usefulness in a private otolaryngology practice. *Arch. Otolaryngol.* 107:40–44, 1981.

Schmitt, G., et al. The diagnostic value of sialography and scintigraphy in salivary gland diseases. *Br. J. Radiol.* 49:326–329, 1976.

Schultz, M. D., and Weisberger, D. The sialogram in the diagnosis of swelling about the salivary glands. *Surg. Clin. North Am.* 27:1156–1161, 1947.

Schvey, M. H., and Polayes, I. M. Diagnosis of facial nerve paralysis. In *Diseases of the salivary glands*, ed. R. M. Rankow and I. M. Polayes. Philadelphia: W. B. Saunders, 1976, pp. 185–201.

Sismanis, A., et al. Diagnosis of salivary gland tumors by fine needle aspiration biopsy. *Head Neck Surg.* 3:482–489, 1981.

Som, P. Computerized tomography of parapharyngeal masses. Paper read at the postgraduate course in Head and Neck Radiology, Department of Radiology, Harvard Medical School, Massachusetts General Hospital and Eye and Ear Infirmary, Copley Plaza Hotel, Boston, Mass., October 2–3, 1980.

Som, P. M., and Biller, H. F. The combined CT-sialogram. *Radiology* 135:387–390, 1980.

Som, P., and Khilnani, M. T. Modification of a butterfly infusion set for sialography. *Radiology* 143:791, 1982.

Sone, S., et al. CT of parotid tumors. *American Journal of Neuroradiology* 3:143–147, 1982.

Sonnabend, E. Sialography. In *Roentgen diagnostics*, vol. I, ed. H. R. Schinz, et al. New York: Grune & Stratton, 1968, pp. 519–525.

Sorsdahl, O. A.; Williams, C. M.; and Bruno, F. P. Scintillation camera scanning of the salivary glands. *Radiology* 92:1477–1480, 1969.

Steinhardt, G. Zur Technik der Speicheldrüsen-sondierung, Zur Sialoskopie und Sialographie. *Dtsch. Zahn-Mund-Kieferheilk* 9:132–145, 1942.

Stone, D. N., et al. Parotid CT sialography. *Radiology* 138:393–397, 1981.

Sucupira, M. S., et al. Salivary gland imaging and radionuclide dacrocystography in agenesis of salivary glands. *Arch. Otolaryngol.* 109:197–198, 1983.

Suzuki, S., and Kawashima, K. Sialographic study of diseases of the major salivary glands. *Acta Radiol.* 8:465–478, 1969.

Tainmont, J.; Dubois, B.; and Hennebert, D. Scinti-graphie salivaire et sialographie comparison des résultats dans quelques affections courantes. *Acta Otorhinolaryngol. Belg.* 33:300–316, 1979.

Talner, L. B., et al. Elevated salivary iodine and salivary gland enlargement due to iodinated contrast media. *Am. J. Roentgenol.* 112:380–382, 1971.

Thackray, A. C. Sialectasis. *Archives of the Middlesex Hospital* 5:151–159, 1955.

Thomas, A. R. The technique of sialography. *Br. J. Radiol.* 29:209–212, 1956.

Trester, P. H. The development and use of contrast media in sialography. *Journal of the Canadian Dental Association* 34:210–213, 1968.

Uslenghi, J. P. Nueva técnica para la investigación radiólogica de las glandulas salivales. *Semana Medica* 41:27, 1925.

Wakely, C. The surgery of the salivary glands. *Ann. R Coll. Surg. Engl.* 3:289, 1948.

Wescott, W. B., et al. Alterations in whole saliva flow rate induced by fractionated radiotherapy. *AJR* 130:145–149, 1978.

Winsten, J.; Gould, D. M.; and Ward, G. E. Sialography. *Surg. Gynecol. Obstet.* 102:315–321, 1956.

Wiskovsky, B. Sialodochografie. *Zentralblatt für Hals-Nasen und Ohrenheilkunde sowie deren Grenzgebiete Berlin* 8:320, 1926.

Wotman, S., and Mandel, I. D. The salivary secretions in health and disease. In *Diseases of the salivary glands,* ed. R. M. Rankow and I. M. Polayes. Philadelphia: W. B. Saunders, 1976, pp. 32–53.

Young, J. A., and Van Lennep, E. W. *The morphology of the salivary glands.* New York: Academic Press, 1978, pp. 72–75.

Yune, H. Y. Sialography and dacrocystography. In *Radiographic contrast agents,* ed. R. E. Miller and J. Skucas. Baltimore: University Park Press, 1977, pp. 485–492.

Yune, H. Y., and Klatte, E. C. Current status of sialography. *Am. J. Roentgenol.* 115:420–428, 1972.

Zijlstra, G., and Ten Bosch, J. J. Sialography with continuous measurement of pressure outside and inside the gland. *Int. J. Oral Surg.* 4:160–167, 1975.

Chapter 2 The Normal Sialogram

Embryology of the Salivary Glands

The parotid, submandibular, and sublingual glands originate and develop in a fundamentally similar fashion (Patten 1968; Hamilton and Mossman 1972; Arey 1974). During the sixth week after conception, the parotid and submandibular glands arise as buds of thickened buccal epithelium (fig. 2.1) that grow into the surrounding parenchyma to form solid epithelial cords. When near their final destination, the buds branch repeatedly and become hollow to form ducts. The tips become more bulbous as they begin to form the secretory acini. The peripheral mesenchyme about the budding duct system condenses to become the capsule, while that between the budding masses of epithelial cells becomes the stroma of the developing gland, so that a pattern of lobules and intervening septa is formed. The initial preponderance of stroma is later reversed so that the gland eventually comes to consist primarily of epithelial elements (Moss-Salentjin and Moss 1976). The sublingual glands arise during the eighth week as a row of 5 to 14 solid buds on the floor of the mouth on each side. The ducts of the most anterior few of these may join together to form Bartholin's duct, which may either join the submandibular duct (fig. 1.14) or may open separately nearby. The remaining more posterior sublingual ducts retain their original openings onto the floor of the mouth.

Definitive epithelial histologic differentiation of the salivary glands occurs after birth, although mucin secretions at least are produced by the fetus (Hamilton and Mossman 1972).

The parotid gland develops in an intimate relationship with the facial nerve. As the proliferating parotid tissue begins to grow dorsally, it is in a plane deep to that of the facial nerve's buccal branches, which have grown ventrally toward it (Gasser 1970). When it reaches the region of the ramus of the mandible it encounters and envelops the already existing facial nerve structures (fig. 2.2). The primordium grows toward the point where the facial nerve bifurcates into the temporofacial and cervicofacial rami. The temporofacial ramus and its branches come to lie in a relatively superficial plane within the primordium, while the cervicofacial ramus and its branches come to lie in a relatively deep plane within the primordium.

Some branches of the proliferating parotid tissue that are deep to the nerve and its divisions, especially those in the cranial portion of the primordium, turn sharply medially directly behind the mandible, forming much of the deep portion of the parotid gland. Those that continue on in a dorsal more superficial course and come to lie entirely lateral to the facial nerve and its branches become the superficial part of the parotid gland. According to Gasser (1970), additional ductules from the superficial branches, especially those in the more dorsal regions of the primordium, pass medially between the facial nerve branches to contribute to the deep portion of the gland. It is rare that ductules from the deep branches grow laterally to contribute to the superficial portion.

Thus, according to Gasser (1970) there is no embryologic evidence that the parotid gland is a bilobed structure as suggested by some (Davis et al. 1956). It has been shown instead to be more accurately described simply as a glandular structure that has developed as an outgrowth of the buccal mucosa and in its posterior migration to its final location has enveloped the facial nerve and its branches (McKenzie 1948; Gasser 1970). McKenzie (1948) likened the encounter of the budding parotid primordium and the facial nerve and its branches to "a creeper weaving itself into the meshes of a trellis-work fence."

The mesenchyme surrounding the submandibular and sublingual glands condenses early, excluding adjacent lymphatic tissue. The capsule around the parotid gland forms later (Chaudhry, Montes, and Cutler 1972), and because lymphatic tissue is forming nearby at the same time, parotid tissue may be found in nearby lymph nodes. Similarly, lymph nodes frequently are included within the parotid capsule and gland (DuPlessis 1957).

Congenital anomalies include absence of a salivary gland, accessory glands, atresia with retention cysts, abnormal location of salivary tissue, inclusion of a branchial cleft or cyst within or in intimate contact with a parotid or submandibular gland (figs. 1.36C, 1.39B,C), vascular malformations, and diverticula (DuPlessis 1957; Arey 1974; Mason and Chisholm 1975).

Heterotopic salivary gland tissue can occur in the upper part of the neck as well as in other locations in the head and neck and even in other regions of the body (Gudbrandsson, Liston, and Maisel 1982).

Histology of the Salivary Glands

The parotid, submandibular, and sublingual salivary glands are tubuloacinar in configuration, consisting of progressively branching duct structures ending in spherical or elongated acini of serous or mucous cells. The general pattern of branching ducts and terminal acini may be likened to a bunch of grapes. The ducts progressing from the acini to the main salivary duct are called, in order, intercalated, secretory (striated), and excretory ducts (fig. 2.3A). The intercalated ducts are quite narrow, and there is a rather abrupt increase in caliber from the intercalated ducts to the secretory ducts. The duct pattern varies among the major salivary glands, with the intercalated ducts being longest in the parotid gland, shorter in the submandibular gland, and almost nonexistent in the sublingual glands (Rauch 1959; Bargmann 1962; Provenza 1964; Weiss and Greep 1977).

Because of the branching nature of the duct system, the parenchyma is naturally arranged in lobules. The intercalated ducts and smaller secretory ducts are intralobular. The larger secretory ducts and the excretory ducts are interlobular (Provenza 1972).

The capsule surrounding the submandibular gland is well defined. The parotid gland is also enveloped in a connective tissue capsule, but it tends to be somewhat less well defined than that of the submandibular gland and is least well developed along the medial aspect of the deep portion of the gland (Gaughran 1961; Anson 1966). The fascia surrounding the salivary glands does not appear to form a rigidly confining capsule since these glands can certainly increase rapidly and markedly in size during distension sialography and with various pathologic processes.

The Acinus

The acinar cells in the parotid gland are almost entirely serous in nature (Weiss and Greep 1977). Those in the submandibular gland are mixed, with both serous and mucous cells, but still predominantly serous (fig. 2.3B). The acini in the sublingual gland are primarily mucous. When acini are of the mixed type, the serous cells are clustered in a crescent at the distal end of the acinus, with the mucous cells located more proximally near the acinar outlet. Clustered serous cells are called a *demilune.*

Flattened stellate shaped cells, called *myoepithelial cells,* can be seen between the secretory cells and their basement membrane. Tendril-like processes extend from these myoepithelial cells around the serous cells. The configuration and arrangement of these cells as well as their ultrastructure is like that of smooth muscle cells, suggesting that these cells have a function in moving the secretions of serous cells (Weiss and Greep 1977).

Tiny intercellular canaliculi are found between the serous cells of the pure serous acini as well as between those of the demilunes. They communicate with the acinar lumens (Weiss and Greep 1977) (fig. 2.3B). Electron microscopy shows these tiny spaces to consist of an intercellular territory continuous with the intercellular space (Provenza 1964, 1972; Young and VanLennep 1978) (fig. 2.3C). They are limited peripherally by the basement membrane of the acinus and laterally by the walls of adjacent cells. According to Provenza (1964), the microvilli shown on electron microscopy indicate that the intercellular territories probably function in the absorption of substances for protein synthesis rather than serving primarily as secretory canaliculi.

The Intercalated Ducts

The intercalated ducts are the terminal ducts leading from the acini. They are entirely intralobular. Their lumens are small, of the same magnitude as those of the acini. The epithelial cells are flattened cuboidal, and on electron microscopy are somewhat similar to the cells of the adjacent acini. Many investigators believe these cells serve as a source for renewal of acinar cells. Basket cells may be found between the secretory cells and the basement membrane. As noted, the intercalated ducts are long and narrow in the parotid gland, shorter and wider in the submandibular gland, and almost nonexistent in the sublingual gland.

The Secretory (Striated) Ducts

The lining cells are low columnar. They have a striated appearance, caused by the basal rows of mitochondria and internal reflections of the basal cell membranes between similar interdigitating cytoplasmic projections of adjacent cells (Provenza 1964; Weiss and Greep 1977).

The primary secretion of the acinar cells has an ionic content similar to that of plasma. The mucosal cells of the striated ducts modify the composition of this secretion by the transport of water and ions (Mason and Chisholm 1975), so that the secretion as it leaves the striated ducts is essentially the final salivary product (Provenza 1964, 1972).

The Excretory Ducts

In the distal portions of the excretory ducts, the epithelium is simple columnar in type. In the larger ducts it becomes pseudostratified columnar, and in the largest excretory ducts, those joining the main duct of the gland, it may become stratified columnar (Weiss and Greep 1977).

The primary function of these ducts is transport, although there is some evidence, at least in the rat, that further transport of ions and water may occur here, converting the saliva from isotonic to hypotonic (Shackelford and Schneyer 1971; Mason and Chisholm 1975; Young et al. 1967; Moss-Salentijn and Moss 1976).

The Main Parotid and Submandibular Duct

The wall of the parotid duct consists of fibrous tissue intermixed with smooth muscle fibers (Anson 1966). The submandibular duct wall consists primarily of fibrous tissue, and the presence of smooth muscle in the wall is the exception rather than the rule (Moss-Salentijn and Moss 1976).

Normal Roentgen Anatomy of the Parotid Gland

The parotid gland, so named because of its location near the ear, is the largest of the salivary glands, weighing 15 to 30 g (Anson 1966). It has a curved triangular shape (fig. 2.4A) and occupies the parotid fossa, where its shape is determined by many musculoskeletal structures. The filling of the parotid bed by the parotid gland has been likened to pouring of liquid paraffin into a mold, the shape of the gland being determined by the shape of the mold and the gland filling many small nooks and corners within the mold (Conley 1975). Posteriorly, the gland is confined by the external auditory canal, the mastoid process and sternocleidomastoid muscle, and the posterior belly of the digastric muscle. Anteriorly, the ramus of the mandible and the masseter and internal pterygoid muscles give the gland a concave shape. The constriction of the middle part of the gland between these anterior and posterior structures may be called the isthmus (Johns 1977). The medial structures that form the floor of the fossa include several muscles as well as the styloid process, the stylomandibular ligament, the internal carotid artery, the internal jugular vein, and the transverse process of the atlas. The pharynx may be in the close proximity to the deep portion of the gland. The superior border of the parotid space is formed by the zygomatic arch. Laterally, the gland is covered only by the parotid fascia, the skin and subcutaneous tissues and, in its lower portion, by the platysma muscle.

The inferior angle of the parotid gland may be closely applied to, or even touch, the adjacent submandibular gland, separated from it only by an interglandular septum (Gaughran 1961; Anson 1966). The normal parotid gland is soft and difficult to identify by palpation. If the gland can be palpated, it usually is abnormal (Diamont 1960).

Although there has been a great deal of controversy about its internal anatomy, the parotid gland is not bilobed but is more accurately described as a single-lobed structure (McKenzie 1948; Gaughran 1961; Rankow and Polayes 1976; Johns 1977). According to the official nomenclature of the *Nomina Anatomica* (International Anatomical Nomenclature Committee 1977), the parotid gland is described in general terms as consisting of a superficial part and a deep part, determined solely by position within the gland. From a practical surgical standpoint, it has been customary to consider the division between the superficial and deep parts of the gland to occur arbitrarily at the location of the facial nerve and its branches (figs. 2.4B,C) (Davis et al. 1956; Patey and Thackray 1957; Anson 1966; Rankow and Polayes 1976), even though these nerve structures are not strictly all arranged in a single sagittal plane (Gaughran 1961). The clinical importance of this concept relates, of course, to the need for preservation of the facial nerve during surgery. While numerous bridges of parotid tissue and ductules pass between the nerve branches to join the deep and superficial portions of the gland (McKenzie 1948), a surgical plane of dissection is easily developed along the nerve and its branches (Hollinshead 1968). The removal of all the parotid tissue superficial to the facial nerve and its branches is termed a *superficial parotidectomy* (figs. 2.12C,D). The superficial portion of the gland is larger and flatter than the deep portion and overlies the deep portion, which extends medially behind the ramus of the mandible. The size and shape of the superficial and deep portions of the gland are quite variable (Anson and McVay 1971). While the facial nerve and its branches within the parotid gland can be seen neither on standard sialography nor by CT, these nerve structures, except for the buccal branches that may accompany the duct, can be shown by surgical dissection (Davis et al. 1950) to be superficial to the main duct (figs. 2.4B,C, 2.15A), consistent with their embryologic development (Gasser 1970), and just lateral to the posterior facial vein and external carotid artery within the gland (figs. 2.22A). The point of entrance of the facial nerve into the posterior margin of the parotid gland can also be determined accurately, since the nerve exits from the stylomastoid foramen, which can be demonstrated by axial radiographs or CT. The short segment of the facial nerve between the stylomastoid foramen and the parotid gland can be demonstrated on axial CT (Curtin, Wolfe, and Snyderman 1983). From these various landmarks, the plane of the facial nerve and its branches within the gland can be fairly accurately localized. Conn and colleagues (1983) state that the position of the facial nerve is determined accurately by an arc of radius 8.5 mm posterior lateral to the most posterior point of the ramus of the mandible. Thus, the position and appearance of a mass within the gland may suggest whether it is likely to be deep or superficial to the facial nerve and thus whether it is likely to displace, splay, or even envelop the facial nerve structures (figs. 1.27, 1.34B,D,E, 1.35, 1.36A, 1.41C). According to Winsten, Gould, and Ward (1956), anatomic lines related to the mandible and to the parotid duct may be drawn to divide the parotid gland into six sections—four superficial and two deep (figs. 2.12A, B). If the plane of the facial nerve is used to divide the gland into superficial and deep portions, however, there may be said to be eight sections—four superficial and four deep (figs. 2.12C,D,E).

Many smaller superficial and deep processes of the gland have been described (Gaughran 1961; Johns 1977). These fill various extensions of the parotid space. Three superficial processes have been described: the condylar, the meatal, and the posterior processes. The first two are small and probably not of radiologic importance. The condylar process is a thin extension of parotid tissue overlying the temporomandibular joint. The meatal process is less common and rests in the incisura of the cartilaginous external acoustic meatus. The posterior process may be larger, varying in length between several millimeters and two centimeters. It originates near the junction of the deep and superficial portions of the parotid gland. It projects dorsally between the mastoid process and the sternocleidomastoid muscle and, more inferiorly, between the digastric muscle and the sternocleidomastoid muscle (figs. 2.15A, 1.34D, 2.21B, 2.22A, 5.5D). It occurs in more than 20% of instances (Gaughran 1961). According to Gaughran (1961), it lies just lateral to the internal jugular vein and so may be of particular clinical significance if it is the site of infection or tumor.

The two deep processes are the glenoid process and the stylomandibular process. The glenoid process is a small projection of parotid tissue resting on the vaginal process of the tympanic part of the temporal bone. The stylomandibular process (figs. 1.27C, 2.15A,B, 2.20, 2.22A, 5.5D), also called the carotid lobe and the pharyngeal extension of the parotid gland, may project anteriorly and medially into the stylomandibular fascia above the superior edge of the stylomandibular ligament. It rests upon the anterior surface of the styloid process and may extend anterior to the internal carotid artery. It may be present to some degree in almost 75% of specimens (Gaughran 1961). A tumor arising in this process may be dumbbell in shape, passing through the stylomandibular membrane or inferior and deep to the stylomandibular ligament, presenting as a pharyngeal mass (McCabe and Work 1969).

In addition to these processes of the main body of the gland, it is common to see one or more accessory processes along the upper margin of the parotid duct anterior to the main portion of the gland. In a series of 100 consecutive sialograms, 38% had one, 7% had two, and 6% had three or more such accessory ducts (Oppenheim and Wing 1960). Enlargement of these processes by inflammation or other pathology may cause a small palpable mass along the parotid duct in the cheek (Polayes and Rankow, 1979).

The parenchyma of the parotid gland consists of multiple lobules between which the connective tissue of the capsule extends. These lobules can be quite prominent radiologically, and the appearance should not be mistaken for an abnormality. Sviridova (1970) has defined a primary lobule as a unit consisting of secretory end pieces, intercalated ducts, and terminal striated ducts, drained by a single second-order striated duct.

The parotid gland varies markedly in size and shape in different individuals. In an autopsy study of 100 glands (Davis et al. 1956), height varied between extremes of 3.9 and 8.0 cm (average 6.0 cm). Width varied between 2.0 and 6.5 cm (average 3.6 cm). Because of the great variation in the size of salivary glands between individuals, measurements of the gland (Ericson 1970) or computation of its volume (Ericson and Hedin 1970) are of little practical value in clinical sialography. Increase in the size of a salivary gland usually is evident clinically if sought for and is often first noted by the patient or associates, although such enlargement is often overlooked by both physician and patient (chapter 7). Furthermore, during sialography the gland size and volume varies considerably according to the amount of contrast material injected and the volume of saliva secreted during performance of the sialogram, and thus sialographic size is difficult to evaluate. The relative size of a gland may be estimated roughly by relating it to other nearby anatomic structures. For example, the gland usually extends from the level of the temporomandibular joint to the angle of the mandible or just below it. Sialographic findings such as increased spacing between the ducts and an appearance of attenuation of the ducts within the gland or increased distance between the main parotid duct and the mandible (figs. 2.8A, 4.5B) may also be used to indicate that the parenchyma of the gland has become enlarged. The size of the salivary glands can probably best be evaluated on plain CT (figs. 2.20–2.23, 2.30).

According to Ericson (1970), there is normally no significant difference in size between the right and left parotid glands of a given patient. He further states that only a weak correlation can be demonstrated between salivary gland size and the sex, age, or weight of an individual. For example, there is a tendency toward some reduction in size of the normal salivary glands with increasing age, especially in men.

The pattern of duct tributaries within the gland is individually variable (Davis et al. 1956; Rauch 1959) (fig. 2.5A). Two or more interlobular tributaries may join to form the main duct (Oppenheim and Wing 1960). Multiple side branches join the main channel or channels, frequently at obtuse or even right angles. As previously noted, in the majority of instances one, two, or three small accessory ducts usually drain into the main duct from above, anterior to the main body of the gland.

The parotid duct thus arises from the confluence of tributaries draining the lobules of the superficial and deep portions of the gland. As the parotid duct leaves the gland at its anterior margin, it lies upon the masseter muscle. It then continues anteriorly and medially, being either horizontal or ascending or descending slightly. At its anterior end it takes a more or less right angle turn as it passes through the buccinator muscle to end on the buccal mucosa opposite the crown of the second upper molar tooth (figs. 1.1, 2.4A, 1.37C). As noted in chapter 1, straightening this bend in the anterior portion of the duct by pulling the cheek forward greatly facilitates cannulation (figs. 1.11, 1.12, 1.27C, 2.15B).

The length of the parotid duct is 3.5 to 5 cm (Anson 1966). The diameter of the normal parotid duct varies considerably (fig. 2.5B). Measurement of the diameter of the parotid duct in healthy patients was studied by Ericson in 1973. The duct usually was straight or gently curved, but some tortuosity did occur in the absence of obstruction or dilatation. The maximum diameter of the duct was always present within the gland, diminishing distally in the gland and also diminishing in the main duct as it passed toward the orifice. The maximum lumen of the parotid duct ranged from 0.9 to 4.0 mm, with a mean of 2.0 mm. The lumens were slightly greater in men (1.0 to 4.0 mm) than in women (0.9 to 3.5 mm). A relatively weak correlation was established between duct diameter and the size of the gland. A difference of greater than 0.7 mm in the diameter of the lumen between the right and left glands was regarded as abnormal. No correlation was found between the duct lumen diameter and the age of the patient or the secretory capacity of the gland.

Lymph nodes are normally present in abundant numbers outside both the submandibular and the parotid glands (fig. 2.6D). They are rarely, if ever, found within the substance of the submandibular gland (Waterhouse 1966), but they are found commonly within the parotid gland (Godwin 1952; Batsakis and Sylvest 1977), where they may be either deep in its substance or in a subaponeurotic location (Mason and Chisholm 1975; Conley 1975; Clark 1953). According to Conley (1975) there are 20 to 30 lymph follicles and lymph nodes within the parotid gland. Such lymph nodes ordinarily are not recognizable by conventional sialography unless they have become abnormally enlarged (figs. 1.32, 2.6A,B,C, 2.13B, 3.42). Enlarged lymph nodes may also be demonstrated by CT (fig. 1.38, 3.45B, 3.46).

The external carotid artery and the posterior facial vein and some of their branches traverse the substance of the parotid gland. These structures can be demonstrated by CT (figs. 2.20, 2.21, 2.22) but are not ordinarily visualized on conventional sialography.

The Normal Parotid Sialogram

Lateral Oblique View

For fluoroscopic examination and spot films of the parotid gland, a basic projection is the lateral oblique view with the head tilted upward and the chin rotated toward the table (fig. 2.7A). The parotid gland is thus projected over the pharyngeal airway, free of the bony structures of the mandible and the cervical spine (figs. 2.7B,C). Masses in the anterior portion of the gland may be best demonstrated by further forward rotation so that this portion of the gland is projected over the maxillary sinus (fig. 2.6B). The posterior part of the gland is normally more opaque than the anterior portion (fig. 2.7C) since the gland is much thicker posteriorly; compare with figure 2.8D.

The Anterior Posterior View

A second basic projection for the parotid gland is the straight anterior posterior (AP) view (figs. 2.8A,B). This provides an overall view of the gland, showing one profile of the superficial and deep parts of the gland and their relationship to the mandible. For comparison with these normal parotid sialogram views, a parotid sialogram in a patient showing a large mass within the deep part of the gland is shown in figures 2.8C,D.

The distance between the lateral margin of the mandible and the main duct in the normal should not exceed 16 mm (fig. 2.8A). A distance greater than this indicates that a mass is present within or outside of the gland or that the gland itself is enlarged (fig. 4.5B, 5.2A, 5.4B, 5.5C). It should be noted that the superficial and deep portions of the gland may vary considerably in size from patient to patient.

As the ducts curve around behind the ramus of the mandible, they may normally have a rounded configuration (fig. 2.9A), which should not be mistaken for a mass such as is shown in figure 2.8C. Furthermore, the normal parotid gland may be deeply grooved anteriorly by the ramus of the mandible and posteriorly by the mastoid process, sternocleidomastoid muscle, and posterior belly of the digastric muscle, causing a narrowed area in the gland, sometimes referred to as the isthmus of the gland. This narrowing may be reflected in the sialogram as a relatively lucent area in the acinar phase of the sialogram (fig. 2.9B).

There are other pitfalls to beware in these views. In some instances, the ducts in the posterior portion of the gland may appear to be "accordioned" or crowded together (fig. 2.10A). This is due to the superimposition of many branches as the gland curves medially behind the ramus of the mandible and in front of the sternocleidomastoid muscle. The transverse process of the atlas sometimes may cause an extrinsic compression on the posterior medial aspect of the gland (fig. 2.10B). This should not be mistaken for an abnormal mass. Also, the external auditory canal may cause a deep impression on the upper posterior portion of the gland which, together with air in the cavum conchae, may cause a well-defined radiolucency that should not be mistaken for an abnormal mass (fig. 2.11).

The six sections of the parotid gland defined by Winsten, Gould, and Ward (1956) are seen in the AP and lateral views of figure 2.12. Such anatomic division is helpful because it provides some reference for location of abnormalities within the gland. Division of the parotid gland into eight sections was described in the section on parotid anatomy. The appearances following superficial parotidectomy are shown in figures 2.12C–E.

Anterior Posterior Oblique Views

It is not always possible to be certain on AP and lateral views whether a mass in the posterior part of the gland is superficial or deep to the facial nerve, because to a great extent the superficial and deep portions of the gland are superimposed on each other in these views. The portions of the gland and the relationship of a mass to the plane of the facial nerve can be better separated in various anterior oblique views. Masses that are in the extreme posterior posterolateral part of the gland may appear to extend quite far medially on the anterior-posterior view and still be in the superficial portion of the gland, that is, lateral to the facial nerve (figs. 1.36A,B, 1.41). Such masses are best demonstrated with the head turned to the contralateral direction (fig. 2.13A). On the other hand, masses in the posteromedial part of the gland immediately behind the mandible are more likely to be deep to the facial nerve (figs. 1.27A,B,C). Very small superficial masses may be demonstrated more accurately in various anteroposterior and oblique tangential views with diminished exposure (55 kV) (figs. 1.20B and 2.13B). Far anterior masses may even be demonstrated in the lateral oblique view with the face over-rotated toward the table to project the mass over the maxillary sinus (fig. 2.6B).

The Water's View

Masses in the tail of the parotid gland may sometimes best be displayed with the Water's view (fig. 2.14).

The Axial (Vertex-Submental) View

The vertex-submental radiograph provides a third perpendicular view of the gland, in addition to the lateral and AP views (fig. 2.15). It is the optimal view for showing the profiles of the superficial and deep portions of the gland separate from each other, since the course of the facial nerve and its branches can be inferred. This view is especially helpful in determining whether a lesion is in the deep portion of the gland (fig. 1.27C, 3.37B) or in the superficial portion.

The Axial-Tangential View

The axial-tangential view (Hettler and Lauth 1961) with soft-tissue technique demonstrates the superficial portion of the parotid gland to good advantage (fig. 2.16), complementing the AP and oblique-tangential views taken fluoroscopically (see also figs. 1.41C and 1.42B).

The Open-Mouth View

The open-mouth projection (Heystek and Hildreth 1958) provides another view of the posterior portion of the parotid gland (figs. 1.41D and 2.17).

The Puffed-Cheek View

This view can be used to demonstrate the presence or absence of opaque calculi in the parotid duct (figs. 2.18, 3.17A, 3.18A, 3.19A, 3.20A).

Panoramic Radiography

Panoramic radiography demonstrates the normal structures of the parotid and submandibular glands (fig. 2.19, 2.19A), as well as pathologic processes involving these glands (figs. 1.31A and 2.19B).

Normal CT Anatomy of the Parotid Glands

The parotid gland is pyramid-shaped, with lateral, anteromedial, and posteromedial surfaces. The external cervical fascia splits into superficial and deep layers that invest the parotid and submandibular glands and the sternocleidomastoid muscle. Anteriorly this fascia fuses with the masseter muscle fascia, and it thickens inferiorly to form part of the stylomandibular ligament, which is attached to the angle of the mandible and forms a septum between the parotid gland and the submandibular gland. Inferiorly, the fascia attaches to the upper margin of the hyoid bone and the lower margin of the mandible and fuses with the fascia of the anterior belly of the digastric muscle. The superficial layer, which is stronger and thicker, attaches superiorly to the cartilage of the external auditory canal and to the zygoma. The deeper thinner layer fuses above with the base of the temporal bone and the styloid process and its muscles, and it also fuses with the fascia of the posterior belly of the digastric muscle.

The normal anatomic relationships of the parotid gland (Kassel 1982) are shown in the straight axial view (fig. 2.20), the semiaxial view with the head extended and the gantry angled craniad (fig. 2.21A,B), the semiaxial view with the head flexed (figs. 2.22A,B), and the coronal view (figs. 2.23A,B,C). The submandibular gland is well demonstrated in the projection shown in figure 2.21B, as well as in a modified axial view with the chin slightly extended and the gantry angled slightly craniad (fig. 2.30). These views correspond with the digital radiographs shown in figures 1.33A,B,C,D,E. The parotid glands shown in figures 2.21A, 2.22A,B, 2.23A,B,C show mild changes of sialosis (chapter 5) and a small mass is present in the left parotid gland, but the appearances are otherwise normal.

The anterior medial wall of the parotid space is formed by the mandible and the masseter and medial pterygoid muscles. On its posterior medial surface the parotid gland lies against the mastoid process, the sternocleidomastoid muscle, the posterior belly of the digastric muscle, and the styloid process and its muscles. The posterior facial vein and the external carotid artery pass directly through the substance of the parotid gland, while the internal carotid artery and the internal jugular vein lie medial to the gland. The facial nerve enters the posterior surface of the parotid gland as it exits from the stylomastoid foramen. Here it may be visualized for a short distance before it enters the parotid gland (Curtin, Wolfe, and Snyderman 1983).

The semiaxial view with the head extended and the gantry angled craniad shown in figures 1.33B and 2.21 is of particular value for CT scanning of the salivary glands. As noted previously, both the submandibular and the parotid glands and their relationship can be imaged in this position without interference from dental amalgam. Also, the anatomic relationships and fascial arrangements described result in formation of a compartment containing the parotid and submandibular gland on each side (fig. 2.21B). This compartment is bordered laterally by the superficial layer of the external cervical fascia and medially by the posterior belly of the digastric muscle. These relationships are best demonstrated in this particular projection, which is parallel with the posterior belly of the digastric muscle and with the styloid process. The higher section shown in figure 2.21A shows the relationship of the parotid gland to the masseter muscle, the medial pterygoid muscle and the mandible anteriorly, and to the styloid process and mastoid process posteriorly. The lower section (fig. 2.21B) demonstrates the parotid and submandibular glands sandwiched between the posterior belly of the digastric muscle and the external layer of the external cervical fascia. Figures 2.21B and 2.30 show the submandibular gland sandwiched between the external cervical fascia laterally and the oropharynx, posterior belly of the digastric muscle, and hyoid bone medially.

The CT density of the parotid glands is variable from patient to patient. According to Sone and colleagues (1982), the density ranges from a slightly higher density than fatty tissue to a slightly lower density than muscle. The density of the submandibular glands normally is in the range of other soft tissues.

Normal Roentgen Anatomy of the Submandibular Gland

The submandibular salivary gland weighs 7 to 10 g and is approximately one-third to one-half the size of the parotid gland. It is also called the submaxillary gland since it lies in the submaxillary triangle. In addition to the main body of the gland, there is a smaller deep, or uncinate, process that extends forward with the submandibular duct, above the mylohyoid muscle (figs. 1.5, 2.4A, 3.5). The gland is covered externally only by skin and subcutaneous tissue and the platysma muscle, and by the superficial cervical fascia, which also forms its capsule. The submandibular gland is separated from the parotid gland by a fascial thickening posteriorly, the stylomandibular ligament.

The submandibular salivary duct arises from the upper medial aspect of the body of the gland near the junction with the uncinate process (Anson 1966). It is about 5 cm in length, passing forward with a further angle upward in its anteriormost portion before ending on the papilla lateral to the frenulum beneath the tongue (fig. 1.13). The orifice of the submandibular duct tends to be much smaller than that of the parotid duct even though the diameter of the duct itself (2 to 4 mm) is larger.

Lymph nodes are not usually found within the submandibular gland but are present outside the capsule, where their enlargement by pathologic processes such as infection, metastases, or lymphoma constitutes a relatively frequent cause of masses in this region (figs. 1.5, 1.21, 1.39A, 1.40A, 3.43, 3.45).

Both the parotid gland and the submandibular gland are exposed to the peripharyngeal spaces (Hollinshead 1968) (fig. 2.24). Thus, infections that commonly arise from the pharynx, tonsils, or teeth can spread to the region of the parotid or submandibular gland either directly or by breakdown of secondarily infected lymph nodes. Such infections may also travel in the reverse direction. The dependent location of the submandibular space, which is the anteroinferior element of the peripharyngeal space and which is limited inferiorly by the superficial layer of the cervical fascia may at least partly account for the fact that abscesses also constitute a relatively frequent cause for masses in the submandibular region (figs. 1.23A, 1.39D,E). Similarly, infected lymph nodes may cause masses that are adjacent to, or actually involve, the deep portion of the parotid gland.

It is clinically recognized that with increasing age the submandibular glands may gradually become slightly more palpable and visible in some patients (fig. 2.25A). This may result from actual enlargement of the glands owing to mild sialosis (see chapter 5) or to unknown causes. Alternatively, apparent enlargement may result from atrophy of the muscular and fascial tissues supporting the floor of the mouth, with resultant sagging of the gland (fig. 2.25B). According to Waterhouse and Winter (1964) the weight of the submandibular gland normally does not vary with age. Under these circumstances the enlargement or apparent enlargement usually is evident bilaterally; such glands normally are of soft consistency and should not be changing in size or consistency. If careful history and physical examination do not reveal any additional findings, only continual observation need be carried out.

The Normal Submandibular Sialogram

The Lateral or Lateral-Oblique View

The lateral or lateral-oblique view similar to that used for examination of the parotid gland may also be used for the submandibular gland (fig. 2.26).

The Anteroposterior Oblique View with the Chin Tilted Up

This view, taken with the ramus and adjacent portion of the body of the mandible perpendicular to the tabletop, provides a second optimal projection for the submandibular gland and duct, also almost bone free (figs. 2.27, 1.6C). In the straight AP view the gland tends to be obscured by the mandible.

The Open-Mouth View

The open-mouth view with the head flexed can be used to demonstrate the submandibular gland and duct, especially the hilar area of these structures (fig. 2.28).

The Axial (Vertex-Submental) View

This view may occasionally be helpful in demonstrating or excluding pathology in or about the submandibular gland (fig. 2.29, 3.6B, 3.43B). An axial view of the floor of the mouth with an intraoral film may be helpful in demonstrating the submandibular duct and gland (figs. 3.1C, 3.2B, 3.9B).

Normal CT Anatomy of the Submandibular Gland

CT, satisfactorily performed in the axial projection, is able to demonstrate the normal submandibular gland and its relationships (fig. 2.30), as well as any masses in or around the submandibular gland (figs. 1.39A,B,E, 1.40A).

CASES

Embryology of the human salivary glands

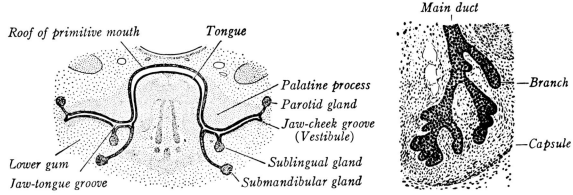

Figure 2.1

Left, the sites of origin of the salivary glands shown by a diagrammatic frontal section across the jaws at about two months (× 15). The close origins of the submandibular and sublingual primordia may explain the fairly common joining of Bartholin's duct with the submandibular duct. *Right*, detail of the branching submandibular gland, at two months (× 70), showing the development of a branching duct system and the capsule. (Arey 1974. Reprinted with permission.)

Embryology of the facial nerve and the parotid gland

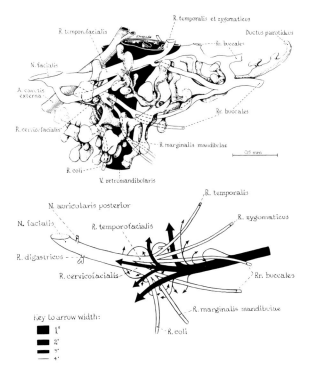

Figure 2.2

Top, the relationship of the facial nerve, the parotid primordium, the retromandibular vein, and the external carotid artery at 37 mm, 10 weeks. Taken from a reconstruction made from liquid stone. The cervicofacial branches are in a deeper position compared with the temporofacial branches. *Bottom*, the general pattern of development. The arrows indicate the direction of growth of the primordium around the facial nerve and its branches. The width of the arrow shows the sequence of development. (Gasser 1970. Reprinted with permission.)

Histology of the salivary glands and ducts

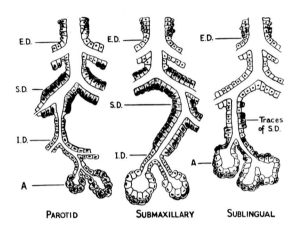

Figure 2.3A

Diagrammatic representation of the duct system of the parotid, the submaxillary, and the sublingual glands: acini (*A*), intercalated ducts (*I.D.*), striated ducts (*S.D.*) and excretory ducts (*E.D.*). (After Jenkins 1966; cited in Mason and Chisholm 1975. Reprinted with permission.)

Figure 2.3B

Reconstruction of the secretory end piece and intralobular ducts of the submandibular gland. *D*, demilune composed of serous cells; *M*, mucous cells; *My*, myoepithelial cells; *SC*, secretory capillaries in a serous acinus; *ID*, intercalated duct; *SD*, striated duct; *A*, cross section through the striated duct; *B*, cross section through the intercalated duct; *C*, cross section through a mucous acinus; *D*, cross section through a serous acinus. (Braus 1924. Reprinted with permission.)

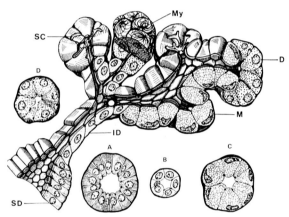

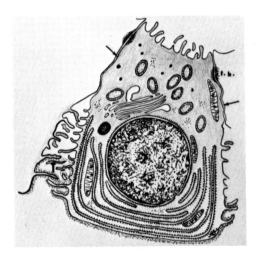

Figure 2.3C

Diagram of a serous acinar cell showing the relationship of the intercellular territory (*T*) and the intercellular space (*arrow*). (Provenza 1964. Reprinted with permission.)

Gross anatomy of the salivary glands

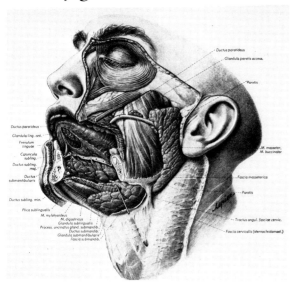

Figure 2.4A

External anatomy of the salivary glands; the body of the mandible has been removed. (Pernkopf 1963. Reprinted with permission.)

Figure 2.4B

Internal anatomy of the parotid gland, surgical concept; the superficial part of the gland has been removed, so-called superficial parotidectomy, to reveal the facial nerve and its branches. The parotid duct as it emerges from the anterior margin of the parotid gland may be accompanied by buccal branches of the facial nerve, but is generally deep to the facial nerve branches posterior to this. A surgical plane of dissection is easily developed along the plane of the facial nerve. (From R. M. Ranko, *Atlas of surgery of the face, mouth and neck* [Philadelphia: W.B. Saunders Co., 1968]. Reprinted with permission.)

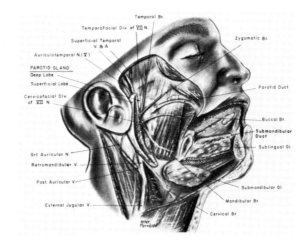

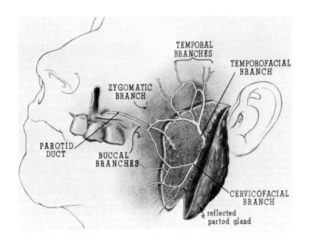

Figure 2.4C

The parotid gland has been fileted to reveal the facial nerve and its branches within the substance of the gland. Note the parotid duct deep to the nerve structures. This figure reflects the internal anatomy of the parotid gland more accurately according to its embryologic development. The parotid gland has been shown to be a single-lobed structure that has enveloped the facial nerve and its branches during its development. Removal of the portion of the gland superficial to the nerve structures, superficial parotidectomy, entails not only dissection through the lobules of the parotid tissue but transsection of ductules, blood vessels, and lymphatics. (Conley 1975. Reprinted with permission.)

Variations in parotid duct size

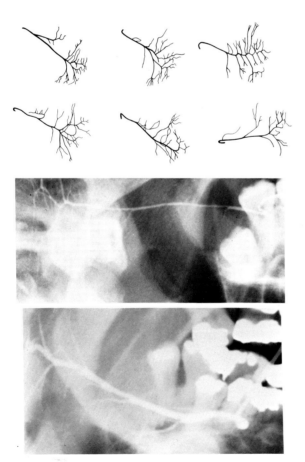

Figure 2.5A

Tracings of parotid ducts, lateral views, taken from sialograms in six different patients to show the variations in the branching patterns that can occur in different patients.

Figure 2.5B

Parotid sialograms, lateral views, in two different patients, to show the variations in size that can occur in normal parotid ducts in different patients.

Lymph nodes as parotid masses

Parotid sialography showing masses in the parotid gland. The patient was a 9-year-old boy with two discrete masses palpable in the right parotid gland, unchanging for two months (only one of the masses is shown here). Superficial parotidectomy was performed. Histologic examination revealed the masses to be lymph nodes that were enlarged and showed marked lymphoid hyperplasia (figs. 2.6A and B).

The patient shown in figure 2.6C was a five-year-old girl with a palpable mass in the parotid gland; histologic examination showed it to be an intraparotid lymph node with inflammatory changes (see also figs. 2.13B). Enlarged lymph nodes outside the submandibular gland are shown in figs. 1.5A,B, and 1.21.

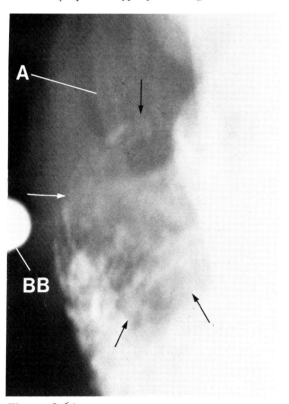

Figure 2.6A

The AP view; the mass (*arrows*) is superimposed upon air in the cavum conchae.

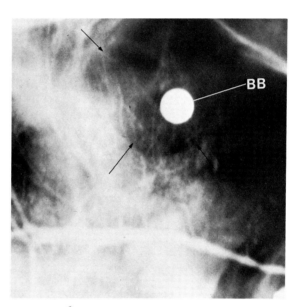

Figure 2.6B

The lateral oblique view with the face rotated forward; the mass (*arrows*) can be seen in the upper anterior quadrant of the gland, superimposed in this projection upon the maxillary sinus.

A = air in the cavum conchae
BB = indicates the palpable mass

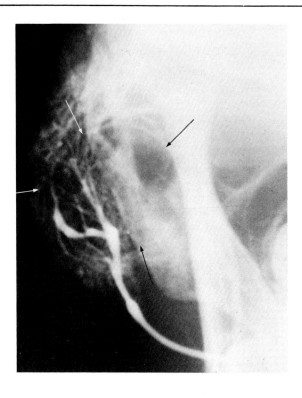

Figure 2.6C

Parotid sialogram, AP view of a mass (*arrows*) in another patient.

Figure 2.6D

Lymph nodes are abundant around both the parotid and the submandibular glands. They are rarely found within the submandibular gland but are numerous throughout the parotid gland, where they may be subaponeurotic or deep within the gland. (Schaeffer 1953. Reprinted with permission.)

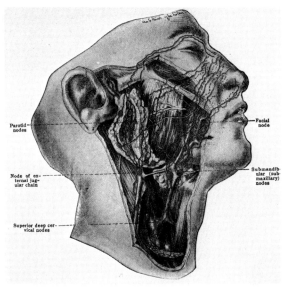

Modified lateral view for fluoroscopic examination and spot films during parotid sialography

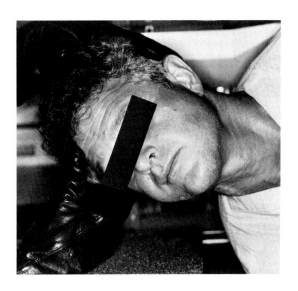

Figure 2.7A

The upper gland, away from the tabletop, is being examined. The head is elevated slightly and the face is rotated slightly toward the table. In this position, much of the parotid gland is free from interfering bony structures, and the posterior part of the parotid gland is superimposed upon the air filled pharynx, as shown in figures 2.7B and C. During exposure of spot films, the patient's head should rest upon the gloved fist of the assistant or upon a bolster to prevent motion.

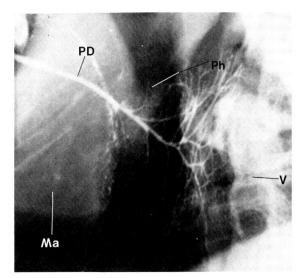

Figure 2.7B

Normal parotid sialogram, positioned as in figure 2.7A, duct-filling phase.

Ma = mandible
PD = parotid duct
PG = parotid gland
Ph = pharynx
V   = vertebrae

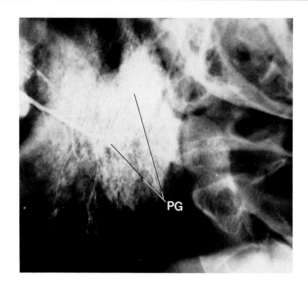

Figure 2.7C

Same patient and position as in figure 2.7B, but taken during the acinar opacification phase. Note that the posterior part of the gland is more opaque than the anterior part in spite of its superimposition upon the pharynx; this is because the posterior part of the parotid gland is much thicker than the anterior part.

Normal parotid sialography, AP view

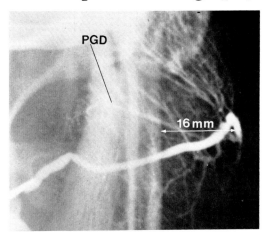

Figure 2.8A

Duct filling phase. The main duct should not be more than 16 mm from the lateral margin of the mandible. A measurement larger than this indicates a mass either within or outside the gland, or enlargement of the gland. Please see also Figure 2.9A. Note the extension of parotid duct branches in the deep part of the gland medially behind the mandible.

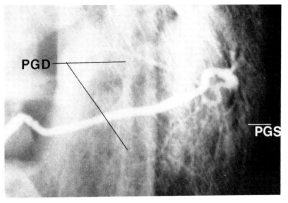

Figure 2.8B

Same patient and position as in figure 2.8A, acinar opacification phase. The superficial part of the parotid gland is usually broader and flatter than the deep part and covers the deep part.

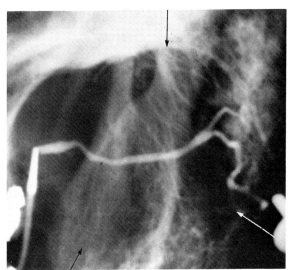

Figure 2.8C

AP view of parotid sialogram in another patient, acinar opacification phase, showing a large mass occupying the deep portion of the gland. Compare with figures 2.8A and B, and 2.9A and B. The tumor, which is outlined by arrows, displaces the superficial part of the gland laterally and markedly thins it.

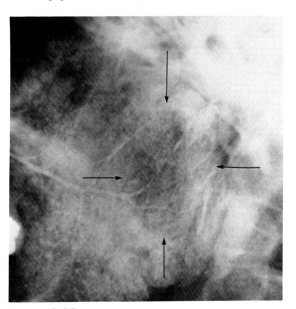

Figure 2.8D

Lateral view of parotid sialogram, acinar opacification phase, same patient as in 2.8C. Note that an area in the posterior portion of the gland is less opaque than the anterior portion of the gland, indicating a mass in this region (*arrows*). Compare with figure 2.7C. Pathologic examination revealed the mass to be a mixed tumor in the deep part of the parotid gland.

Normal parotid gland versus mass

Ma = mandible
PD = parotid duct branch curving around the ramus of the mandible
PG = parotid gland

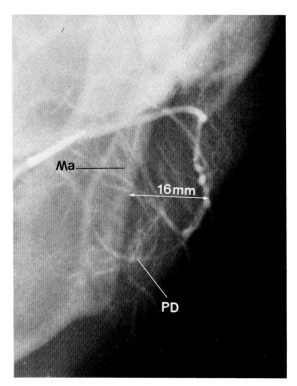

Figure 2.9A

Normal parotid sialogram, AP view, duct filling phase, to show the normal curvature of a parotid duct branch around the ramus of the mandible and the masseter muscle. This normal appearance is seen occasionally and should not be mistaken for a mass. Compare with figures 2.8A and 2.8C. Note that the parotid duct is not more than 16 mm lateral to the lateral margin of the mandible.

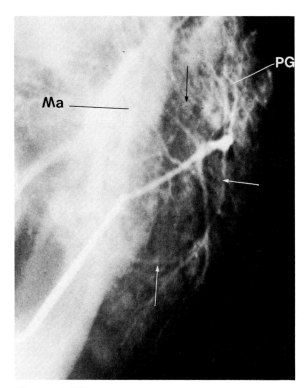

Figure 2.9B

Normal parotid sialogram, acinar opacification phase, to show the relative lucent central part of the gland (*arrows*) caused by thinning of the gland in the region between the ramus of the mandible anteriorly and the mastoid process, sternocleidomastoid muscle, and posterior belly of the digastric muscle posteriorly. This narrowed area is sometimes referred to as the isthmus of the parotid gland (see figs. 2.15A,B, 2.22A). This appearance should not be mistaken for a mass. Please compare with figure 2.8C.

Normal transverse process versus mass

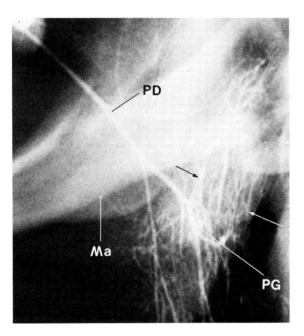

Figure 2.10A

Modified lateral view of normal parotid sialogram, positioned as in 2.7A, with the face rotated slightly more toward the table. Note the appearance of crowding together of the parotid duct branches (*arrows*). This appearance is due partly to the curve of the gland behind the mandible so that more branches are superimposed on each other and partly to external compression of the gland by the large transverse process of the first cervical vertebra, as shown in 2.10B.

Ma = mandible
PD = parotid duct
PG = parotid gland
Tr = transverse process of the first cervical vertebra

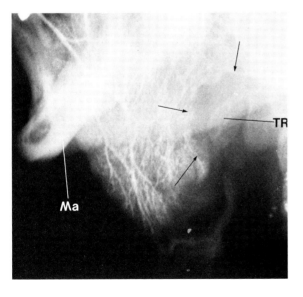

Figure 2.10B

Same patient as in figure 2.10A, but with the face rotated further toward the tabletop. The postero-medial margin of the parotid gland is deformed (*arrows*) by the large transverse process of the first cervical vertebra. This appearance is normal and should not be mistaken for a mass.

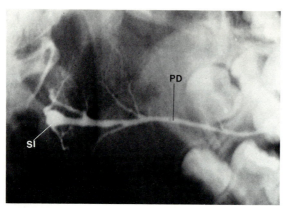

Figure 2.12C

Lateral view, right parotid sialogram.

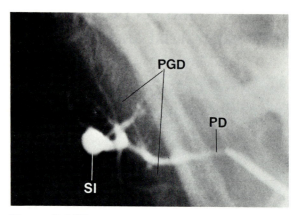

Figure 2.12D

AP view, right parotid sialogram; the entire superficial portion of the gland has been removed. The remaining visualized ducts are in the deep part of the gland. The clublike dilatation and deformity of the remaining posterior portion of the main duct and the slight deformity of the remaining branches in this region could be postoperative in nature or could be due to preexisting abnormal changes in the ducts.

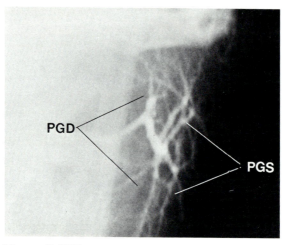

Figure 2.12E

AP view of left parotid sialogram performed at the same time, showing an essentially normal appearance. Note the normal superficial portion of the parotid gland lateral to the main parotid duct, in contradistinction to the appearance on the right side, where the superficial tissue has been removed and none remains lateral to the main duct.

The patient in figures 2.12C–E was a 9-year-old boy who had an eight-month history of bilateral parotid swelling; the swelling on the left had disappeared, but a tender mass that varied somewhat in size had remained in the tail of the right parotid gland; so that a superficial parotidectomy had been performed on this side. Pathologic examination of the removed superficial portion of the right parotid gland showed severe chronic active sialadenitis.

It can be seen from figures 2.12C and D and from figures 2.4B and C that parotid tissue is present deep to the facial nerve far anteriorly as well as in the retromandibular location. Thus, if the plane of the facial nerve is accepted as separating the deep from the superficial part of the gland (figs. 2.15A), there may be said to be four deep quadrants as well as four superficial quadrants, or eight parotid sections.

Superficial parotid mass

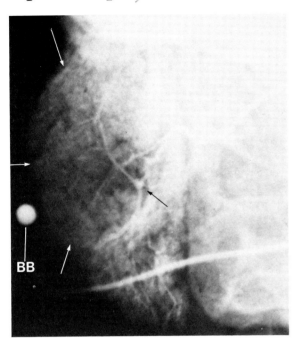

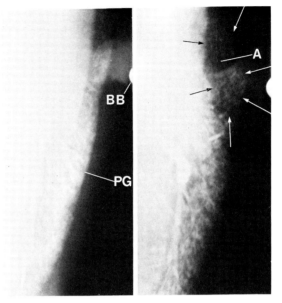

Figure 2.13B

A = air in the cavum conchae
BB = marker indicating the clinically palpable mass
PG = parotid gland

Figure 2.13A

Parotid sialogram, distention sialography, ocinar opacification phase, anterior oblique view with the head turned toward the opposite side, showing a mass in the superficial posterior portion of the gland (*arrows*). Arrows outline the mass, underlying the BB. A mass in such a location would be expected to be superficial to the facial nerve structures. AP view showed the mass to be superimposed over the ramus of the mandible, and lateral view showed it to be posterior, findings similar to those seen in figures 1.41A and B. Similar clinical and sialographic findings were present in the opposite parotid gland, not shown. Superficial parotidectomy was performed, removing the mass. Pathologic examination revealed it to be a Warthin's tumor. Please refer to figures 2.15A and 2.22A for the position of the facial nerve in the parotid gland.

Parotid sialogram late acinar opacification phase showing a mass (*arrows*) in the anterior-superior quadrant of the gland. The patient was a 27-year-old man with a palpable mass in the parotid gland. *Left*, straight AP view of the superficial portion of the parotid gland. A mass can be suspected in the superficial part of the gland beneath the BB, but is not clearly visualized. The margin of the parotid gland is normally smoothly outlined as shown here in its mid and lower portions. See also figure 1.22 for normal gland margin. *Right*, the face has been rotated toward the side of the sialogram, and a lenticular shaped mass can now be seen in the superficial portion of the gland (*arrows*), beneath the BB, and superimposed upon air in the cavum conchae. Pathologic examination showed a bulging deformity in the area shown by sialography. Cut section revealed a well-defined ovoid mass measuring 1.9 cm in diameter. Microscopic examination revealed this to be an area of nodular lymphoid hyperplasia.

Water's view

BB = marker
Ma = mandible
PG = parotid
gland

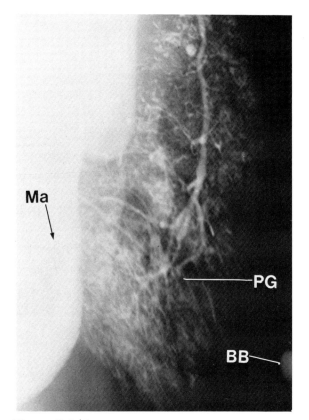

Figure 2.14A

Normal parotid gland, Water's view, late in the examination, showing some breakup of the sialogram. The parotid gland is somewhat enlarged due to pent-up salivary secretions and contrast material. The tail of the parotid gland, underlying the BB, is completely filled. Same patient as shown in figures 1.23D and 1.50.

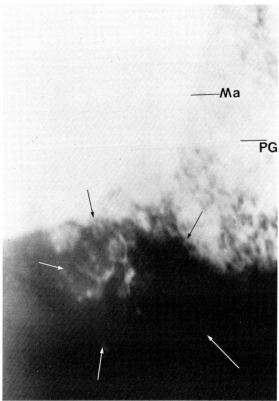

Figure 2.14B

Water's view, somewhat magnified, in another patient. The tail of the parotid gland could not be filled with contrast material because it has been replaced by a large mass. Pathologic examination revealed a Warthin's tumor. Arrows outline the large mass replacing the tail of the parotid gland.

Axial view

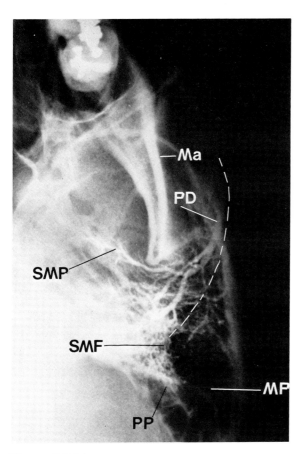

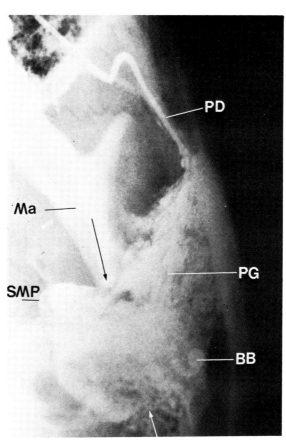

BB   = BB
Ma = mandible
MP = mastoid process
PD = parotid duct
PG = parotid gland
PP = posterior process of the parotid gland
SMF = location of the stylomastoid foramen
SMP = stylo-mandibular process

Figure 2.15A

Axial view of the normal parotid gland, duct-filling phase. The ducts curve medially around the posterior edge of the ramus of the mandible. The duct extending the farthest medially drains the so-called stylomandibular process. Note that the mandibular ramus and the mastoid process impinge upon the midportion of the parotid gland causing narrowing of the midportion of the gland, sometimes referred to as the isthmus.

The anatomic course of the facial nerve through the parotid gland is indicated by the dotted line. See also figure 2.22A.

Figure 2.15B

Parotid sialography, axial view, acinar opacification phase. A mass, not well seen in this view, is present in the posterior-inferior portion of the gland beneath the BB; same patient as in figure 2.14B. The isthmus is indicated by the arrows. It is partially obliterated by enlargement of the gland associated with distention sialography.

Axial-tangential view

BB = BB
Ma = mandible
PD = parotid duct
PG = parotid gland
Z = zygomatic arch

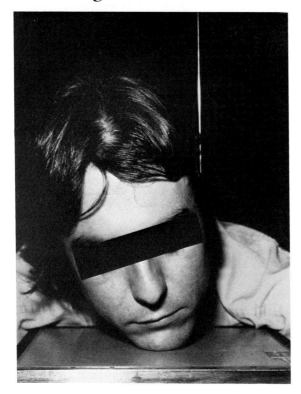

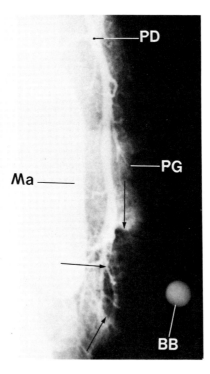

Figure 2.16A

The head is positioned as for a vertex-submental axial view and then tilted approximately 15 to 20 degrees away from the side being examined.

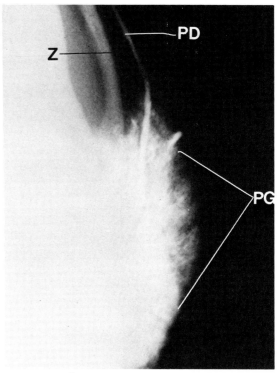

Figure 2.16B

Normal axial-tangential view shows the margin of the parotid gland to be smooth and regular.

Figure 2.16C

Axial-tangential view in a patient with a small, superficially located mass (*arrows*), underlying the BB. Pathologic examination revealed a small mixed tumor.

Open-mouth view

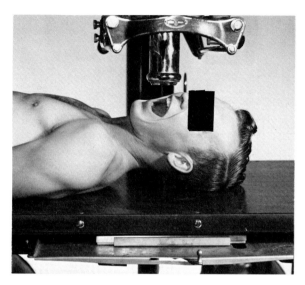

Figure 2.17A

The open-mouth view was originally described for the demonstration of submandibular calculi such as shown in figure 1.6B. The head is turned 30 degrees toward the side being examined. The x-ray beam is vertical. This view is also useful for demonstrating the submandibular duct and gland, best seen with the head flexed. The posterior portion of the parotid gland can also be well seen in this projection if the head is somewhat extended as shown in fig. 2.17B. (Heystek and Hildreth 1958. Reprinted with permission.)

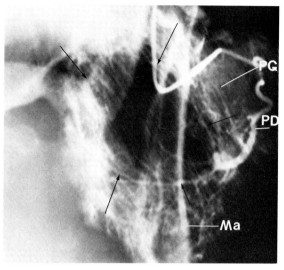

Ma = mandible
PD = parotid duct
PG = parotid gland

Figure 2.17B

Open-mouth view in a patient with a large tumor (*arrows*) of the parotid gland.

The patient was a 76-year-old woman with an egg-shaped mass posterior to the angle of the jaw. At surgery the mass was found to occupy the superficial portion of the parotid gland. It displaced the upper facial nerve division laterally and upward and the lower division medially. Superficial parotidectomy was performed. Pathologic examination revealed the mass to be a Warthin's tumor. See also figure 1.41D.

Puffed-cheek view

A = air in the puffed out cheek
Ma = mandible

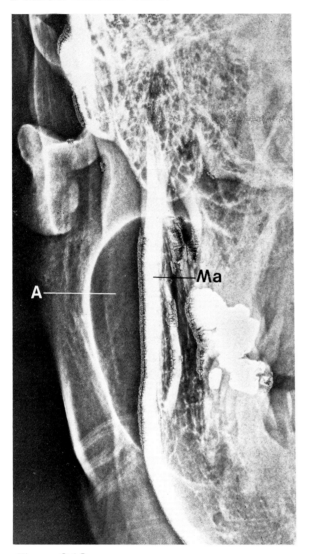

Figure 2.18

The puffed-cheek view, normal examination, xerox film. The patient is instructed to puff out the cheek on the side being examined and the head and face are rotated approximately 25 degrees toward the same side. This view can be used to demonstrate opaque calculi in the anterior portion of the parotid duct. (See also figures 3.17A, 3.18A, 3.19A, 3.20A.)

Panoramic radiography

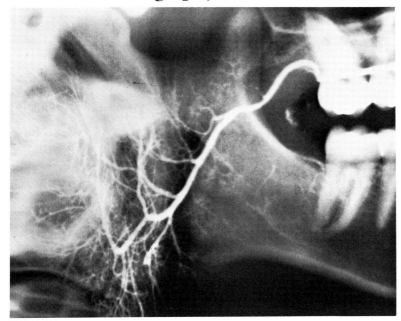

BB = marker
PD = parotid duct
PG = parotid gland

Figure 2.19A

Normal orthopantomogram, duct-filling phase.

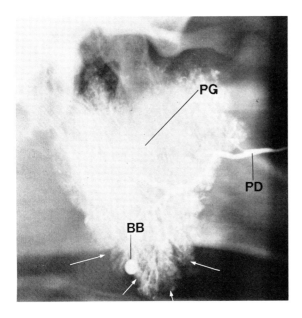

Figure 2.19B

Orthopantomogram, acinar opacification phase, another patient. A mass was palpable underlying the BB. Acinar filling is slightly deficient in this region. The findings were due to invasion of the inferior margin of the parotid gland by metastatic tumor (*arrows*) in adjacent lymph nodes, most of the mass being extrinsic to the gland; same patient as in figure 1.18.

CT of the salivary glands

CAB = Corpus adiposum buccae
ECA = external carotid artery entering the parotid gland
ICA = internal carotid artery
IJV = internal jugular vein
Ma = mandible
MM = masseter muscle
MPM = medial pterygoid muscle
PBD = posterior belly of the digastric muscle
PFV = posterior facial vein
PG = parotid gland
SCM = sterno-cleidomastoid muscle
SMP = stylo-mandibular process
St = styloid process

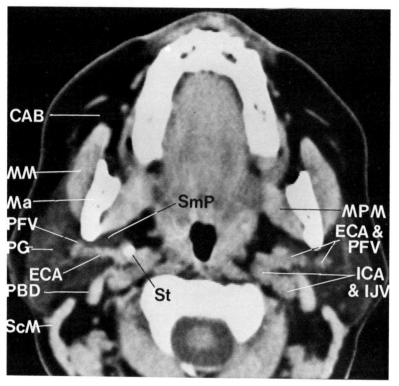

Figure 2.20

Straight CT section through the midportion of the parotid glands, corresponding with the projection shown in the digital radiograph, figure 1.33A. Normal examination. (Rabinov, Kell, and Gordon 1984. With permission.)

Semiaxial CT of the salivary glands

The head is extended and the gantry angled 20 degrees craniad, corresponding with the digital radiograph shown in figure 1.33B. This projection is routinely the most useful to image the entire parotid and submandibular glands free of artifact from dental amalgam.

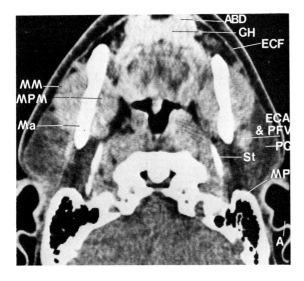

Figure 2.21A

Section through the upper midportion of the parotid glands. The parotid glands are slightly enlarged due to sialosis of unknown cause in this patient; same patient as in figure 1.33B.

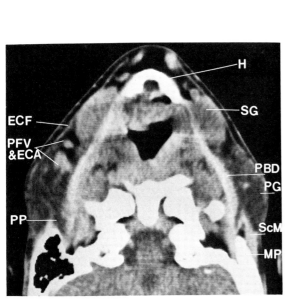

Figure 2.21B

Section through the lower portions of the parotid glands and the submandibular glands in another patient; normal examination. Note the compartment formed laterally by the superficial layer of the external cervical fascia and medially by the posterior belly of the digastric muscle. This compartment contains the parotid and submandibular glands on each side. (Rabinov, Kell, and Gordon 1984. With permission.)

A = air in the cavum conchae
ABD = anterior belly of the digastric muscle
ECA = external carotid artery
ECF = external cervical fascia, superficial layer
GH = genio-hyoid muscle
H = hyoid bone
Ma = man-dible
MM = masseter muscle
MP = mastoid process
MPM = medial pterygoid muscle
PBD = posterior belly of the digastric muscle
PFV = posterior facial vein
PG = parotid gland
PP = posterior process of the parotid gland
SCM = sterno-cleidomastoid muscle
SG = sub-mandibular gland
St = styloid process

CAB = corpus
adiposum buccae
ECA = external
carotid artery
I   = isthmus
of the parotid
gland
ICA = internal
carotid artery
IJV = internal
jugular vein
LPM = lateral
pterygoid muscle
LPP = lateral
pterygoid plate
M   = mass
Ma   = man-
dible
MM   = masseter
muscle
MPM = medial
pterygoid muscle
MPP = medial
pterygoid plate
PBD = posterior
belly of the
digastric muscle
PG   = parotid
gland
PP   = posterior
process of the
parotid gland
SCM = sterno-
cleidomastoid
muscle
SMP = stylo-
mandibular
process of the
parotid gland
St   = styloid
process
TM   = tem-
poralis muscle

Semiaxial CT view with the head flexed and the gantry angled 10 degrees craniad

The parotid glands are slightly enlarged and of somewhat low density, owing to sialosis of unknown cause; same patient as in figure 2.21A; same patient and position as shown in figure 1.33C. The facial nerve is not visualized by CT but the approximate anatomic course of the facial nerve in the right parotid gland, just lateral to the posterior facial vein and external carotid artery, is indicated by the broken line. (Mason and Chisholm 1975; Blount and Lachman 1953; Pernkopf 1963; Larsell 1953; Mancuso and Manafee 1982). See also figure 2.15A (Rabinov, Kell, and Gordon 1984. With permission.)

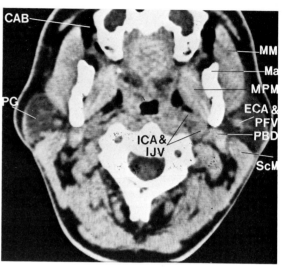

Figure 2.22B

CT section through the lower portion of the parotid glands.

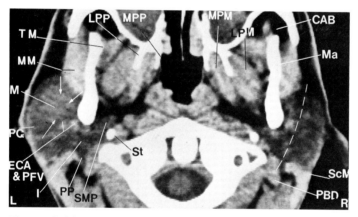

Figure 2.22A

CT section through the upper portions of the parotid glands. A small mass (*arrows*) is poorly visualized in the anterior part of the left parotid gland. Note the narrow isthmus of the parotid gland between the ramus of the mandible anteriorly and the muscles posteriorly.

Direct coronal CT examination

Parotid examination of same patient as in figure 2.22; same position and patient as in figure 1.33D.

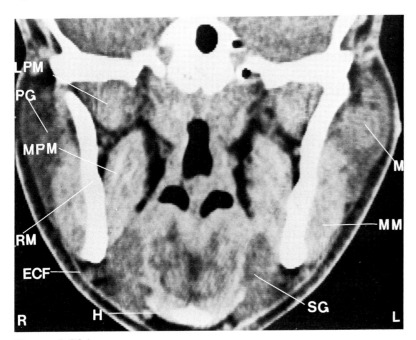

Figure 2.23A

CT section through the anterior portion of the parotid glands. The small mass within the left parotid gland was a benign cystic mixed tumor. The mass was folded about a branch of the facial nerve, and thus a portion of the mass was in the superficial part of the gland and a portion was in the deep part.

Con = con-
dyloid process of
the mandible
EAC = external
auditory canal
ECF = external
cervical fascia,
superficial layer
H = hyoid
bone
LPM = lateral
pterygoid muscle
M = mass
MM = masseter
muscle
MPM = medial
pterygoid muscle
PBD = posterior
belly of the
digastric muscle
PG = parotid
gland
RM = ramus of
the mandible
SG = sub-
mandibular gland
St = styloid
process

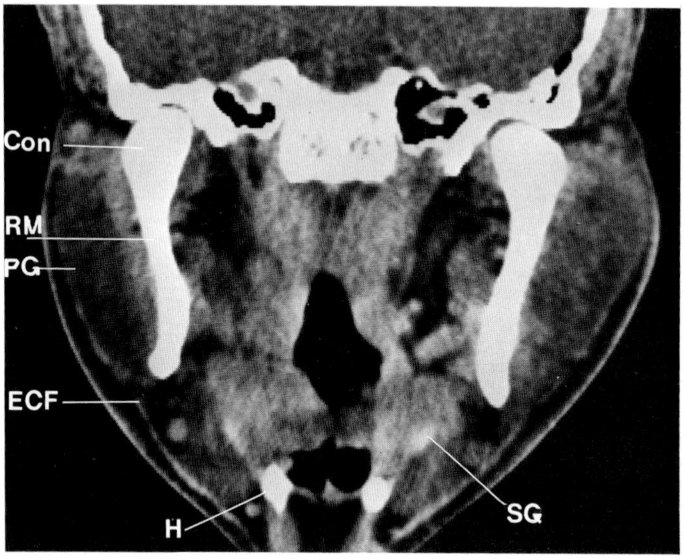

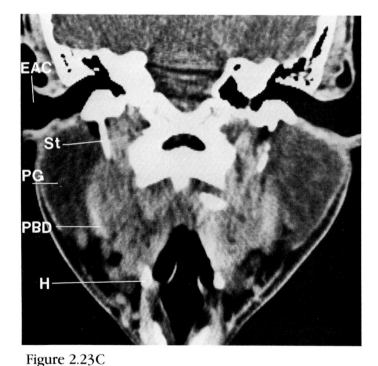

Figure 2.23B

CT section through the midportion of the parotid
glands and ramus of the mandible.

Figure 2.23C

CT section through the posterior portion of the
parotid glands, dorsal to the mandible. (Rabinov,
Kell, and Gordon 1984. With permission.)

The peripharyngeal spaces

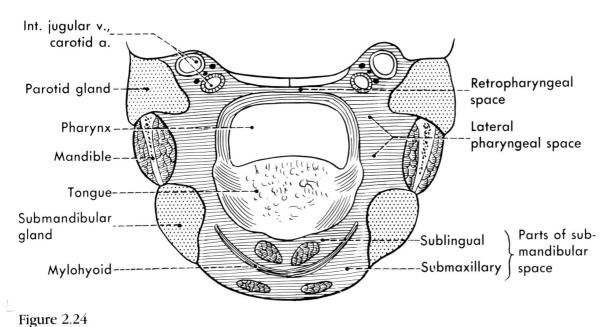

Figure 2.24

Oblique section, showing the general relations of
peripharyngeal spaces and their continuity with
each other. (Hollinshead 1968. Reprinted with
permission.)

Normal submandibular sialography

BB = marker
Ma = mandible
SG = submandibular gland

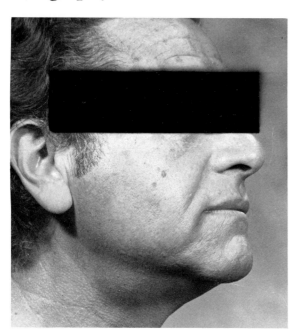

Figure 2.25A

Prominence of submandibular glands. The gland was normally soft in consistency possibly owing to mild sialosis. This appearance was present bilaterally; same patient as in figure 7.5. The submandibular glands may show a gradual, slight increase in prominence with increasing age. This finding is usually present bilaterally; such glands are soft and normal in consistency and do not change over a long period of observation.

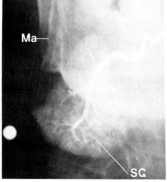 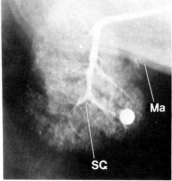

Figure 2.25B

Left, AP view; *right,* lateral view. Another patient. The contrast material is Ethiodol. The examination is within normal limits except that the submandibular gland has descended to a slightly lower position than usual. Soft masses were palpable in the submandibular region bilaterally. The BB indicates that the palpable mass is the submandibular gland. It had sagged and become more prominent, perhaps owing to atrophy or relaxation of the musculofascial tissues that normally support it.

Submandibular sialography, lateral view

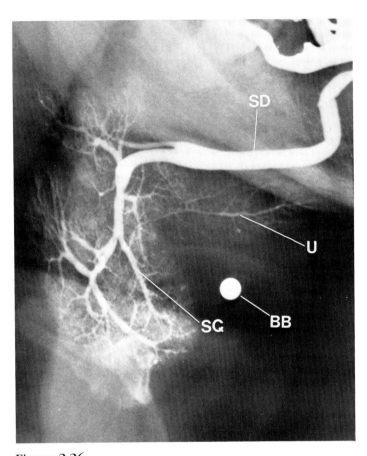

BB = marker
SG = body of the submandibular gland
SD = submandibular duct
U = uncinate process of the submandibular gland

Figure 2.26

Same patient as in figure 1.5. The submandibular gland itself is normal; there is a mass of enlarged lymph nodes anterior to the gland, indicated by the BB.

Position for submandibular sialography

C   = calculus
Ma = mandible
MP = mastoid process
SD = submand-ibular duct
SG = submand-ibular gland

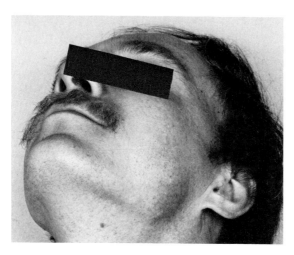

Figure 2.27A

AP oblique view; the chin is tilted up and the head is extended and rotated approximately 45 degrees toward the side to be examined so that the ramus and adjacent part of the body of the mandible are perpendicular to the tabletop.

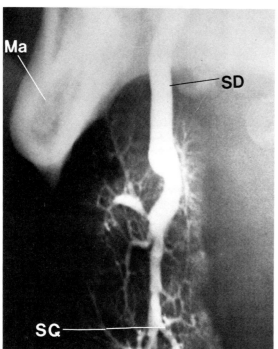

Figure 2.27B

Sialogram performed with Ethiodol, in position shown in 2.27A. This view provides a relatively bone-free projection of the gland. The medial margin of the gland may normally be concave in some patients (please see fig. 2.30) although this appearance could be due to the mass in this instance; same patient as in figure 2.26.

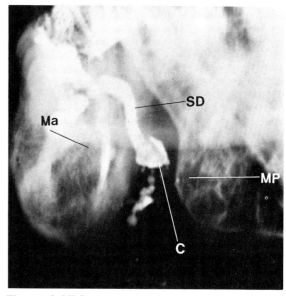

Figure 2.27C

Another patient (shown in figs. 1.6A,B, 2.28), same projection, but with the chin tilted higher. A calculus can be seen at the junction of the submandibular duct and gland, projected between the mandible and the mastoid process.

Submandibular sialography

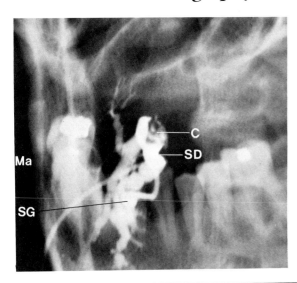

C = calculus
Ma = mandible
SD = submandibular duct
SG = submandibular gland

Figure 2.28

Open mouth view; same patient as in figures 1.6A,B, and 2.27C.

Submandibular sialography

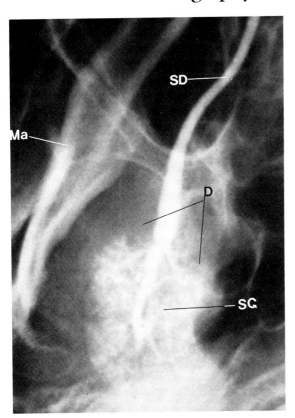

Figure 2.29

Axial view, performed with Ethiodol; the submandibular gland is pushed slightly posteriorly and its anterior margin is deformed by a mass of unknown nature.

The patient was a 57-year-old woman with a mass of moderate size palpable anterior to the right submandibular salivary gland. This examination was performed prior to the availability of CT. CT examination is now the preferable method for the study of such masses. Please see figure 1.39A,B,E, 1.40A. Surgery was not performed.

D = deformity of the anterior margin of the submandibular gland
Ma = mandible
SD = submandibular duct
SG = submandibular gland

CT of the submandibular glands

Ca = common or internal carotid artery
ECF = external cervical fascia, superficial layer
H = hyoid bone
IJV = internal jugular vein
PG = parotid gland lower tip
Ph = pharynx
SCM = sterno-cleidomastoid muscle
SG = submandibular gland

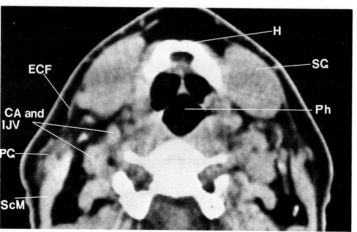

Figure 2.30

Head extended and the gantry angled 20 degrees craniad; this CT image was taken at a somewhat higher angle than shown in figure 1.33E. In this view, the submandibular gland can be seen to lie between the external layer of the external cervical fascia laterally and the hyoid bone and oropharynx medially.

References

Anson, B. J. *Morris' human anatomy,* 12th edition. New York: McGraw-Hill, 1966, pp. 1251–1261.

Anson, B. J., and McVay, C. B. *Surgical anatomy,* 5th edition. Philadelphia: W. B. Saunders, 1971, pp. 183–210.

Arey, L. B. *Developmental anatomy,* 7th edition. Philadelphia: W. B. Saunders, 1974, pp. 226–227.

Bargmann, W. *Histologie und mikroskopische Anatomie des Menschen.* Stuttgart: Georg Thieme Verlag, 1977, pp. 411–424.

Batsakis, J. G., and Sylvest, V. *Pathology of the salivary glands.* Chicago: American Society of Clinical Pathologists, 1977.

Blount, R. F., and Lachman, E. The digestive system. In *Morris' human anatomy,* 11th edition, ed. J. P. Schaeffer. New York: McGraw-Hill, 1953, pp. 1304–1312.

Braus, H. *Anatomie der menschen.* Berlin: Springer-Verlag, 1924.

Chaudhry, A. P.; Montes, M.; and Cutler, L. S. Structural and functional maldevelopment of salivary glands. In *Salivary glands and their secretion: proceedings of a symposium,* ed. N. H. Rowe. Ann Arbor, Mich.: University of Michigan, 1972, pp. 59–93.

Clark, E. R. The lymphatic system and the spleen. In *Morris' human anatomy,* 11th edition, ed. J. P. Schaeffer. New York: McGraw-Hill, 1953.

Conley, J. *Salivary glands and the facial nerve.* Stuttgart: Georg Thieme Verlag, 1975.

Conn, I. G.; Wiesenfeld, D.; and Ferguson, M. M. The anatomy of the facial nerve in relation to CT/sialography of the parotid gland. *Br. J. Radiol.* 56.901–905, 1983.

Curtin, H. D.; Wolfe, P.; and Snyderman, N. The facial nerve between the stylomastoid foramen and the parotid: computed tomographic imaging. *Radiology* 149:165–169, 1983.

Davis, R. A., et al. Surgical anatomy of the facial nerve and parotid gland based upon a study of 350 cervicofacial halves. *Surg. Gynecol. Obstet.* 102:385–412, 1956.

Diamont, H. Enlargement of the parotid gland. *Acta Otolaryngol.* 52:299–310, 1960.

DuPlessis, D. J. Some important features in the development, structure and function of the parotid salivary glands. *S. Afr. Med. J.* 31:773–781, 1957.

Ericson, S. The normal variation of the parotid size. *Acta Otolaryngol.* 70:294–300, 1970.

Ericson, S. Width of the parotid main duct in healthy subjects. *Acta Radiol. (Diagn.)* 14:17–25, 1973.

Ericson, S., and Hedin, M. A clinical roentgenologic method of calculating the volume of the parotid gland. *Oral Roentgenol.* 29:536–543, 1970.

Gasser, R. F. The early development of the parotid gland around the facial nerve and its branches in man. *Anat. Rec.* 167:63–78, 1970.

Gaughran, G. R. L. The parotid compartment. *Ann. Otol. Rhinol. Laryngol.* 70:31–51, 1961.

Godwin, J. T. Benign lymphoepithelial lesion of the parotid gland. *Cancer* 5:1089–1103, 1952.

Gudbrandsson, F. K.; Liston, S. L.; and Maisel, R. A. Heterotopic salivary tissue in the neck. *Otolaryngol. Head Neck Surg.* 90:279–282, 1982.

Hamilton, W. J., and Mossman, H. W. *Hamilton Boyd and Mossman's human embryology.* Baltimore: Williams & Wilkins, 1972, p. 311.

Hettler, M., and Lauth, G. Die gezielte Sialographie. *Furtschr. Rontgenstr.* 95:493–495, 1961.

Heystek, H. D., and Hildreth, R. C. *Med. Radiogr. Photogr.* 34:20–22, 1958.

Hollinshead, W. H. *The head and neck. Anatomy for surgeons,* vol. 1, 2nd edition. New York: Harper & Row, 1968, pp. 347–357.

International Anatomical Nomenclature Committee. *Nomina anatomica,* 4th edition. Amsterdam: Excerpta Medica, 1977.

Johns, M. E. The salivary glands: anatomy and embryology. *Otolaryngol. Clin. North Am.* 10:261–271, 1977.

Kassel, E. E. CT sialography, part I: introduction, technique, anatomy and variants. *J. Otolaryngol. (suppl.)* 1982 Dec., 11 (12 Suppl.), pp. 1–10.

Larsell, O. The nervous system. In *Morris' human anatomy,* 11th edition, ed. J. P. Schaeffer. New York: McGraw-Hill, 1953, p. 1103.

Mancuso, A. A., and Hanafee, W. N. *Computed tomography of the head and neck.* Baltimore: Williams & Wilkins, 1982, pp. 168–202.

Mason, D. K., and Chisholm, D. M. *Salivary glands in health and disease.* Philadelphia: W. B. Saunders, 1975, pp. 18–33, 83–91.

McCabe, B. F., and Work, W. P. Disorders of the salivary glands. In *Otolaryngology, IV,* ed. W. H. Mahoney. Hagerstown, Md.: Harper & Row, 1969.

McKenzie, J. The parotid gland in relation to the facial nerve. *J. Anat.* 82:183–186, 1948.

Moss-Salentijn, L., and Moss, M. L. Developmental and functional anatomy. In *Diseases of the salivary glands,* ed. R. M. Rankow and I. M. Polayes. Philadelphia: W. B. Saunders, 1976, pp. 17–31.

Oppenheim, H., and Wing, M. Sialography and surface anatomy of the parotid duct. *Arch. Otolaryngol.* 71:80–83, 1960.

Patey, D. H., and Thackray, A. C. The pathological anatomy and treatment of parotid tumors with retropharyngeal extension (dumb-bell tumors) with a report of 4 personal cases. *Br. J. Surg.* 44:352–358, 1957.

Patten, B. M. *Human embryology,* 3rd edition. New York: McGraw-Hill, 1968, pp. 385–387.

Pernkopf, E. *Atlas of topographical and applied human anatomy.* Vol. 1, *Head and neck.* Philadelphia: W. B. Saunders, 1963.

Polayes, I. M., and Rankow, R. M. Cysts, masses and tumors of the accessory parotid gland. *Plast. Reconstr. Surg.* 64:17–23, 1979.

Provenza, D. V. *Oral histology, inheritance and development.* Philadelphia: J. B. Lippincott, 1964, pp. 412–438.

Provenza, D. V. *Fundamentals of oral histology and embryology.* Philadelphia: J. B. Lippincott, 1972, pp. 71, 222–231.

Rabinov, K.; Kell, T.; and Gordon, P. H. Computed tomography of the salivary glands. *Radiol. Clin. North Am.* 22:145–159, 1984.

Rankow, R. M. *Atlas of surgery of the face, mouth, and neck.* Philadelphia: W. B. Saunders, 1968.

Rankow, R. M., and Polayes, I. M. Surgical anatomy and diagnosis. In *Diseases of the salivary glands,* ed. R. M. Rankow and I. M. Polayes. Philadelphia: W. B. Saunders, 1976, pp. 156–184.

Rauch, S. *Die speicheldrusen des menschen. Anatomy, physiologie und klinische pathologie.* Stuttgart: Georg Thieme Verlag, 1959.

Schaeffer, J. P. *Morris' human anatomy.* New York: Blakiston, 1953.

Shackelford, J. M., and Schneyer, L. H. Ultrastructural aspects of the main excretory duct of rat submandibular gland. *Anat. Rec.* 169:679–696, 1971.

Sone, S., et al. CT of parotid tumors. *American Journal of Neuroradiology* 3:143–147, 1982.

Sviridova, I. K. Intraorganic lymphatic bed of the human parotid salivary gland. *Arkh. Anat. Gistol. Embriol.* 59:10–18, 1970.

Waterhouse, J. P. Inflammation in the salivary glands. *Br. J. Oral Surg.* 3:161–171, 1966.

Waterhouse, J. P., and Winter, R. B. Evidence for a trend of replacement of functional secreting cells by fat and connective tissue in human submandibular salivary glands through adult life. *J. Dent. Res.* 43:965–966, 1964.

Weiss, L., and Greep, R. O. *Histology.* New York: McGraw-Hill, 1977, pp. 652–659.

Winsten, J.; Gould, D. M.; and Ward, G. E. Sialography. *Surg. Gynecol. Obstet.* 102:315–321, 1956.

Young, J. A., et al. Micropuncture and perfusion studies of fluid and electrolyte transport in the rat submaxillary gland. In *Secretory mechanisms of salivary glands,* ed. L. H. Schneyer and C. A. Schneyer. New York: Academic Press, 1967. pp. 11–31.

Young, J. A., and Van Lennep, E. W. *The morphology of the salivary glands.* New York: Academic Press, 1978, pp. 72–99.

Chapter 3

Calculi and Inflammation; Interventional Procedures; Trauma

Sialolithiasis

Sialolithiasis is second in frequency only to mumps in diseases of the salivary glands, and probably it is the most frequent disease in persons beyond the second decade of life, occurring in men twice as often as in women (Rauch 1959a). Stones form in patients from the first decade to old age, with a peak incidence between 30 and 50 years. Cases in infants as young as three weeks have been reported (Rauch 1959b).

The submandibular gland is the most common site of involvement, followed by the parotid gland and, rarely, the sublingual gland. In a series of 180 cases reported by Levy and colleagues (1962), 80% of stones occurred in the submandibular gland, 19% in the parotid gland, and 1% in the sublingual gland. In the majority of cases the stones are single, but 32% of multiple stones developed in the parotid gland, while only 22% were located in the submandibular gland; bilateral stones were present in 2.2% of cases (Levy, ReMine, and Devine 1962). Eighteen percent of patients had passed stones or had other stones removed previously.

Of patients with recurrent chronic sialadenitis 65% have had sialolithiasis. The size of the stones varies from small grains in smaller ducts to large stones in the main duct, especially Wharton's duct. Most often only one gland is affected (König 1951). A combination of stones in the salivary glands, gallbladder, and kidneys is rare, but five such cases were reported by Perint (1948). Most stones are round to oval or elliptical in shape. The surface is smooth or slightly irregular and rough; roughness is caused by short, sharp projections from the surface.

Stones in the parotid gland often are irregular in size and shape, with pointed projections that may cause considerable pain (Rauch 1959a). Although stones vary in size and weight, the average ranges are about 0.1 to 20 mm and 0.1 to 3.0 g (Rauch 1959a). Large stones several centimeters in size and weighing from 6 to 182 g have been reported (Rauch 1959b; König 1951). The color of stones is yellowish white to brown; the consistency ranges from soft and friable to a hard mass. Stones in the major ducts usually are hard, while intraglandular stones are soft. The cross section of a stone may be homogeneous or layered. The centrum usually consists of a hard anorganic mass or, less often, of epithelial debris or a foreign body. The main components of a stone are calcium carbonate and phosphate.

Etiology

The etiology and pathogenesis of salivary stone formation are related to several factors. The pathogenesis of salivary gland calculi appears to be related to the pH of the saliva. The salivary pH in the alkaline submandibular gland is 6.8 to 7.1, as opposed to the more acidic product of the parotid gland, which has a pH of 6.3 to 7.4. This difference in pH may explain the greater incidence of stone formation in the submandibular gland. In a relatively alkaline medium with elevation of salivary bicarbonate and alteration of salivary calcium phosphorus ratio, the solubility of salivary apatite is exceeded with consequent precipitation. Owing to stasis from obstruction by stones, infection is superimposed and results in precipitation of proteinaceous debris, sloughed epithelium, and leukocytes. These products form an organic or resinous layer, which alternates with the calcareous layer of apatite.

Certain secondary factors may facilitate stone formation: the mucus content of the submandibular gland may become more viscous, thus promoting stone formation; Wharton's duct follows an uphill course that encourages stagnation of saliva, and stagnation leads to calculus formation. Some evidence suggests that submandibular calculi form first and infection follows as a consequence of obstruction. Parotid calculi, however, form secondarily as a result of infection.

Salivary gland calculi have a laminated structure. Calcium phosphates and carbonates comprise the major inorganic substances. Superimposed on the nucleus are alternate layers of white calcareous mineral and organic, brownish yellow resinous material; the latter substance also forms the outer layer of the stone.

Lithiasis of the Submandibular Gland

(Figs. 3.1–3.15, 3.48, 3.50–3.52, 3.54)
Thirty percent of stones of the submandibular gland are in the proximal portion of Wharton's duct or in the hilum of the gland. The mucous consistency of the saliva and the ascending course of the submandibular duct may contribute to stone formation. The asymptomatic period for submandibular stones is longer than that for parotid stones ranging from one month to 10 years, with an average of 1–1½ years; this may be related to the larger size of Wharton's duct and smoothing out of sharp edges of stones by a mucous coating (Rauch 1959a).

As in the parotid gland, intraglandular stones can be differentiated from extraglandular stones. Rauch (1959b) determined the location of submandibular stones as follows: 30% near the ostium, 20% in the middle third of the duct, 35% at the right-angle bend of the submandibular duct, and 15% proximal to the right-angle bend and hilum of the submandibular gland.

Lithiasis of the Parotid Gland

(Figs. 3.16–3.21, 3.49, 3.53, 3.55)
Stones of the parotid gland are located most frequently in Stenson's duct and usually are smaller than submandibular stones (Rauch 1959b). The incidence of intraglandular versus extraglandular stones has a reported ratio of 1:35 (Rauch 1959b). The intraglandular stones are situated in the smaller ducts and rarely in the parenchyma of the gland. The pressure from flow of the serous secretions and the descending course of Stenson's duct probably are responsible for the location of stones in the distal portion of the main duct. The absence of mucus in parotid secretions prevents precipitation of mucus on the stone surface, thereby retarding enlargement of the stone. Stones within the duct cause painful swelling after meals; the swelling may subside spontaneously after several hours. Intraglandular stones are less painful and may cause a localized swelling that simulates a tumor. Parotid stones generally are diagnosed one to two months following the onset of symptoms as opposed to about one and a half years for submandibular stones (Rauch 1959a).

Signs and Symptoms

The duration of symptoms varies considerably from one acute episode to repeated attacks extending over many years. Sialolithiasis is characterized by a dull or sharp colicky pain and periodic swelling in the region of the submandibular and parotid glands and occurring with eating. The swelling may be acute or insidious and usually lasts two to three hours. In some patients, the glands remain swollen and indurated. The enlargement of the gland may occur with each meal or as seldom as once or twice yearly. The glands may be tender and painful. The severity of symptoms depends on the degree of obstruction related to the size and location of the calculus. Stones within the gland tend to cause less severe symptoms and may lead to formation of a tender inflammatory mass. In a small percentage of patients, stones induce a discrete asymptomatic mass simulating a tumor. Stones sometimes are discovered in asymptomatic patients; incidental stones have been found in 1% of autopsies performed (Rauch and Gorlin 1970). Complete ductal obstruction may result in a continually swollen gland with severe pain, swelling in the floor of the mouth or cheek, and pus emanating from the duct orifice. Localized cellulitis and fever may be present. Bimanual palpation of either Wharton's or Stenson's duct may indicate sialolithiasis if the stone is of sufficient size.

Radiographic Evaluation of Salivary Gland Calculi

(Figs. 3.1–3.21)

Radiologic investigation of patients with suspected salivary gland calculi consists of preliminary plain films usually followed by sialography (Rubin and Holt 1957; Garusi and Sassi 1963; Ollenshaw and Rose 1951; Yune and Klatte 1972; Eisenbud and Cranin 1963). For evaluation of parotid calculi, AP puffed-cheek, lateral, and oblique views are obtained; and occlusal, oblique, lateral, and basal views are indicated for examination of the submandibular gland. The intraoral occlusal view should encompass the entire floor of the mouth back to the molar area. This projection usually demonstrates the entire Wharton's duct, including the right-angle bend near the hilum of the gland. The central beam is parallel to the lingual surface of the symphysis of the mandible. Any slant of the lingual surface of the mandible may obscure small stones near the duct orifice. Radiopaque stones must be distinguished from opaque densities outside the salivary glands and ducts. The most common calcific densities that can simulate calculi are osteomas, calcified lymph nodes, phleboliths, and foreign bodies. Osteomas lack lamination and remain in a constant relationship to the mandible on films with different degrees of rotation. Fluoroscopic spot films may be useful to secure the proper projection. Calcified lymph nodes are mottled and irregular in outline and often are multiple. Phleboliths have a dense ring with a radiolucent center; knowledge of the anatomic location of the salivary glands and ducts usually projects these densities outside the confines of the glands and ducts.

Sialography with water-soluble contrast material usually is the only means of ruling out salivary calculi. Salivary calculi manifest different sizes and shapes. The radiographic density is a reflection of the mineral composition of the calculus. According to one report (Levy, ReMine, and Devine 1962), salivary gland calculi are radiolucent in 20% of cases, while in another report (Rubin and Holt 1957), radiolucent stones are found in 20% in the submandibular gland and in 40% in the parotid gland. Sialography in clinically suspected sialolithiasis can be expected to:

1. Detect radiolucent calculi.
2. Differentiate various calcific densities in the area of the salivary duct and gland (radiographic density indicates mineral composition of calculi).
3. Determine the position of a known stone and aid in its surgical removal.
4. Determine the presence of multiple stones.
5. Determine the status of salivary ducts and gland proximal to the stone.

6. Evaluate sialodochitis and sialectasia.

7. Assess impairment of drainage of contrast material caused by a stone, mucus block, or stricture in the main duct or branches.

Sialography is done under fluoroscopic control. Spot films are obtained during the procedure to document the anatomy of the ducts and gland and record abnormalities. Postevacuation films, often fluoroscopic spot films, are required in all patients with no obvious abnormality. Following removal of the cannula, evacuation of contrast material from Wharton's or Stenson's ducts proceeds uninterrupted. Any delay in evacuation from within the main duct or branches may indicate obstruction by a radiolucent stone. Large stones may completely obstruct the main duct. The interface between the stone and contrast column is characterized by a crescent-shaped defect. In most instances, however, contrast material will bypass the stone, which causes a filling defect of varying shape and size. Variable degrees of dilatation of the main duct and/or intraglandular branches proximal to the stone are associated findings. A localized stricture or multiple strictures associated with segments of dilated ducts are the usual sequelae to infection, and the presence of stones contributes to this outcome. Sialodochiectasis with or without strictures occur in a large variety of different patterns as illustrated. The dilatation of the ducts may be of a slight degree, or large saccular dilatation may involve the main duct and the intraglandular branches.

Smaller stones may be completely obscured by the contrast material during the filling phase, although fluoroscopy may reveal a temporary holdup in the flow of the contrast agent at the location of the stone. Postevacuation films after introduction of contrast material may demonstrate a complete or partial obstruction at the site of the stone. This is preferably observed at fluoroscopy and documented with spot films. Blockage of contrast material caused by small stones may be the only radiographic finding on the postevacuation film. Small stones are often missed near the orifice of the duct, where they are obscured by the inlying cannula. Moreover, contrast material usually does not fill the distal portion of the duct because of the cannula. Small stones that are not embedded in the mucosa often move proximally within the duct during the introduction of the contrast material. Intraparenchymal stones may be situated in sialectatic cavities. Diverticulum, like outpouchings of the main duct, may contain one or several small stones. Rarely, stones perforate the duct system and form a fistula into the oral cavity or skin.

Sialadenitis

Inflammatory disorders of the major salivary glands caused by bacterial or viral infections are the most common salivary gland diseases. Mixed infection usually ascends from the mouth, whereas specific infections often are blood borne. Predisposing factors include reduction of salivary flow of various etiologies (e.g., surgery, radiation, and drugs). Inflammatory disorders may be classified as follows:

I. Nonobstructive
   A. Viral (mumps)
   B. Bacterial
      1. Acute
      2. Subacute
      3. Chronic
   C. Postsurgical
   D. Postirradiation
   E. Pneumoparotitis
II. Obstructive
   A. Stones
   B. Strictures
III. Recurrent parotitis
   A. Children
   B. Adults
IV. Granulomatous diseases
   A. Tuberculosis
   B. Fungus
   C. Sarcoid
   D. Cat scratch fever
   E. Syphilis
   F. Toxoplasmosis
V. Sjögren's syndrome

Mumps and Other Viral Infections

Mumps is the most common of all salivary gland diseases (Rankow and Polayes 1976). It is an acute, contagious, and generalized viral disease occurring predominantly in children. The incubation period ranges from two to three weeks. The illness is characterized by pain and swelling of one (30%) or both (60%) parotid glands, with displacement of the ear lobe upward and outward. These findings are associated with systemic symptoms such as fever, muscular pain, headache, and malaise. The duct orifice is swollen and red but no pus exudes. The parotid gland is involved in 85% of cases, but swelling of the submandibular gland does occur occasionally.

Other viral agents that cause parotitis are parainfluenza viruses I and III, coxsackievirus A (herpangina), echovirus, and choriomeningitis virus.

Neonatal Suppurative Parotitis

This disease predominantly afflicts premature infants (35% to 40%) with dehydration as a predisposing condition (Leake and Leake 1970). The presenting signs and symptoms consist of fever and parotid gland swelling with tender or nontender and firm or fluctuant glands. The disease is clinically apparent 7 to 14 days after delivery. The clinical findings include erythema of the overlying skin. The disease often becomes bilateral. The swelling usually disappears in three to six days. Staphylococci are responsible for the infection in most patients, but other types of bacteria, such as *Pseudomonas aeruginosa,* streptococci, pneumococci, and *Escherichia coli,* have been implicated. The infecting organisms advance via the ascending route through the parotid duct or by the hematogenous route.

Potential complications, reported chiefly in the preantibiotic era, included salivary fistulas, facial palsy, perforation into the external canal, and mediastinitis. Because of the acute and transitory nature of the disease, sialography usually is not performed.

Acute Nonspecific Parotid Sialadenitis

This type of inflammation usually is bacterial in origin and is caused by an ascending ductal infection. In the pediatric age group, predisposing factors include fever and dehydration from respiratory infection, systemic viral illnesses, acute glomerulonephritis, immunosuppression states, failure to thrive, respiratory distress syndrome, previous mumps or parotitis, and trauma to the gland (Kaban, Mulliken, and Murray 1978).

Symptoms of acute parotid sialadenitis in children and adults are characterized by fever, general malaise, and painful swelling of the gland with local tenderness. There is purulent exudate from the buccal stoma of Stensen's duct. In addition to these features, the edema may involve the cheek, periorbital region and neck, and may be accompanied by trismus. In some patients local swelling and induration may persist for weeks before gradually subsiding. In a small number of cases, small abscesses may form and eventually coalesce into a larger abscess. If the infection is inadequately treated, the abscess may extend into the parapharyngeal or masticator fascial spaces. If an abscess has formed, surgical drainage, in addition to antibiotic therapy, is indicated. A concomitant finding in sialadenitis is lymph gland adenitis of the intraparotid and/or periparotid lymph nodes.

Acute Postoperative Parotitis

Postoperative parotitis is most often encountered in debilitated patients suffering from dehydration, suppression of salivary secretions, vomiting, and mouth breathing (Lary 1974; Speirs and Mason 1972). A dry mouth is a precipitating factor. The inflammation starts in the ducts and by means of periductal infiltration penetrates the glandular tissue. The causative organisms, in order of frequency, are *Staphylococcus aureus, Staphylococcus pyogenes, Streptococcus viridans,* and *Pneumococcus.* The incidence of the infection ranges from about 0.004% to 0.74% in patients that have had major surgical procedures. The infection occurs at any age, but the majority of patients are in the third, fourth, or fifth decade of life. Postoperative parotitis occurs bilaterally in about 20% of cases. The first symptoms manifest between the second and the twentieth postoperative days, most often between the second and fifth days.

The symptoms are caused by acute inflammation and are manifested by swelling in front of the ear lobe spreading to the entire gland during the evolution of the disease. The onset is rapid and accompanied by severe pain and tenderness over the gland. In addition to swelling, the skin becomes red, and in severe cases, the edema may involve the cheek, periorbital region, and neck. The patient may have difficulty opening the mouth. The temperature rises from 102° to 104° F and is accompanied by headache, malaise, and leukocytosis. The opening of Stensen's duct is swollen and red, and purulent material exits from the orifice when gentle pressure is applied along the duct toward the orifice. The history usually reveals a recent operation, extensive trauma, or a prolonged illness. The incidence of the disease has declined in recent years because of improved anesthesia, shortened operative time, advanced surgical technique, informed management of electrolyte and fluid balance, wider use of blood transfusions, improved oral care, and antibiotic control of systemic and local infections.

Chronic Recurrent Parotid Sialadenitis

This is usually a disease of adults but may occur at any age. Predisposing factors are strictures and stones within the ducts (Eisenbud and Cranin 1963; Travis and Hecht 1977; Blatt 1966; Keenan, Beahrs, and Devine 1958; Hemenway and English 1971; Bigler 1946). The disease is characterized by recurrent inflammation over a period of months or years with pain, intermittent swelling, and persistent drainage of pus from Stensen's duct. There may be intermittent acute exacerbations. The recurrent inflammatory process leads to fibrosis and destruction of the glandular and ductal tissues. These various changes cause a multitude of sialographic patterns.

The infectious process may be low grade with no significant clinical findings. In such cases a localized inflammatory mass, simulating a tumor, may develop within the parotid gland.

Sialadenitis of the Submandibular Gland

Submandibular gland sialadenitis, either acute or chronic, is less common than parotid sialadenitis. The greater parotid susceptibility to retrograde infection has been explained by the tendency of parotid secretions to have less bacteriostatic activity (Spratt 1961) and a slower flow rate at rest. In submandibular sialadenitis there is a high incidence of associated sialolithiasis, which is an important factor in the etiology of submandibular sialadenitis (Rauch 1959a). The symptoms are characterized by submandibular pain, swelling, and localized tenderness. In chronic sialadenitis, a mass may be palpable in the submandibular area and may mimic a tumor mass. Lymphadenitis in submandibular lymph nodes adjacent to the gland often cannot be differentiated from chronic submandibular sialadenitis or a submandibular tumor. In these instances, conventional sialography with tomography or CT sialography may provide the answer.

Specific Infections

The salivary glands are seldom involved in specific inflammatory disorders such as tuberculosis, cat-scratch fever, syphilis, actinomycosis, or toxoplasmosis (Rauch 1959a; Rauch 1959b; Hopkins 1973; Allen-Mersh and Florsyth 1958; Sazama 1965; Patey and Thackray 1954). These granulomatous infections usually appear clinically as mass lesions. They arise from intra- and periparotid lymph nodes or in lymph nodes in juxtaposition to the submandibular gland. Sialography combined with conventional tomography or CT can locate these lesions and determine the size. A final diagnosis, however, is established by bacteriologic and histologic examination after the mass has been excised.

Tuberculosis of the Salivary Glands

(Fig. 3.43)
According to Anthony and Fisher, 70% of cases of tuberculosis of the salivary glands occur in the parotid, 27% occur in the submandibular gland, and 3% are in the sublingual gland (Allen-Mersh and Florsyth 1958; Patey and Thackray 1954). Tuberculosis may appear in a disseminated-infiltrative form or a circumscribed nodular form. The infiltrative form, which occurs in two-thirds of cases, is characterized by a painless induration without fever and no significant swelling. No pus exudes from the duct orifice. The sialographic features are nonspecific and manifest inflammatory changes as seen in bacterial sialadenitis. In the nodular form, swelling is encountered occasionally with palpation of a mass. This form is caused by tubercle bacteria that probably enter from the oral and/or nasal cavity and are transmitted to the salivary gland via the lymphatic system.

Syphilis

Syphilis has a distribution in the salivary glands similar to that reported for tuberculosis (Alpern 1935) (Rauch 1959a; Rauch 1959b). An infiltrative and nodular form affects the salivary glands. A painless swelling or a palpable mass usually is encountered.

Actinomycosis

This fungus disease (Hopkins 1973; Sazama 1965) usually invades the salivary glands from neighboring structures. The submandibular gland is more frequently involved. The disease appears clinically in acute or chronic form. The chronic form is characterized by induration of the overlying skin with a slight painful sensation.

Toxoplasmosis and Cat-Scratch Fever

(Fig. 3.46)

These entities may involve the salivary glands (Rauch 1959a). Enlarged lymph nodes are one of the manifestations of salivary gland involvement.

Parotid Gland Sarcoidosis

(Fig. 3.44)

Sarcoidosis is characterized by noncaseating granulomas involving multiple organ systems (Som, Shugar, and Biller 1981; Batsakis 1979; Greenberg et al. 1964). Clinically detectable parotid gland involvement occurs in 10% to 30% of patients with the systemic disease (Batsakis 1979). On occasion, it may be the first manifestation of sarcoidosis. Bilateral parotid involvement has been reported in 83% of cases, even though one side may be affected more than the other (Greenburg et al. 1964). Most of the cases do not need treatment and regress spontaneously. In some patients, parotid gland enlargement is accompanied by uveitis and facial paralysis. The combination of these findings is known as Heerfordt's syndrome (Rankow and Polayes 1976; Miglets, Viall, and Kataria 1977). The following patterns of radiographic abnormalities either demonstrated by conventional sialography with tomography and/or CT have been observed:

1. Diffuse enlargement of the parotid glands with no distinct mass lesion identified.
2. Multiple small nodular densities distributed throughout the gland; the size of these nodules vary so that filling defects in the parenchyma or displacement of smaller ducts are seen.
3. Solitary parotid mass.

The following disease entities must be differentiated from sarcoidosis of the salivary glands: (1) tuberculosis, (2) atypical microbacterial infections, (3) cat-scratch fever, and (4) actinomycosis and tumors.

Clinically, xerostomia may be encountered and mimic Sjögren's disease. Xerostomia and sarcoid are caused by involvement of the minor salivary glands of the mouth rather than involvement of the major salivary glands.

Postirradiation Sialadenitis

Postirradiation sialadenitis is characterized by acute swelling, tenderness, and pain, which subsides within a few days (Kashima, Kirkham, and Andrews 1965). Xerostomia, gland tenderness, and enlargement all appear within 24 hours. Gland enlargement usually subsides within three days. The clinical manifestations are associated elevation of salivary amylase component of serum and urine.

Radiographic Evaluation of Sialadenitis

Sialodochitis, Sialectasia, and Stricture

(Figs. 3.22–3.33, 3.56, 3.57)
Early inflammatory changes in the parenchyma are characterized by slight dilation of the main ducts, intraglandular branches, and sialectasia (Rubin and Holt 1957; Ollenshaw and Rose 1951; Carter, et al. 1981). Recurrent infection is followed by progressive dilation of the ductal system with irregularity of the lumen. In advanced cases, the main duct and major branches reveal a sausage shape caused by a sequence of dilated and narrowed segments. When the ducts are filled with pus and intraluminal debris, the terminal intraparenchymal branches do not fill, imparting a "pruned tree" appearance to the intraglandular ductal system. The debris and pus can cause intraluminal filling defects simulating stones. Dilatation of tertiary duct branches is referred to as *sialectasia*. Sialectasia within the gland is seen in inflammatory conditions caused by a variety of bacteria. An even distribution of small to medium sized sialectatic cavities throughout the parotid gland is encountered in recurrent parotitis in childhood, recurrent parotitis in women, and in Sjögren's syndrome. In recurrent sialadenitis, mainly of the submandibular gland, the parenchyma shrinks, with consequent decrease in size and sparse ramification of dilated and distorted intraglandular ducts.

Abscess Cavity

(Figs. 3.34–3.39)
A large single abscess or smaller abscesses are other findings encountered in sialadenitis. If the intraglandular inflammatory process penetrates the capsule, periglandular inflammation results. The inflammatory mass may encroach upon the nasopharynx, oropharynx, and hypopharynx and dissect along fascial planes in the neck. Breakdown of inflammatory tissue with perforation through the capsule is followed by an abscess in the periglandular tissue. The abscess will fill with contrast material if connected with the parotid or submandibular duct system.

Inflammatory Mass

(Figs. 3.40–3.47)
Low-grade subclinical infections are manifested as a localized inflammatory mass. Such an inflammatory mass may be located within the gland and may simulate a tumor, especially when there are no clinical signs of inflammation. Lymph node inflammation of various etiology, adjacent to the parotid or submandibular glands, causes marginal filling defects.

CT in Inflammatory Lesions

Inflammatory disease produces a diffuse irregular radiodense lesion in an enlarged salivary gland (Bryan et al. 1982). Inflammatory tissue within a salivary gland may be localized and mimic a mass lesion. Inflammatory tissue that involves a gland diffusely may mimic a malignant neoplasm on CT. The clinical findings, in conjunction with conventional sialography, are usually conclusive in determining the underlying etiology of the salivary gland abnormality. If sialectasia and inflammatory tissue are present within the gland, there may be high- and low-density images on the CT scan within an enlarged gland. Stones are easily demonstrated by CT. The sensitivity in detecting stones is slightly greater with CT when compared with conventional radiography. Duct changes secondary to strictures and dilatations are usually not seen by CT, however. Enlarged lymph nodes extrinsic to the salivary gland can easily be shown by CT. This is particularly relevant in the submandibular region, where lymph node disease is seen as an extrinsic mass in juxtaposition to the submandibular gland. Enlarged lymph nodes within the parotid gland, however, are difficult to differentiate from primary neoplasm as these nodes produce within the parenchyma discrete high-density lesions that mimic tumors. Such well-defined enlarged lymph nodes most frequently are caused by granulomatous infections, including tuberculosis, cat-scratch fever, toxoplasmosis, and sarcoid.

CT is of particular value in demonstrating abscesses within the intra- and extraglandular soft-tissue structures. A pathognomonic finding is a low-density area surrounded by an enhancing rim. The location of an abscess, as outlined by CT, provides the surgeon undertaking a drainage procedure with useful information. The extent of inflammatory tissue in fascial planes of the neck (masticator, parapharyngeal, and retropharyngeal spaces) can be accurately depicted by CT. The success of antibiotic therapy, with change in size of the inflammatory process, is readily monitored by CT.

Therapy

(Figs. 3.48–3.57)

Therapeutic procedures play a relatively minor role in the practice of sialography. Nevertheless, the removal of calculi near the duct orifice may sometimes be accomplished by certain maneuvers (figs. 3.48, 3.49). The treatment varies with the duration and severity of symptoms and the number and location of calculi. Mild, infrequent episodes require conservative management with removal of the offending stone if it is in an accessible location. Sometimes a small surgical nick at the duct orifice (figs. 1.24, 3.50, 3.51), using a number 11 pointed surgical blade or a tiny scissors, will suffice. Large stones or those further back in the duct may sometimes be removed or partly removed using a Dormia wire basket (figs. 3.52–3.54), 4-French size, identical to those used for removal of ureteral calculi. The procedure is carried out under fluoroscopic monitoring. Contrast material may be injected into the duct to visualize the calculus if necessary. The duct orifice may be enlarged by dilators or by making a small nick in the wall of the duct orifice. The basket instrument should then be introduced to a point beyond the calculus. The catheter should then be partially withdrawn, allowing the basket to open within the duct, engaging the stone. The basket, stone, and catheter are then withdrawn together. Stones located in a far posterior position, near the junction of the duct and the gland, cannot be removed by this method since the device cannot be advanced beyond the stone to engage it by the basket. It is not always possible to remove large stones by this method, despite an advantageous location, and complications may ensue (fig. 3.55).

Strictures may be easily dilated by various instruments such as probes, dilators, closed-end cannulas (figs. 1.2, 1.3, 1.11B, 3.56, 3.57, 3.66), or catheters or coaxial catheters (fig. 3.56) of various sizes.

Trauma and Surgical Changes

The submandibular glands are well protected from external trauma. On the other hand, the parotid gland and duct are exposed to both penetrating injuries and blunt trauma. Conventional sialography may be helpful in demonstrating the precise nature of the injury (Yune and Klatte 1972). The most common causes of penetrating injuries are automobile accidents with shattering of windshield glass and knife wounds (Joffe 1967); these injuries often are associated with damage to facial nerve branches. Laceration of a main duct or large branch duct may lead to scarring and duct stricture or occlusion or to a communicating saliva-filled cavity (sialocele) within the gland or in the surrounding tissues (fig. 3.58). The sialocele may be associated with an internal or external fistula.

Direct blunt trauma may result in a hematoma of the parotid gland (fig. 3.59A). This may calcify (fig. 3.59B). Bleeding into a salivary gland as a result of treatment with anticoagulants has also been reported by DeCastro, Hall, and Glasser 1970.

Surgical entry of salivary ducts may occur intentionally or unintentionally, so that fistulas often are iatrogenic (Ananthakrishnan and Parkash 1982). If a fistula results, it may drain internally into the mouth (figs. 3.60, 3.63A) or externally (figs. 3.64, 3.65). Fistulas may occur as a complication of calculi or infection in the salivary gland (fig. 3.60, 3.61), in association with tumor (fig. 3.64), or from undetermined causes (fig. 3.62) (Mason and Chisholm 1975).

The most common injury to the submandibular duct is postsurgical scarring in the floor of the mouth with occlusion of the duct orifice, preventing successful cannulation. If a fistula is present, it may be cannulated directly (fig. 3.63A,B). If the anatomic duct orifice is patent, a long cannula may be inserted into the duct beyond the fistula (fig.

1.14C). Demonstrable postsurgical changes include ligation of the submandibular duct and removal of the superficial portion of the parotid gland (figs. 2.12C,D).

Recurrent infection may develop in the residual ligated submandibular duct following the standard surgical procedure for removal of the submandibular gland for calculous disease. Calculi may be retained (fig. 3.63B,C). Complete surgical removal of these retained structures may be required. Bacteria may enter the ligated duct from the mouth and establish infection because of the absence of salivary flow to cleanse the duct.

It is possible for the parotid papilla or adjacent portion of the duct to be traumatized by being nipped between loose-fitting dentures and the alveolar ridge or by an adjacent sharp tooth or protecting clasp, or it may be inadvertently bitten (Wakeley 1948; Hutchinson 1954; Rose 1954; Furstenberg and Blatt 1958; Blatt 1964; Banks 1968; DeCastro, Hall, and Glasser 1970; Mason and Chisholm 1975; Wilson, Eavey, and Lang 1980) (figs. 3.66, 3.67). The papilla is particularly vulnerable to being traumatized by chewing during eruption of new teeth, following installation of new dental prostheses, or following dental extraction (Ollerenshaw and Rose 1957).

CASES

Two stones in the right submandibular duct with sialadenitis

This 71-year-old man noted swelling of the right submandibular area exacerbated with meals. A similar episode occurred four years ago when he passed a 2-cm-long calculus. Examination revealed a tender and terse right submandibular gland. Under local anesthesia, the duct was opened and a stone 0.75 cm long was removed.

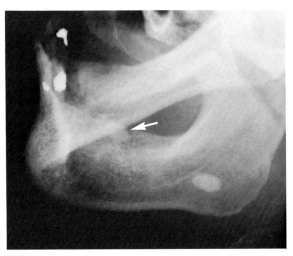

Figure 3.1B

Oblique view of the mandible reveals an oval stone over the mandible near the angle. A second stone is noted anteriorly overlying the alveolar portion of the mandible (*arrow*).

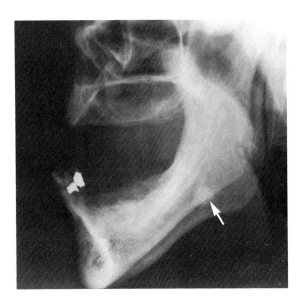

Figure 3.1A

Lateral view of the mandible reveals an opaque stone at the inferior margin of the body of the mandible (*arrow*). A stone anteriorly near the orifice is not demonstrated on this projection.

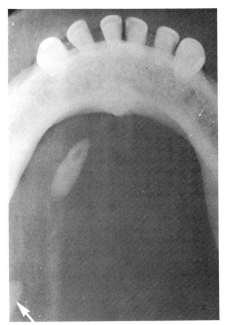

Figure 3.1C

Occlusal view shows the elliptical anterior stone. A second more proximal stone is incompletely demonstrated on this occlusal projection (*arrow*).

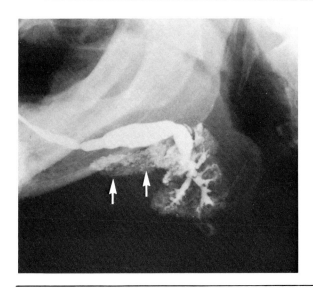

Figure 3.1D

Submandibular sialogram shows dilatation of the main duct and major branches within the submandibular gland. The stones are obscured by the contrast material. Note accessory glandular tissue anteriorly below main duct (*arrows*).

Right submandibular duct stone

A 34-year-old man complained six or seven times over the past 18 months of recurrent right submandibular swelling with eating. Physical examination revealed a palpable stone near the hilum of the submandibular gland. He underwent excision of the right submandibular gland and the duct calculus.

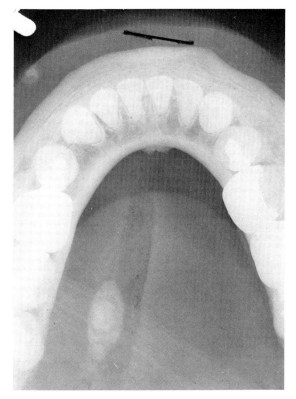

Figure 3.2B

Occlusal view shows an oval stone within the proximal portion of the right submandibular duct.

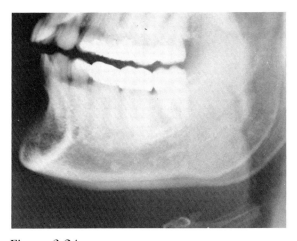

Figure 3.2A

Lateral view of the mandible reveals no stone.

Three faceted stones in the right submandibular duct

A 46-year-old man had onset of right submandibular swelling and pain about two months ago. He had a similar problem 15 years ago with spontaneous remission. He underwent excision of the right submandibular gland and duct, including stones. Pathologic examination revealed chronic sialadenitis with duct ectasia.

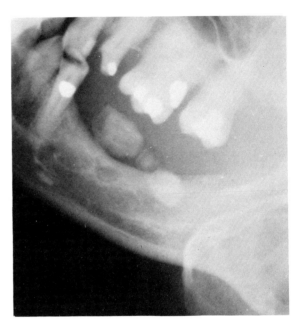

Figure 3.3

Oblique view of the mandible demonstrates three faceted calculi in the proximal submandibular duct.

Right submandibular stone in the hilum of the gland

A 32-year-old man complained of persistent pain and swelling of the right submandibular gland of several months' duration. Calculus was palpable through the mouth. He underwent excision of the gland and duct, including stone.

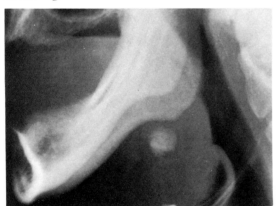

Figure 3.4A

Round, slightly irregular stone below the angle of the mandible.

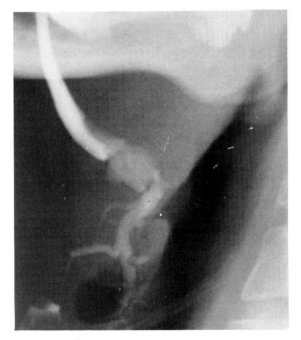

Figure 3.4B

Submandibular sialogram with water-soluble contrast material shows slight dilatation of the duct with coating of the stone in the proximal duct. There is slight dilatation of the duct system proximal to the stone.

Large stone in the hilum of the right submandibular gland

This 31-year-old man had intermittent swelling and pain in the right submandibular area over a period of six to seven years. He never had any signs of infection. He passed numerous stones from the right submandibular duct in the past seven years. He noted increasing pressure and swelling associated with meals, and especially with spicy foods. He underwent excision of the right submandibular gland and duct. A small abscess cavity, not demonstrated on the sialogram, was noted proximal to the stone.

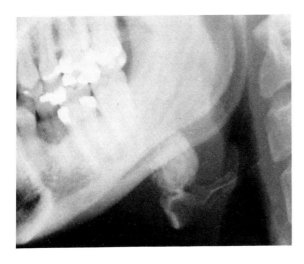

Figure 3.5A

Large mottled laminated irregular stone below the body of the mandible.

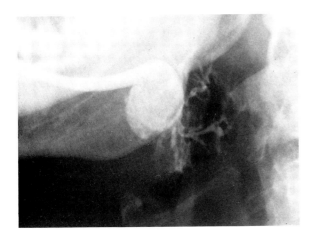

Figure 3.5B

Right submandibular sialogram reveals the stone in the hilum of the gland. Contrast material surrounds the stone and fills slightly dilated ducts within the gland.

Stone in the right submandibular duct at the hilum of the gland

A 40-year-old man noted recurrent right submandibular swelling about one year ago. In the past three months, he has had several painful episodes and passed stones. He underwent a right submandibular gland excision. Pathologic examination revealed chronic sialadenitis with marked fibrosis.

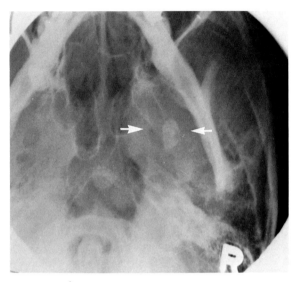

Figure 3.6B

Base view shows the stone in the region of the hilum of the submandibular gland medial to the right mandible (*arrows*).

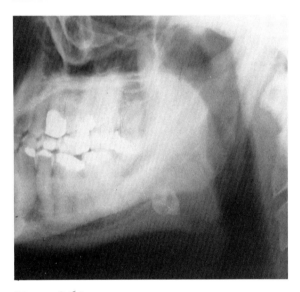

Figure 3.6A

Lateral view of the mandible reveals a partially opaque stone below the angle of the mandible.

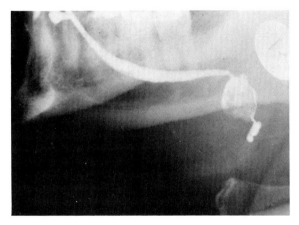

Figure 3.6C

Right submandibular sialogram shows coating of the stone and a small amount of contrast material within a small, dilated, deformed duct within the gland. The duct system of the gland is not completely visualized.

Stones in the hilum of the right submandibular gland with sialodochiectasis and demonstration of a small submandibular gland

A 26-year-old man with a one-year history of repeated episodes of right submandibular sialadenitis. There was no pain or tenderness. Examination revealed a mass, 1 cm in diameter, in the right submandibular gland, indicating chronic sialadenitis with fibrosis.

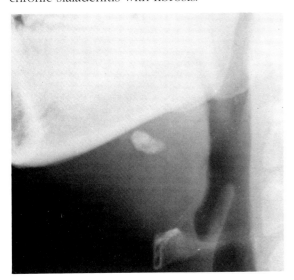

Figure 3.7A

Calculus below the body of the right mandible within the hilum of the gland.

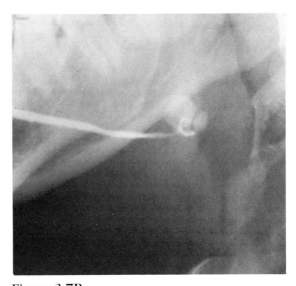

Figure 3.7B

Right submandibular sialogram reveals a normal duct. There is a hemispherical filling defect in the duct at the junction with the stones.

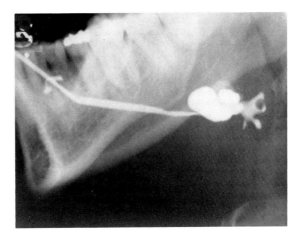

Figure 3.7C

Additional contrast material shows slight narrowing of the main duct in the region of the hilum of the gland along with marked dilatation of duct structures within a small shrunken gland.

Large stone in the right submandibular gland

Patient complained of recurrent swelling with pain and a mass in the right submandibular gland.

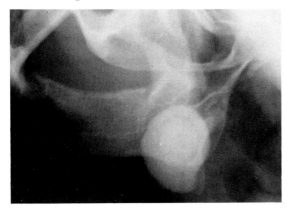

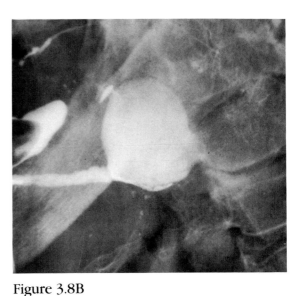

Figure 3.8A

Large, homogeneous, sharply marginated stone over the angle of the mandible.

Figure 3.8B

Right submandibular sialogram demonstrates a normal Wharton's duct with some contrast material at the inferior margin of stone.

Stones at the orifice of the right submandibular duct causing obstruction

This 48-year-old woman had intermittent pain and swelling in the right submandibular gland region.

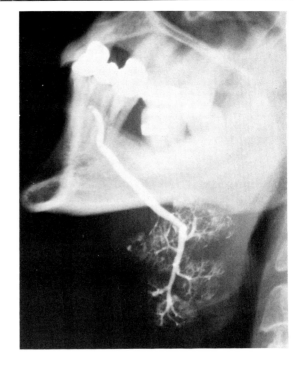

Figure 3.9A

Lateral postevacuation view of a submandibular sialogram reveals obstruction in the outflow of contrast material at orifice.

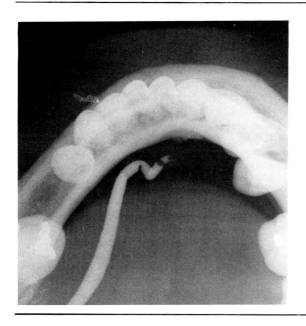

Figure 3.9B

Occlusal view shows two defects in the terminal portion of the duct, secondary to two stones. These stones cause complete obstruction.

Nonopaque stone at the duct orifice causing obstruction

A 20-year-old man with a history of swelling in the left submandibular gland of several months' duration; he passed a stone spontaneously.

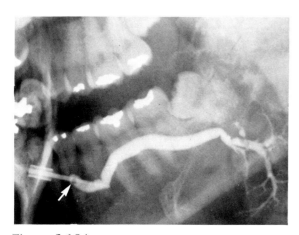

Figure 3.10A

Left submandibular sialogram reveals slight dilatation of the main duct. The stone is adjacent to the inserted cannula (*arrow*).

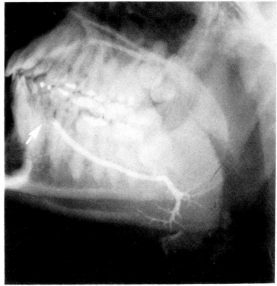

Figure 3.10B

Lateral postevacuation view following removal of cannula reveals a filling defect in the contrast column at the orifice secondary to nonopaque stone. There is obstruction of the duct at the orifice (*arrow*).

Small stone in the hilum of the right submandibular gland

A 53-year-old man with recurrent pain and swelling in the region of the right sub-mandibular gland.

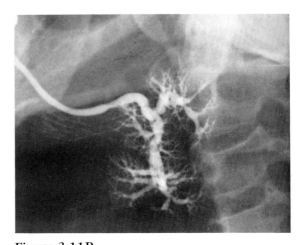

Figure 3.11B

Right submandibular sialogram reveals slight dilatation of the major ducts within the gland. The hilar stone is obscured by the contrast material.

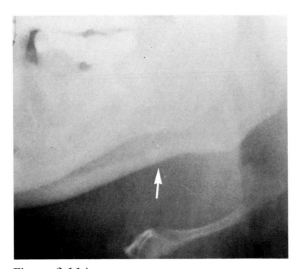

Figure 3.11A

Lateral view of the mandible demonstrates a small opaque stone overlying the inferior cortex of the right mandible (*arrow*).

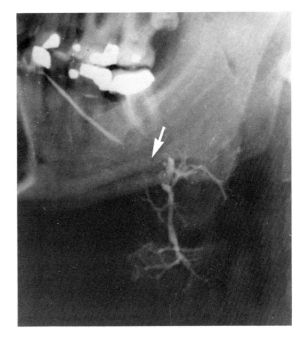

Figure 3.11C

Lateral postevacuation film reveals a filling defect in the duct at the hilum of the gland, causing obstruction (*arrow*). Note some residual contrast material in the mid- and distal portion of the normal-appearing duct.

Stone in the proximal portion of the right submandibular duct causing partial obstruction

This 29-year-old man had a two-day history of left submandibular swelling with pain, especially when eating. A stone was palpated in the floor of the mouth.

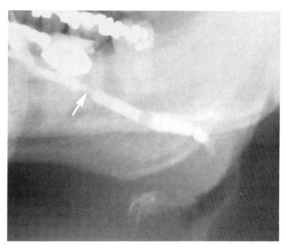

Figure 3.12B

Lateral projection of the submandibular sialogram demonstrates a filling defect in the slightly dilated duct. Note slight stricture in the mid- to distal portion of the duct (*arrow*).

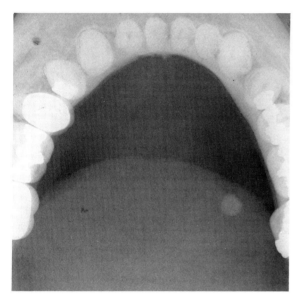

Figure 3.12A

Occlusal view reveals a calculus in the right submandibular duct.

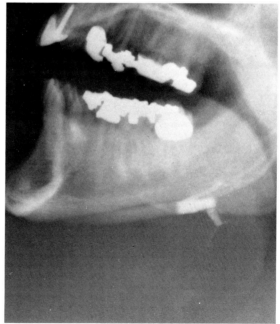

Figure 3.12C

Lateral postevacuation film reveals retained contrast material proximal to the stone, indicative of partial obstruction.

Stone in right submandibular duct

A 45-year-old woman with a one month history of a right submandibular mass with incomplete resolution with antibiotics.

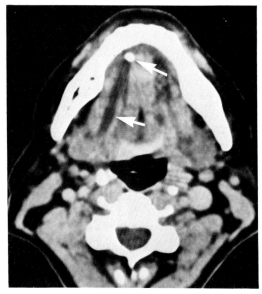

Figure 3.13A

Axial contrast CT scan illustrates an opaque stone at the right submandibular duct orifice (*top arrow*) with a slightly dilated duct indicated by a low density tubular area (*bottom arrow*). The gland is normal.

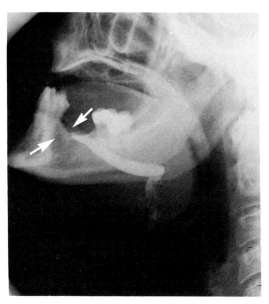

Figure 3.13B

Lateral postevacuation view of the right submandibular sialogram demonstrates a nonopaque stone at the orifice (*arrow*) with dilatation of Wharton's duct.

Calcified lymph node in the submandibular region on the right and a stone at the duct orifice of the left submandibular gland

A 54-year-old woman complained of swelling of the left submandibular gland.

Figure 3.14A

There is an irregular calcific density, secondary to a calcified lymph node, below the right mandible.

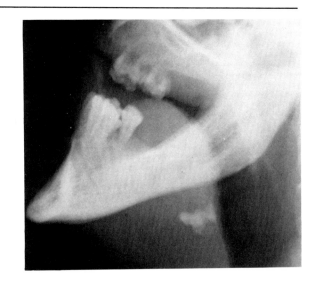

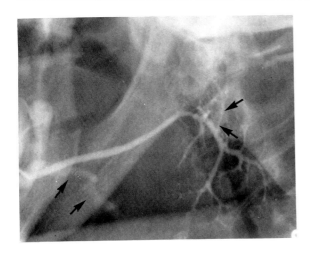

Figure 3.14B

Right submandibular sialogram reveals a normal Wharton's duct, intraglandular branches and gland. The calcified lymph node is superimposed on the gland (*left arrows*). Note retained contrast material in left duct from an obstructing stone at the orifice (*arrows*).

Submandibular stones with a fistula into the oral cavity

This 61-year-old man has had recurrent submandibular swelling and tenderness over a period of 8 to 10 years. These attacks have worsened in the last two to three weeks, lasting for two hours, especially after ingestion of fruit.

During a clinic visit, one stone was removed from the duct measuring $1.7 \times 1 \times 1$ cm in size. The pain disappeared, but the swelling decreased only by about one-third.

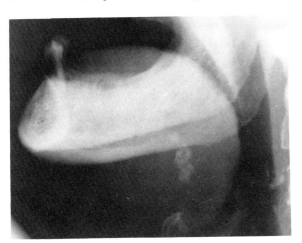

Figure 3.15A

Several irregular, mottled stones in the right submandibular gland at and below the body of the mandible.

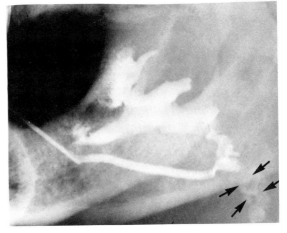

Figure 3.15B

A left submandibular sialogram demonstrates filling of the upper portion of the gland, above the stones, with a fistula that extends into the oral cavity. Note extravasated contrast material in the oral cavity and stones in the submandibular gland below the upper opacified portion (*arrows*).

Two calculi in the midportion of the right parotid duct

This 67-year-old man has a three- to four-year history of right parotid swelling, which has become frequent and constant in the last few months. His discomfort is worse at mealtime.

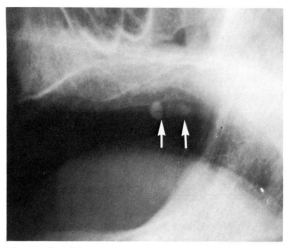

Figure 3.16B

Lateral projection reveals the same stones below the posterior portion of the hard palate (*arrows*).

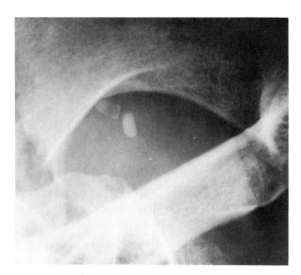

Figure 3.16A

Oblique view of the mandible reveals two oval, sharply marginated calculi.

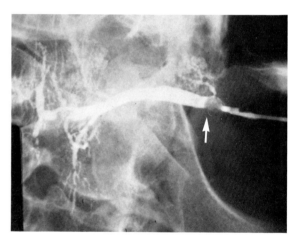

Figure 3.16C

Right parotid sialogram demonstrates a filling defect in the midportion of the parotid duct secondary to the stones (*arrow*). There is slight dilatation of the main duct, proximal to the stones and branches.

Opaque stone in the proximal portion of the right parotid duct

This 48-year-old man noted recurrent swelling at the angle of the right mandible associated with eating and slight pain.

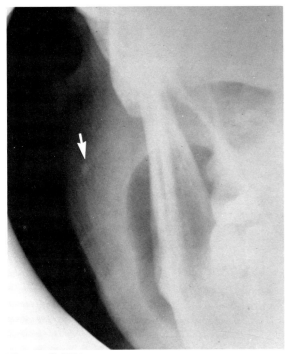

Figure 3.17A

AP puffed-cheek view demonstrates a calculus in the soft tissues of the right cheek (*arrow*).

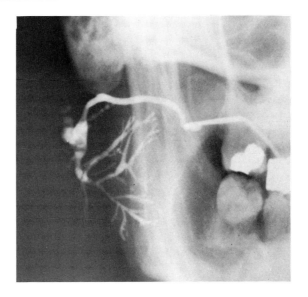

Figure 3.17B

Right parotid sialogram (AP view) demonstrates a filling defect in the proximal portion of the duct, which is slightly dilated.

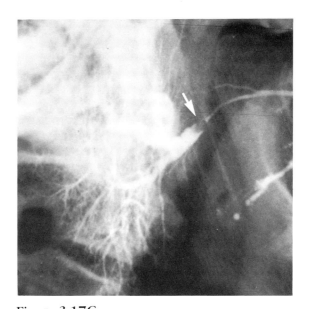

Figure 3.17C

Lateral view of the parotid sialogram reveals an oval filling defect from the described stone (*arrow*) with associated slight dilatation of the ducts proximal to the stone.

Opaque stone in the right parotid duct causing obstruction

This 24-year-old woman had occasional intermittent swelling and pain in the right parotid region with an acute onset of swelling in the right parotid gland for two days before admission.

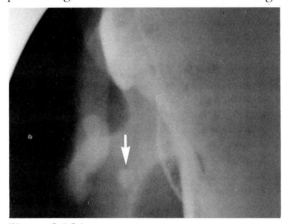

Figure 3.18A

AP puffed-cheek view demonstrates a calculus in the soft tissue structures (*arrow*).

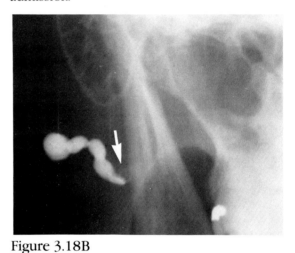

Figure 3.18B

AP postevacuation film shows the same stone causing obstruction in the outflow of contrast material (*arrow*).

Multiple left parotid stones with chronic left parotitis

This 48-year-old woman complained of left-sided, intermittent parotitis occurring three to five times yearly. In the last four or five months she had three episodes associated with pain and swelling. She underwent a superficial parotidectomy. The pathologic diagnosis was chronic sialadenitis. At surgery, there was a small abscess cavity in the inferior portion of the parotid gland.

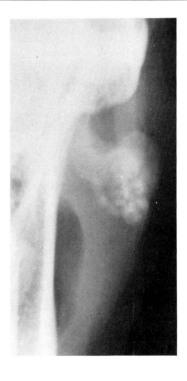

Figure 3.19A

AP puffed-cheek view shows multiple, irregular calculi in the soft tissue structures of the cheek.

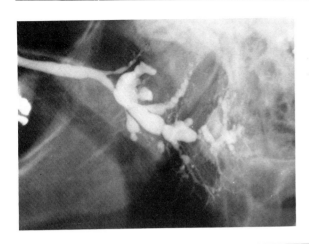

Figure 3.19B

Sialogram shows considerable ectasia of the visualized ducts in the parotid gland. There is also slight dilatation of the main duct. The peripheral branches, within the gland, are poorly visualized. The stones are obscured by the contrast material.

Small sialectatic cavities with stones

This 55-year-old woman complained of pain in the region of the left parotid gland with intermittent swelling after eating. Physical examination revealed a tender, slightly enlarged left parotid gland.

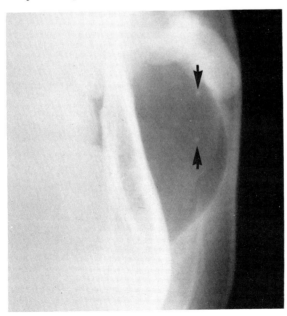

Figure 3.20A

AP puffed-cheek view revealed small calculi in the left parotid gland best seen through the aerated portion of the cheek (*arrows*).

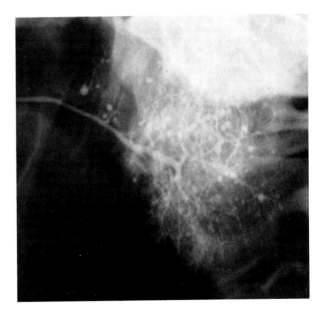

Figure 3.20B

Lateral view of the parotid sialogram shows small, round-to-oval sialectatic cavities throughout the gland.

Multiple bilateral parotid stones with sialectasis

This 55-year-old woman complained of intermittent swelling in the region of both parotid glands.

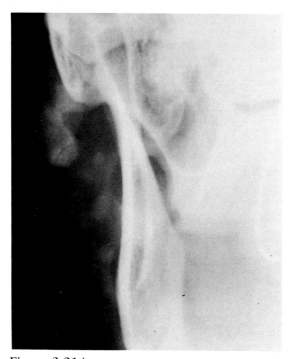

Figure 3.21A

AP view of the right parotid gland demonstrates multiple stones within the gland.

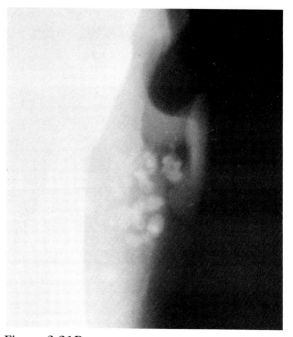

Figure 3.21B

AP view of the left parotid gland also shows multiple, irregular stones in the parotid gland.

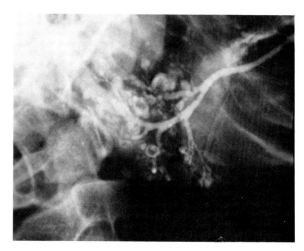

Figure 3.21C

Left parotid sialogram demonstrates slight dilatation of the ducts and sialectatic cavities, which contain stones. These stones cause filling defects within the opacified cavities.

Sialodochiectasis of the proximal main duct and major branches in the hilum of the right parotid gland

This 49-year-old woman complained of a lump in front of her right ear when eating. She had had an infected gland two months previously.

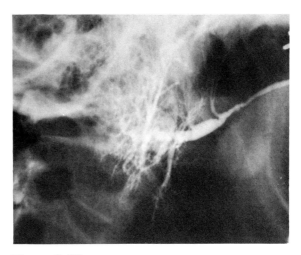

Figure 3.22

Right parotid sialogram shows diffuse, slightly irregular dilatation of the proximal third of the Stensen's duct, along with some dilatation of the major branches in the hilum of the gland.

Sialodochiectasis secondary to stones and infection

This 65-year-old man complained of left lower parotid swelling of two months' duration.

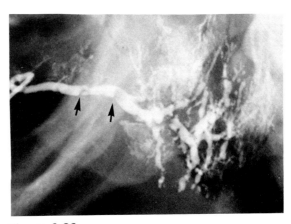

Figure 3.23

Left parotid sialogram reveals diffuse dilatation of the main parotid duct and the intraparotid branches. The ducts are irregular, probably secondary to retained inflammatory exudate. Two oval filling defects in the proximal third of the main duct are secondary to stones (*arrows*).

Stricture with dilatation of the proximal right Stensen's duct and major branches

This 45-year-old woman had swelling in the right parotid gland for about one week. The gland increased in size during eating. She had had two previous episodes of swelling in the parotid region, three and five years ago.

Figure 3.24

There is slight diffuse narrowing of the anterior two thirds of the right parotid duct with an area of dilatation proximal to this stenotic segment. There is slight dilatation of major branches within the gland.

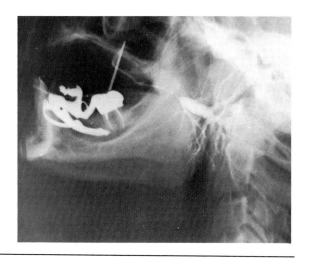

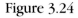

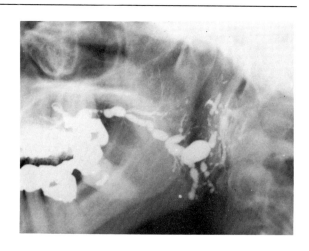

Sialodochiectasis with strictures

This 30-year-old woman had intermittent swelling of the right parotid gland.

Figure 3.25

There is dilatation of the main parotid duct and branches. There are some strictures in between the dilated segments.

Sialodochiectasis with strictures

This 66-year-old woman had pain and swelling in the region of the left parotid.

Figure 3.26

There is dilatation of the main duct and branches within the parotid gland. There are also some areas of narrowing between the dilated segments.

Sialodochiectasis with multiple strictures

This 61-year-old woman had intermittent swelling in the right parotid region for several years. She had no tenderness or enlarged lymph nodes.

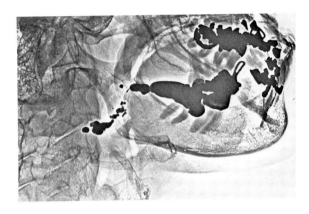

Figure 3.27

Xerosialogram, oblique view, shows marked dilatation of the main duct with strictures between the dilated segments. There is incomplete filling of branches within the gland.

Stricture in the proximal portion of the parotid duct with dilatation of the major intraparotid branches

This 80-year-old man developed a right parotid mass with pain and tenderness of two weeks' duration. Examination revealed a mass, 2 × 3-cm, in the right parotid gland. Biopsy revealed fibroadipose tissue.

Figure 3.28

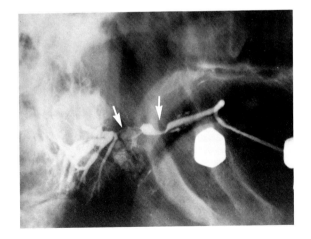

Right parotid sialogram demonstrates a stricture in the proximal portion of the Stensen's duct (*left arrow*) with some dilatation of the major branches within the hilum of the parotid gland. There is a hemispherical defect in the midportion of the parotid duct, which may represent a nonopaque stone (*right arrow*). The mass is not demonstrated within the parotid gland.

Sialodochiectasis with strictures of the right parotid duct

This 29-year-old woman was seen in the emergency ward for swelling and tenderness of both parotid glands, greater on the left, of two weeks' duration. Physical examination revealed swelling and tenderness of the superficial lobes of both parotid glands. She improved considerably on antibiotic therapy but continued to have pain and swelling of both parotids following meals.

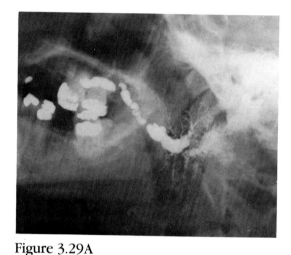

Figure 3.29A

Right parotid sialogram, lateral view, reveals marked dilatation of the main duct and major branches within the hilum of the gland, with multiple strictures.

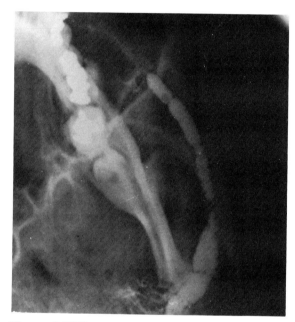

Figure 3.29B

Base view of area shown in figure 3.29A.

Marked sialodochiectasis of Stensen's duct and intraglandular branches

This 62-year-old man complained of recurrent swelling in the region of the right parotid gland.

Figure 3.30

Right parotid sialogram reveals marked dilatation of the main duct and dilatation of all branches within the parotid gland.

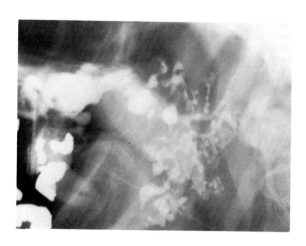

Sialodochiectasis with sialectasis and strictures in the right parotid duct and gland

This 72-year-old woman has a 10-year history of recurrent swelling of the right parotid gland postprandially. Symptoms became more severe in the past year, occurring after every meal. On physical examination, a cystic, soft right parotid gland was palpated. She had a right tympanic neurectomy and ligation of the right Stensen's duct. Because of persistent symptoms, a superficial parotidectomy was carried out two years after the first surgical intervention. Pathologic examination revealed nerve and fibrous tissue fragments.

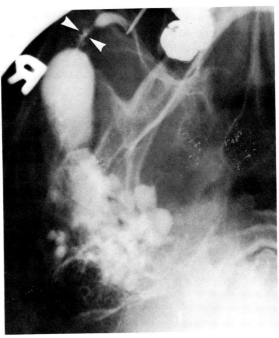

Figure 3.31B

The base view demonstrates marked dilatation of the main duct and branches within the gland. Note stricture in the middle third of Stensen's duct (*arrows*).

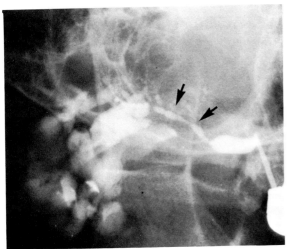

Figure 3.31A

Lateral view of a parotid sialogram reveals marked dilatation of the right parotid duct with a stricture in the middle third of the duct (*arrows*). There is marked sacular dilatation of all branches within the right parotid gland.

Pneumoparotitis of the left parotid gland

This 25-year-old man, a trumpet player, had recurrent pain and swelling of the left parotid duct for a period of 15 months while playing the trumpet. He also had a similar problem with the right parotid gland, but of shorter duration. He also complained of swelling of the left parotid gland following eating.

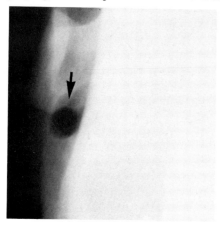

Figure 3.32A

AP view of the right parotid gland reveals air in a dilated parotid duct (*arrow*).

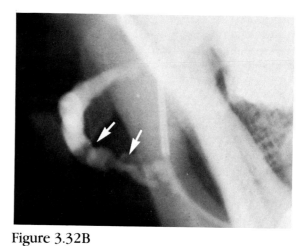

Figure 3.32B

Right parotid sialogram (AP view) reveals dilatation of the main duct with some air proximally (*arrows*).

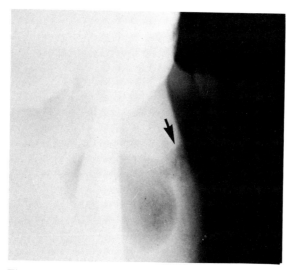

Figure 3.32C

AP view of the left parotid gland reveals air in a dilated duct (*arrow*).

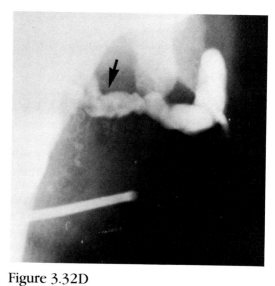

Figure 3.32D

AP view of a left parotid sialogram reveals dilatation of the main duct and some air interspersed in the contrast material (*arrow*).

Dilatation of Wharton's duct and major branches within the left submandibular gland

This 57-year-old man had recurrent swelling in the left submandibular gland region for the past several weeks. This generally occurred following eating, and each episode subsided gradually. On physical examination there was slight to moderate swelling and tenderness in the region of the submandibular gland.

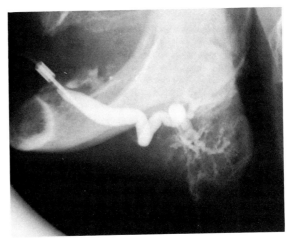

Figure 3.33

There is slight to moderate dilatation of the main left submandibular duct and major branches within the left submandibular gland.

Abscess in the right submandibular gland with stones

This 53-year-old man complained of pain in the right jaw of five days' duration. Surgery was performed and the right submandibular gland and duct were excised. A large abscess and some stones were found within the right submandibular gland.

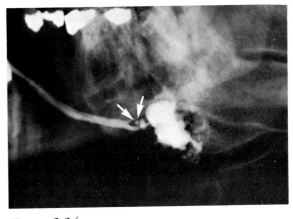

Figure 3.34

Right submandibular sialogram demonstrates an irregular cavity from an abscess in the gland. A filling defect in the Wharton's duct adjacent to the abscess is consistent with stones (*arrows*).

Abscess adjacent to the right submandibular gland

This 26-year-old man noted the onset of a nontender, small nodule in the right submandibular area one month before admission. This persisted unchanged until five days before admission, when it became tender and enlarged. On physical examination, there was a tender right submandibular mass. An incision and drainage of an abscess was carried out.

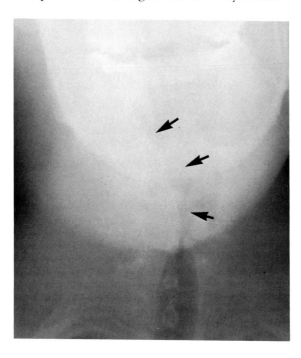

Figure 3.35A

AP view of the neck shows a large mass in the right submandibular area indenting the right oropharynx and hypopharynx (*arrows*).

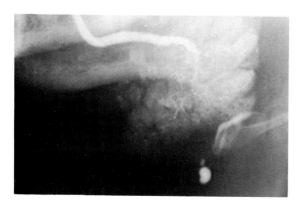

Figure 3.35B

A right submandibular sialogram reveals indentation of the inferior portion of the gland with extravasation of contrast material into an abscess.

Two abscesses in the left parotid gland

This 20-year-old man developed an upper respiratory infection three weeks before the development of the abscess. Prior to admission, he noted an asymptomatic lump, about the size of a peanut, in the left preauricular region. He then developed discomfort over the left parotid area with a diffuse, nonfluctuating swelling. He also had some ear discomfort when opening his mouth, tenderness in the parotid region, and generalized lethargy. He had been treated with antibiotics for the last three weeks as an outpatient and the swelling had decreased slightly. After fluctuance developed, he underwent drainage of a left parotid abscess. Three weeks postoperatively, the parotid gland began to swell slightly more posteriorly than on his first admission. He also had tenderness and pain over the parotid region on movement of the neck. He underwent a second drainage procedure for an abscess that had developed in the posterior inferior portion of the parotid gland.

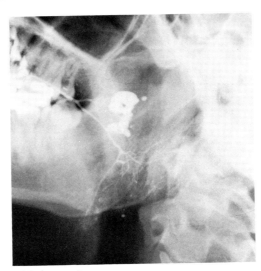

Figure 3.36B

Left parotid sialogram reveals an irregular abscess in the anterior superior portion of the parotid gland.

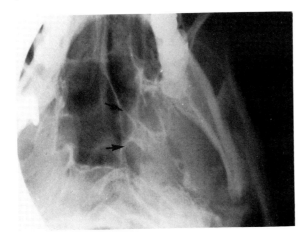

Figure 3.36A

Base view of the skull shows increased density in the left parotid region and parapharyngeal space with slight displacement of the lateral pharyngeal wall medially (*arrows*).

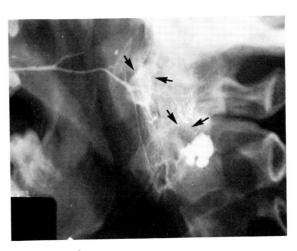

Figure 3.36C

Repeat left parotid sialogram three weeks post-surgery reveals a second abscess in the posterior inferior portion of the gland, with an inflammatory mass causing an ill-defined filling defect (*bottom arrows*). Note residual contrast material in the previously drained abscess cavity in the anterior superior portion of the gland (*arrows*).

Abscesses and inflammatory mass in the left parotid gland

This 66-year-old woman complained of a throbbing, steady pain in the left side of her face along with swelling over the left parotid area. On physical examination the left parotid was tender and swollen but not grossly inflamed. The patient improved with conservative management.

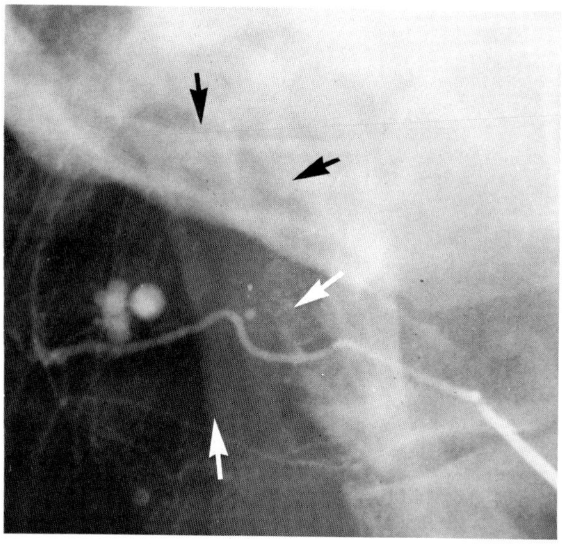

Figure 3.37A

Oblique view of a left parotid sialogram reveals an inflammatory mass and small abscesses in the medial portion of the left parotid gland (*arrows*).

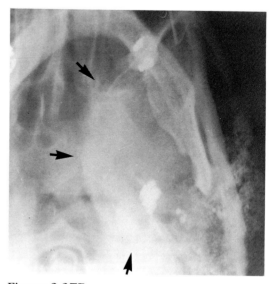

Figure 3.37B

A base view sialogram reveals an inflammatory mass in the parapharyngeal space and deep portion of the parotid (*arrows*). Note abscess cavities within the inflammatory mass.

Inflammatory mass with small abscess cavities

This 61-year-old man noted a painless mass in the right parotid region.

Figure 3.38A

A right parotid sialogram reveals a small collection of contrast material in the mid to inferior portion of the parotid gland (*top left arrow*). Note two smaller collections posteriorly within the gland (*bottom arrows*).

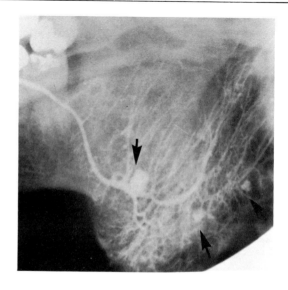

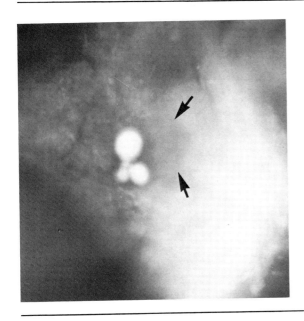

Figure 3.38B

Lateral tomographic section reveals a filling defect in the left parotid gland secondary to the inflammatory mass (*arrows*). There are some irregularly shaped abscesses within the anterior aspect of the inflammatory mass.

Infected left branchial cleft cyst

This 55-year-old man noted the onset of recurrent swelling of the left parotid gland associated with slight tenderness. Superficial parotidectomy was carried out, and an infected branchial cleft cyst was excised. The mass measured 3 × 2 cm, appeared cystic, and contained 10 cc of purulent material. The mass was adherent to the anterior portion of the sternocleidomastoid muscle.

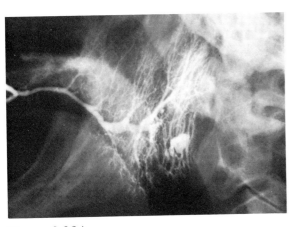

Figure 3.39A

A left parotid sialogram reveals a collection of contrast material within the posterior inferior portion of the gland with slight stretching of ducts.

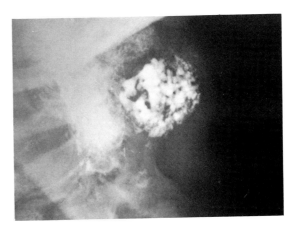

Figure 3.39B

Parenchymal phase of the left parotid sialogram shows filling of a round, sharply defined branchial cleft cyst that causes indentation of the posterior border of the parotid gland.

Inflammatory mass in the posterior left submandibular gland

This 54-year-old woman had a two-month history of an enlarging nontender mass in the left submandibular triangle. On physical examination a nonpulsatile mass, 2 × 3 cm, was palpated in the left upper neck. An excision of the mass and left submandibular gland was carried out. The pathologic report was chronic sialadenitis with marked fibrosis.

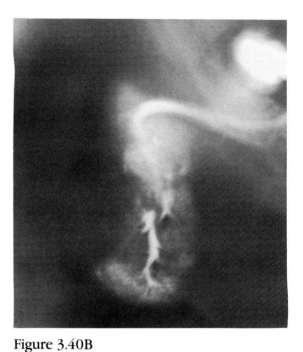

Figure 3.40B

A lateral tomographic section reveals a sharply marginated indentation of the posterior glandular tissue. The visualized ducts appear normal.

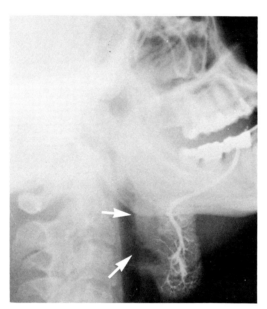

Figure 3.40A

Lateral submandibular sialogram reveals poor definition of the posterior border of the gland with suggestion of a filling defect (*arrows*).

Inflammatory mass in the left parotid gland

This 21-year-old man had a three- to four-month history of a painless mass in the anterior superior portion of the left parotid gland. He had no other symptoms. A left superficial parotidectomy was performed with excision of a tumorlike mass in the superficial lobe that measured 2 × 2 × 2 cm in greatest diameter. Part of the mass was cystic on gross examination. Pathologic examination revealed chronic sialadenitis, duct ectasia, myoepithelial proliferation, and nodular lymphoid infiltration.

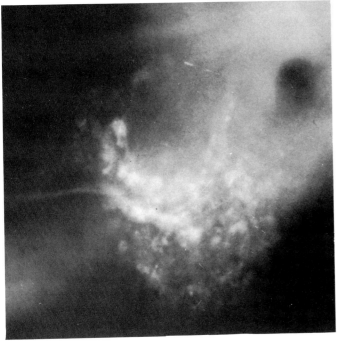

Figure 3.41

Lateral tomogram performed after a left parotid sialogram reveals a sharply defined, oval mass in the anterior superior portion of the parotid gland.

Inflammatory mass in a lymph node of the left parotid gland

This 33-year-old woman had a five-month history of a slowly enlarging left parotid mass, which caused some intermittent pain. A left parotidectomy was performed and revealed a mass in the tail of the parotid gland. Pathologic examination revealed chronic sialadenitis with focal duct ectasia within a parotid lymph node.

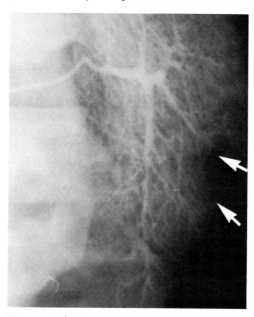

Figure 3.42A

Oblique view of a left parotid sialogram reveals an ill-defined defect in the posterior inferior portion of the parotid gland (*arrows*).

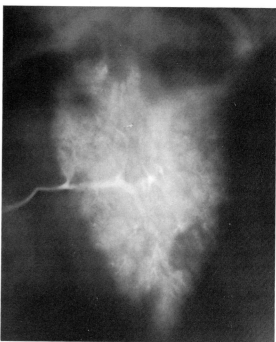

Figure 3.42B

Lateral tomogram in the parenchymal phase reveals a sharply marginated, oval filling defect in the posterior inferior portion of the left parotid gland.

Tuberculosis of a lymph node in the right submandibular area indenting the submandibular gland

This 49-year-old woman noted the onset of right submandibular swelling. She had no fever, chills, or night sweats; there was no pain or tenderness. Biopsy of the node revealed caseating granulomas in a submandibular lymph node.

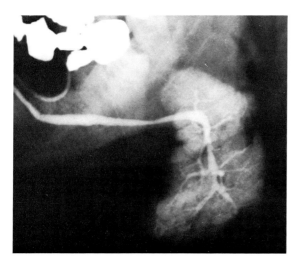

Figure 3.43A

Right submandibular sialogram reveals indentation of the gland anteriorly.

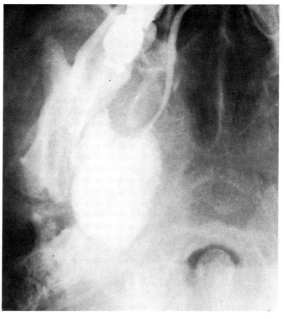

Figure 3.43B

A basal view of the submandibular gland reveals a sharply marginated defect in the anterior portion of the gland with slight medial displacement of the proximal half of the right submandibular duct.

Sarcoid of the right parotid gland

This 60-year-old man had a history of a mass in the right parotid region. On examination there was some fullness of the right parotid in the upper half posteriorly. He underwent a superficial parotidectomy, and the pathologic examination revealed chronic inflammation with numerous noncaseating granulomas consistent with sarcoidosis.

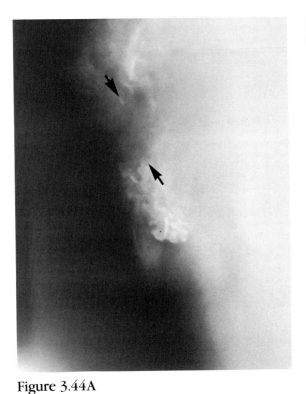

Figure 3.44A

AP tomographic section of the parotid gland in the parenchymal phase reveals an oval filling defect in the superficial midportion of the right parotid gland (*arrows*).

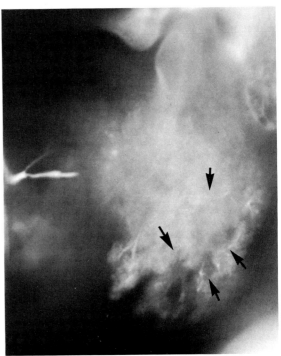

Figure 3.44B

Lateral tomographic sections suggest several filling defects in the posterior inferior portion of the parotid gland (*arrows*).

Wharthin's tumor in a patient with sialadenitis of the parotid gland

This 66-year-old man has had enlargement of the parotid gland with pain postprandially for many years. In the last three months he noted an increase in the size of the parotid gland secondary to an enlarging mass. There was no facial weakness. Patient underwent a superficial left parotidectomy, and a papillary cyst-adenoma lymphomatosum (Warthin's tumor) was removed from the tail of the left parotid gland. The mass measured $5 \times 4 \times 2$ cm in greatest diameter.

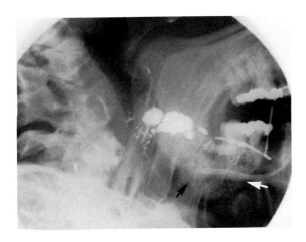

Figure 3.47A

Left parotid sialogram reveals strictures and dilatation of the main duct and branches within the hilum of the gland. Note aberrant glandular tissue along the upper portion of the main parotid duct (*arrows*).

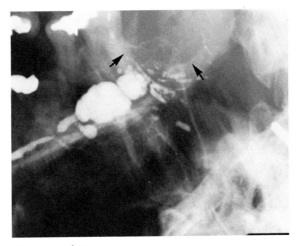

Figure 3.47B

The dilatation and stricture of the duct and major branches are seen again. A posterior and superior mass is indicated by stretching and displacement of intraglandular ducts (*arrows*).

Right submandibular sialogram evacuation phase

C   = calculus
Can= cannula
SD = submandibular duct
SG = submandibular gland

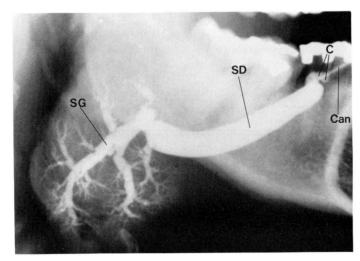

Figure 3.48A

Lateral view; contrast material was Sinografin. The main duct is somewhat larger than average. Mild sialectasia is seen in the intraglandular branches. One or two tiny, ill-defined lucent shadows are present in the duct near the orifice, bypassed by the cannula.

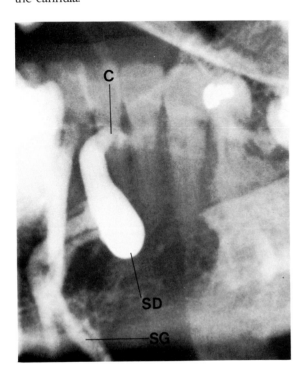

Figure 3.48B

Anterior posterior view, evacuation phase; it was noted fluoroscopically and on film that the contrast material did not evacuate from the gland. A small, ill-defined lucent calculus can be seen impacted at the duct orifice; on direct inspection, the stone was discernible at the orifice. Dilation was accomplished with a metal dilator, and the stone escaped from the duct with copious flow of saliva upon removal of the cannula.

The patient is a 41-year-old woman with enlargement of the right submandibular salivary gland, particularly with eating. The stone that was removed was approximately 1.5 mm in diameter.

Right parotid sialogram, evacuation phase and stone extraction

C = calculus
PD = parotid duct
S   = stricture

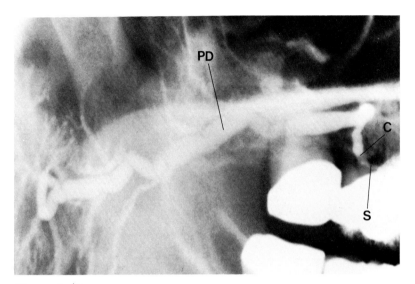

Figure 3.49

A small stone is impacted at the duct orifice preventing evacuation of the contrast material. Cannulation of the parotid duct at another institution had been unsuccessful. Inspection at this time revealed no saliva coming from the right parotid duct orifice, but a tiny opening was identified and was dilated with probes and a 27-gauge cannula was put in place. Injection of Sinografin demonstrates moderately advanced sialectasia. Upon withdrawal of the cannula, evacuation did not occur, and direct inspection of the parotid duct orifice revealed a tiny 2-mm calculus impacted at the duct orifice. This was easily teased out with two tongue blades. Saliva then flowed fairly freely from the duct orifice. A short stricture is present just posterior to the duct orifice; this was subsequently dilated with probes.

The patient was a 55-year-old woman with a history of several bouts of swelling of the right side of the face.

Right submandibular sialogram and stone extraction

C   = calculus
Can = cannula
SD = submand-
ibular duct

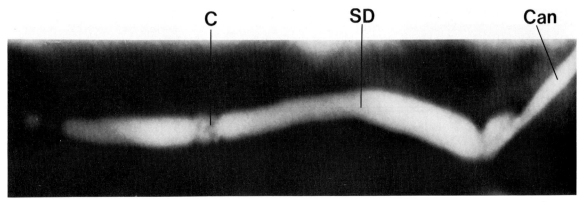

Figure 3.50

Under fluoroscopy, a tiny calculus was visible moving back and forth in the duct system. This was maneuvered far anteriorly and, by making a small nick in the duct orifice, the stone readily popped out. Contrast material was Ethiodol.

The patient was a 60-year-old woman with a history of swelling in the submandibular region on the right side with eating.

Left submandibular sialogram and stone extraction

C   = calculus
Can= cannula
SD = submand-
ibular duct
SG = submand-
ibular gland

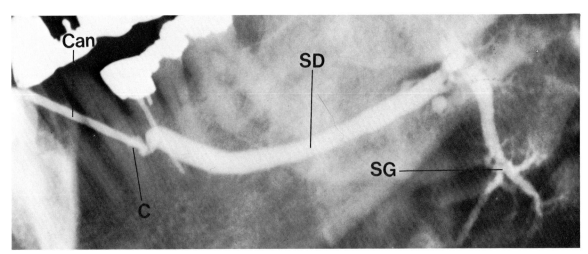

Figure 3.51

Lateral view; a tiny calculus is visible near the tip of the cannula. A tiny nick was made at the duct orifice and the tiny stone was delivered into the mouth without difficulty. The contrast material was Renografin-76.

Left submandibular sialogram and stone extraction

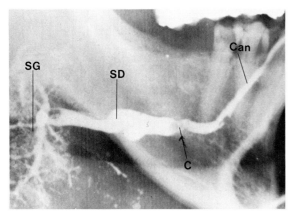

Figure 3.52A

Lateral view of a calculus in the mid-anterior portion of the main salivary duct, which is moderately dilated.

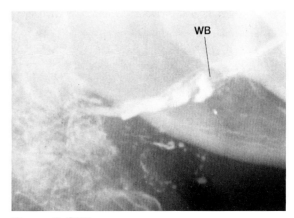

Figure 3.52B

A slit has been made in the margin of the salivary duct orifice under local anesthesia. The wire basket that was passed into the duct beyond the calculus has been pushed out of its sheath, allowed to expand, and is being withdrawn. The calculus exited the duct with the basket.

C   = calculus
Can = cannula
SD = submand-
ibular duct
SG = submand-
ibular gland
WB = wire
basket

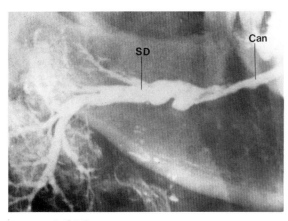

Figure 3.52C

Sialogram performed after withdrawal of the basket shows no calculi to be present. The patient was a 28-year-old man with a history of swelling in the left side of the neck, especially during eating. Contrast material is Ethiodol.

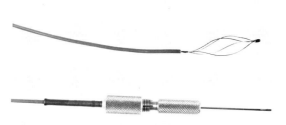

Figure 3.52D

Four French Dormia wire basket apparatus used for extracting stones from the salivary duct.

Right parotid sialogram and stone extraction

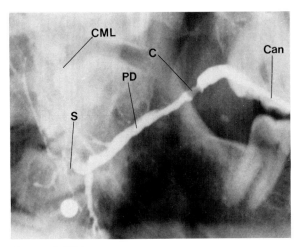

Figure 3.53A

Right parotid sialogram, lateral view, performed with Ethiodol. A moderate sized calculus is visible in the anterior midportion of the duct. There is no acinar opacification in the central portion of the body of the gland, but there is evidence of a lobular pattern of extravasation in the upper and lower portions of the duct. A stricture is present in the posterior part of the duct.

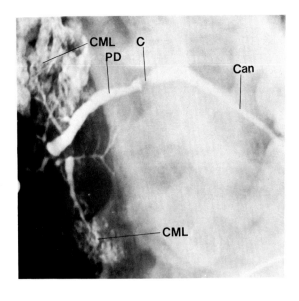

Figure 3.53B

AP view.

The patient was a 57-year-old man with a mass palpable in the parotid region; purulent secretions had been seen coming from the duct orifice and the patient was being treated with antibiotics for an abscess. The calculus is causing only partial obstruction of the duct and the contrast material could be expressed manually from the duct. Because of the history of recent infection, stone extraction was delayed several weeks.

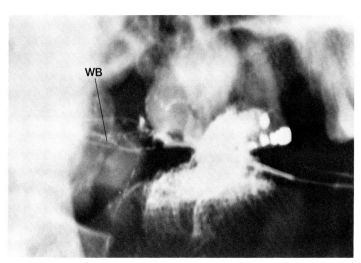

C   = calculus
Can = cannula
CML = contrast material in a lobular pattern in the parotid gland, presumably extravasated, a common finding in diseased glands.
PD = parotid duct
S   = stricture
WB = wire basket

Figure 3.53C

Parotid sialogram, lateral view during stone extraction. The basket extractor was easily passed into the parotid duct orifice after it had been dilated. The basket has been passed beyond the calculus and allowed to open. Numerous particles of grumous material, thought to be pieces of the calculus that had been broken up, were withdrawn with the basket. The large collection of contrast material is in a gauze in the mouth.

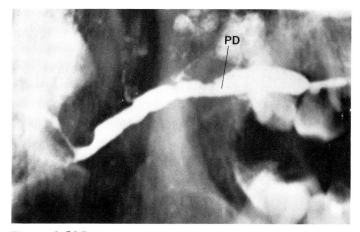

Figure 3.53D

Parotid sialogram, lateral view; immediately after withdrawal of the basket and flushing out of the duct with contrast material; the calculus is no longer visible. Three years later the patient had a recurrent abscess in the parotid gland; it was treated successfully with antibiotics.

Right submandibular sialogram and stone manipulation

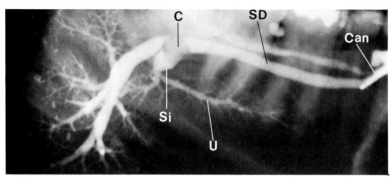

Figure 3.54A

Right submandibular sialogram, lateral view, performed with Ethiodol; a large calculus is present in the submandibular duct. There is dilatation of the origin of a large branch just behind the calculus.

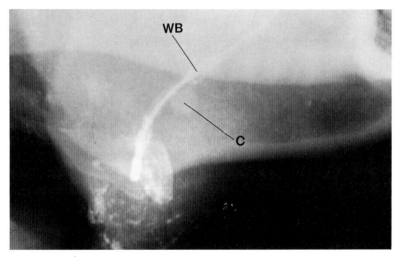

Figure 3.54B

Lateral view of the submandibular region during attempted stone extraction; a submandibular block has been performed for anesthesia, and the duct orifice has been enlarged by a small surgical neck at the margin of the duct orifice. The basket has been passed beyond the calculus and is partially open. The calculus could not be entirely removed but portions of its puttylike material were extracted with the basket.

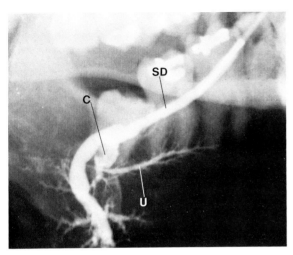

C   = calculus
Can = cannula
SD = submandibular duct
Si = dilatation of the origin and first part of the uncinate duct
U   = uncinate duct
WB = wire basket

Figure 3.54C

Sialogram following withdrawal of the basket shows the calculus to be slightly smaller than before and the remainder of the calculus to be displaced into the dilated side branch. Follow-up seven years later revealed that the patient has had no further symptoms or signs related to this calculus.

Right parotid sialogram, and attempted stone removal

Figure 3.55

Lateral view; a large calculus is seen in the midportion of the duct. The duct orifice was progressively dilated, and the wire basket apparatus was easily inserted without any incisions. The stone was so large that the basket could not pass beyond it, and the stone was gradually pushed into the posterior-most portion of the duct and could not be removed. Approximately four weeks later partial parotidectomy was performed because of recurrent infection in the gland.

The patient was a 60-year-old man with a history of chronic infection in the right parotid gland; the sialogram was performed initially to see if any calculi were present.

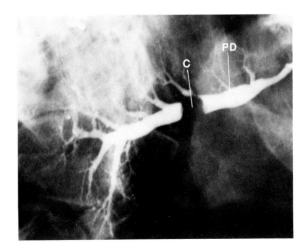

C = calculus
PD = parotid duct

Left submandibular sialogram with dilatation of stricture

Cath = catheter
S = stricture
SD = submandibular duct

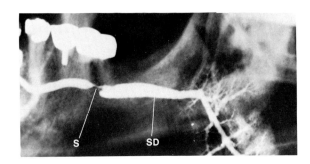

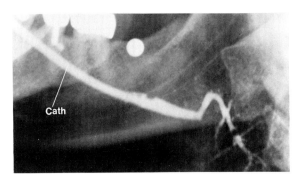

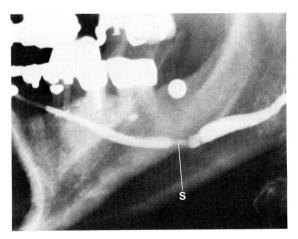

Figure 3.56A

Left submandibular sialogram, lateral view, performed with Ethiodol; a short area of very narrow stricture formation is present in the midportion of the duct with mild dilatation beyond the stricture.

Figure 3.56B

Successive dilations of the duct orifice were accomplished using progressively larger probes through the orifice and subsequently through the stricture. A tiny incision was then made in the margin of the duct orifice and a number 5 and finally a number 6.3 French catheter was passed through the stricture and left in place for several minutes. The BB was taped on the skin to indicate the location of the stricture during the dilatation.

Figure 3.56C

Sialogram performed immediately following dilation shows the stricture to be less narrow than previously, although moderate narrowing is still present.

The patient was a 47-year-old woman with a history of swelling in the left submandibular gland region; the sialogram was requested to determine whether a stone or stricture was present. Follow-up over the next several months revealed the patient to be asymptomatic. She was told to return if further symptoms appeared but the patient has not returned for further therapy, now seven years later.

Left parotid sialogram and stricture dilatation

Can = cannula
PD = parotid duct
S = strictures
LT = long tapered cannula used as a dilator

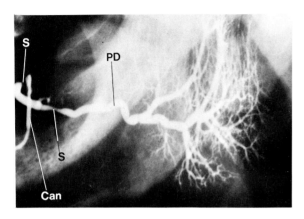

Figure 3.57A

Left parotid sialogram, lateral view, using Ethiodol; two strictures are present in the anterior portion of the duct: one is just behind the duct orifice and a second one is approximately 1.5 cm beyond this.

Figure 3.57B

Taken during the dilatation of the strictures, the long tapered cannula (21 LT) shown in figure 1.3 has been passed through the several strictures.

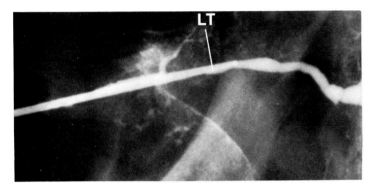

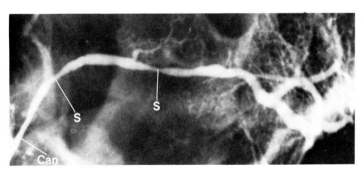

Figure 3.57C

Repeat sialogram following withdrawal of the long cannula shows the anterior-most of the two strictures to be considerably improved, while the one behind it appears only slightly improved. Nevertheless, evacuation through these two strictures was much more free than before the stricture dilation procedure.

The patient was a 64-year-old man with pain and swelling in the left parotid region. There was a history of carcinoma of the palate, treated with radiation therapy. Large metastatic lymph nodes were subsequently demonstrated deep to the left parotid gland.

Sialocele, left parotid sialogram

BB = marker for large palpable mass
Can = cannula
CM = globules of contrast material in the sialocele
PD = parotid duct

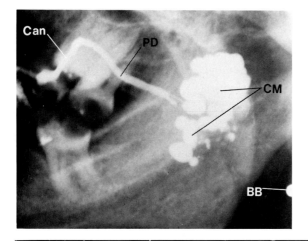

Figure 3.58

Lateral view, performed with Ethiodol; globules of Ethiodol can be seen collected in a sialocele.

The patient is a 24-year-old woman who received a stab wound with a kitchen knife in the left cheek approximately one and one-half months earlier. The laceration had been sutured but a large swelling developed under the wound. No external fistula had developed.

Hematoma of the parotid gland

M = mass with flattened edge against the parotid parenchyma
Ma = mandible
MP = mastoid process
PD = parotid duct
PG = parotid gland with flattened lateral margin
SC = subcutaneous tissue

The patient was a 12-year-old boy who had been struck in the right cheek by a sister's elbow. A large mass was present in the parotid region by the following day. Old blood had been drained out surgically on two occasions but the mass had recurred, and the question of underlying tumor or other abnormality was raised. On the basis of the sialographic findings shown here and the clinical findings, a tentative diagnosis of subcapsular hematoma was suggested. The mass eventually disappeared spontaneously.

Figure 3.59A

Parotid sialography performed with Ethiodol, slightly tilted Water's position, xerox film; the lateral surface of the parotid gland is flattened by a half spindle-shaped soft tissue mass (*arrows*) lateral to it, deep to the subcutaneous tissues. The appearance shown on this xerox film suggests that the mass had arisen in the superficial portion of the parotid gland and was compressing the parotid gland.

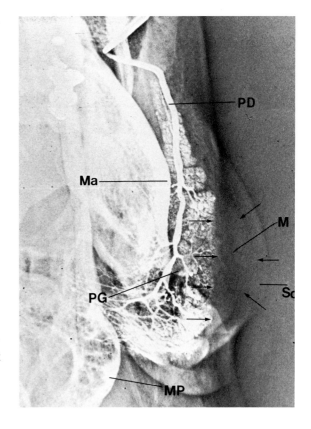

Myositis ossificans in the masseter muscle

The patient was a 34-year-old man who had been struck on the left side of the face with a fist two months earlier. The next morning the area was swollen but the patient could open his mouth normally. Trismus developed over the next two weeks. He was struck again in the same area one month later by a baseball. Over the next 2 to 4 weeks the patient experienced progressive inability to open his mouth until, at the time of the CT examination, only 15 degrees of opening could be accomplished. Over the next month, the patient kept straining to open his mouth as hard as he could, and suddenly felt a snap; he has been able to open normally since that time.

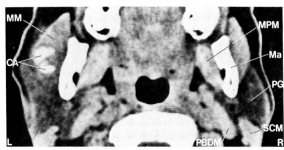

Figure 3.59B

Axial CT performed without contrast material. The left masseter muscle is larger than the right one and contains several contiguous areas of calcification.

C = calcifications in the masseter muscle
Ma = mandible
MM = enlarged masseter muscle
MPM = medial pterygoid muscle
PBDM = posterior belly of digastric muscle
PG = parotid gland
SCM = sternocleidomastoid muscle

Stone and fistula of the salivary gland

This 61-year-old man underwent drainage of a left submaxillary "abscess" 25 years previously. For the past 8 to 10 years he has had recurrent left submaxillary swelling and tenderness, particularly exacerbated more recently. A left submaxillary stone was removed from the duct six weeks prior to this sialogram. The stone measured 1.7 × 1 × 1 cm. Swelling decreased, but a firm, tender, irregular mass persisted.

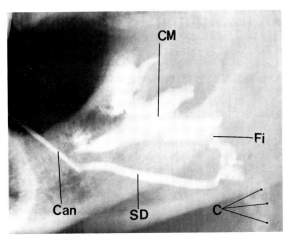

Figure 3.60

Left submandibular sialogram, lateral view; a fistula is present between the posterior portion of the submandibular duct and the floor of the mouth. Calculi can be seen within the submandibular gland.

C = calculi
Can = cannula
CM = contrast material that spilled through the fistula into the glossoalveolar sulcus
Fi = fistula
SD = submandibular duct

Chapter 4   Sjögren's Syndrome

This disease process is also referred to as autoimmune sialosis, benign lymphosialadenopathy, benign lymphoepithelioma of the parotid gland, chronic lymphoepithelial sialadenopathy, nonobstructive sialectasis, Mikulicz's disease, recurrent parotitis, punctate parotitis, and by many other terms (Kelly, Spiegel, and Maves 1975).

History

The individual components of Sjögren's syndrome have been recognized for many years. Thus, filamentous keratitis was reported by Leber in 1882, xerostomia by Hadden 1888, and lacrimal and salivary gland enlargement by Mikulicz in 1888. The generalized nature of Sjögren's syndrome was noted in 1925 by Gougerot, who described dryness not only of the eyes and mouth but also of the nose, larynx, and vulva in association with progressive atrophy of the salivary glands. The association of filamentary keratitis with chronic arthritis was reported by Houwer in 1927.

In 1933 Sjögren published a comprehensive description of the local and systemic findings that comprise the syndrome that bears his name, with further reports following in 1937, 1948, 1951, and 1971.

Sjögren's syndrome is a benign, chronic systemic disorder of unknown etiology (Hardin and Bloch 1978). It has the characteristics of a disorder of immune regulation (Whaley and Buchanan 1980). Sjögren's syndrome appears to involve a lymphocyte-mediated destruction of the acinar tissue of exocrine glands such as the lacrimal glands and the major and minor salivary glands, as well as those exocrine glands located in the upper and lower respiratory tract, the esophagus and stomach, the vagina and vulva, and possibly the skin, leding to absent glandular secretions and mucosal dryness (Moutsopoulos et al. 1980; Bloch 1983).

Clinical Findings

Sjögren's syndrome occurs in all decades of life, but the greatest incidence is between 40 and 60 years of age (Shearn 1971; Hardin and Bloch 1978; Whaley and Buchanan 1980). It occurs in children only rarely (Shearn 1971). Approximately 90% of cases of Sjögren's syndrome occur in females.

Classically, Sjögren's syndrome consists of a triad of kerato-conjunctivitis sicca (with or without lacrimal gland enlargement), xerostomia (with or without salivary gland enlargement), and a connective tissue disease, usually rheumatoid arthritis and less commonly systemic lupus erythematosus, progressive systemic sclerosis, periarteritis nodosa, or polymyositis (Bloch et al. 1965; Hardin and Bloch 1978; Whaley and Buchanan 1980). While there is no absolute definition of Sjögren's syndrome, and while no single clinical feature is absolutely diagnostic of Sjögren's syndrome, the combination of such features is characteristic. The presence of at least two of these three components, especially the first two, is sufficient to establish the diagnosis of Sjögren's syndrome on clinical grounds (Bunim 1961; Bloch et al. 1965; Whaley and Buchanan 1980). According to Shearn (1971), two of the salient features of Sjögren's syndrome—kerato-conjunctivitis sicca and the histologic appearance of the lacrimal and salivary glands—are highly characteristic and virtually specific for the diagnosis of Sjögren's syndrome.

Multiple system involvement is frequent, with abnormalities of the cutaneous, respiratory, genitourinary, gastrointestinal, neuromuscular, and articular systems (Bunim 1961; Bloch et al. 1965; Shearn 1971; Whaley et al. 1973a; Hardin and Bloch 1978; Moutsopoulos et al. 1980; Epstein, Thomas, and Sherlock 1980).

Much past confusion in terminology can be traced to the great variability in the presence and sequence of appearance of any of the major features of Sjögren's syndrome in a given patient. It is not unusual for the patient to present with a single abnormality that may even remain the sole manifestation of the disease for some time (Shearn 1971). According to Hardin and Bloch (1978), Sjögren's syndrome usually develops either concomitantly with or as a late complication of rheumatoid arthritis, and it is unusual for rheumatoid arthritis to develop long after the sicca complex appears. In about 10% of instances, however, the eye and mouth symptoms may precede the arthritis (Cummings et al. 1971). It is also known that any one or many of the particular components of Sjögren's syndrome, such as keratoconjunctivitis sicca, xerostomia, or rheumatoid arthritis, may never appear in the course of the disease (Shearn 1971). Shearn (1971) further states that the belief that any given manifestation must be present for the diagnosis of Sjögren's syndrome to be made has led to reports of an unrepresentatively high incidence of that particular manifestation in some series and in other series has led to the exclusion of the diagnosis in some patients who have the disease.

The term *Mikulicz's disease* (Mikulicz 1888, 1892, 1937) has been used clinically for instances in which parotid and lacrimal gland enlargement, keratoconjunctivitis sicca, and xerostomia are present, but without systemic symptoms. Morgan and Castleman (1953) and Morgan (1954) showed that the histologic changes in Mikulicz's disease and Sjögren's syndrome are identical and the clinical findings similar. These authors concluded that "Mikulicz's disease is not a distinct clinical and pathologic disease entity as previously believed but rather is merely one manifestation of a more generalized systemic symptom complex known as Sjögren's syndrome" (Morgan and Castleman 1953). For this and other reasons, it has been suggested by some authors that Mikulicz's disease be abandoned as a diagnostic term (Godwin 1952; Patey and Thackray 1955; du Plessis 1958; Kelly, Spiegel, and Maves 1975).

The use of the terms *Mikulicz's disease* for the salivary gland enlargement, *recurrent parotitis* for repeated episodes of inflammation of the parotid glands, keratoconjunctivitis sicca for the ocular manifestations and the "sicca syndrome" for dryness of the eyes and mouth and other tissues as well has tended to obscure the concept of a multisystem disease process with protean manifestations. To avoid these pitfalls, it was suggested by Waterhouse (1966) and Shearn (1971) that the term *Sjögren's syndrome* should be applied to the total entity without regard to the nature of the presenting manifestations. Perhaps the term should also be applied without regard to the nature of the predominant manifestations.

It has been customary to recognize two groups of patients with Sjögren's syndrome. If the abnormalities are limited to the ocular and oral manifestations only, the descriptive term *sicca syndrome* has been used, whereas if rheumatoid arthritis or associated connective tissue disease is also present, the diagnosis of Sjögren's syndrome with the particular connective tissue disease specified has been made (Hardin and Bloch 1978; Whaley and Buchanan 1980).

Currently, on the basis of certain genetic and clinical distinctions, two major types of Sjögren's syndrome are recognized: primary Sjögren's syndrome and secondary Sjögren's syndrome (Moutsopolous et al. 1980; Bloch 1983). When only the ocular and oral components of this syndrome are present, (the sicca syndrome), the term *primary Sjögren's syndrome* is applied. If these components of Sjögren's syndrome are accompanied by rheumatoid arthritis or other auto-immune disease, *secondary Sjögren's syndrome* is said to be present. The histologic changes in the salivary glands and many of the clinical and laboratory findings are the same in both groups, although many clinical and genetic similarities and differences have been demonstrated

(Bloch 1983). Bloch noted that among the clinical differences between the two groups, a higher incidence of recurrent parotid enlargement has been recognized in patients with primary Sjögren's syndrome.

The risk of developing lymphoma or pseudolymphoma is higher in patients with parotid swelling than in those without it (Chused 1980; Bloch 1983), so that parotid swelling is an indication of increased risk of developing lymphoma.

The diagnosis of Sjögren's syndrome can be established with a high degree of probability based upon a constellation of clinical and serological findings (Bloch 1983).

Salivary Gland Involvement

Although arthralgia, arthritis, and ocular symptoms are the most common initial symptoms of Sjögren's syndrome, recurrent parotid swelling may occur as the initial symptom, as in 15 of 80 patients (18%) reported by Shearn (1971). While most patients with Sjögren's syndrome eventually suffer from dryness of the mouth, xerostomia is an uncommon presenting complaint, occurring in only 4 of the 80 patients in Shearn's (1971) report. According to Whaley et al. (1980b), xerostomia was present in half of the patients in their series. According to Ericson (1968), of all the salivary glands, the parotid glands are not only the most frequently involved in systemic disease, but also have the most marked lesions both clinically and by biopsy.

Thus, the parotid gland is by far the most commonly enlarged of the salivary glands in Sjögren's syndrome. Parotid gland enlargement is reported to occur in 26%, 30%, 32%, 50%, and 55% of cases reported (respectively, Whaley and Buchanan 1980; Chisholm and Mason 1973; Shearn 1971; Bunim 1961; Bloch et al. 1965). According to Moutsopoulos and colleagues (1980), intermittent unilateral or bilateral parotid gland enlargement or other major salivary gland enlargement occurs in 80% of patients with Sjögren's syndrome.

Bloch and co-workers (1965) and Shearn (1971) state that the parotid gland enlargement usually is bilateral. Most commonly it is symmetrical, but it may be asymmetrical. It usually involves the entire gland, although it may present as a more discrete mass. Whaley and Buchanan (1980), on the other hand, stated that in a series of 171 patients with Sjögren's syndrome, contrary to popular belief, salivary gland enlargement was usually unilateral and episodic. In the series reported by Morgan (1954) and Maynard (1965), slightly more than half the patients had only unilateral enlargement.

According to Shearn (1971) and Whaley and Buchanan (1980), parotid swelling may occur suddenly, reaching maximum enlargement within several days, or it may be insidious in onset and persist for several months, in some instances becoming chronic. Multiple discrete episodes of recurrent swelling and detumescence may occur, so-called recurrent parotitis (Payne 1933; Pearson 1935; Patey and Thackray 1955; Blatt et al. 1956; Blatt 1964; Patey 1965; Maynard 1965). Except during the acute phase when it may be accompanied by pain and tenderness that is further aggravated by eating, the enlargement is otherwise neither painful nor tender.

According to Bloch and associates (1965) and Bloch (1983), three clinical patterns of salivary gland abnormalities have been identified: "Acute recurrent swelling of the parotid or submaxillary glands; chronic enlargement with superimposed acute episodes of swelling (the most common pattern); and mild enlargement first detected during examination" (Bloch 1983).

The swelling of the salivary glands in Sjögren's syndrome is presumed to be caused by increased immunologic activity and inflammation within the glands (Whaley and Buchanan 1980). The clinical presentation of the disease process as it affects the parotid glands most commonly suggests a diffuse inflammatory-obstructive process, but less commonly, when a particular part of the gland is more involved than the rest of the gland, the presentation may suggest a tumor (Godwin 1952; Patey and Thackray 1955; Patey 1965) (figs. 4.4, 4.9). The accessory processes attached to the upper margin of the main parotid duct may also be involved by the process (figs. 4.3, 4.7A, 4.14) and become enlarged, causing a palpable mass in the cheek anterior to the main gland (Katzen and DuPlessis 1964). Because the nature of the parotid gland enlargement seen in Sjögren's syndrome has not always been recognized, many of these glands have been removed surgically (Morgan and Castleman 1953; Blatt 1964; Shearn 1971), although sialography or biopsy of a salivary gland might have led to the correct diagnosis.

Submandibular gland enlargement (fig. 4.20C) is much less common than enlargement of the parotid gland, occurring in only 1 of 19 patients reported by Payne (1933), in 1 of 40 cases reported by Patey (1965), in 5 of 80 patients reported by Shearn (1971), in 10 of 62 patients reported by Bloch and colleagues (1965) (it was questionably enlarged in 4 others), and in 1 of 10 cases (bilateral) reported by Kelly, Spiegel, and Maves (1975).

Submandibular gland enlargement was accompanied by parotid gland enlargement in all 10 patients in the series reported by Bloch and associates (1965) but existed without parotid enlargement in 3 of the 5 patients reported by Shearn (1971). Lacrimal gland enlargement was noted in 3 of 80 patients (Shearn 1971) and in 2 of 62 patients (Bloch et al. 1965).

Recurrent parotitis in children (Pearson 1935, 1961; Thackray 1955; Patey and Thackray 1956; Katzen and DuPlessis 1964; Blatt 1966; Touloukian 1976; Konno and Ito 1979) has similar clinical, pathologic and radiologic findings to those seen in the adult form of recurrent parotitis as a component of Sjögren's syndrome. As opposed to the adult form, however, the age of onset of attacks is in childhood, varying between 8 months and 15 years, most commonly starting between the ages of 3 and 6 years. The sex incidence is also different from the adult form, recurrent parotitis in childhood being somewhat more common in boys than in girls (Katzen and DuPlessis 1964; Patey 1965; David and O'Connell 1970). Furthermore, in childhood the disease process usually is self-limited, with the signs and symptoms decreasing with age, the attacks usually ceasing spontaneously at puberty (Katzen and DuPlessis 1964; Blatt 1966). In a report of 52 patients by Konno and Ito (1979), none of their cases progressed to Sjögren's syndrome in adult life. Other authors, however, have reported some instances in which recurrent parotitis that started in childhood continued beyond puberty or even into adult life (see also figs. 4.12, 4.15). Maynard (1965) reported that 5 of 12 patients continued to have attacks after the onset of puberty, and David and O'Connell (1970) reported that 8 of 30 patients continued to have recurrences after the age of 15.

Furthermore, accompanying systemic abnormalities are apparently much less common in recurrent parotitis in children than in Sjögren's syndrome, being noted in only 4 of 21 cases reported by Blatt (1966) and in none of 44 cases reported by Katzen and DuPlessis (1964). The etiology of this condition is unknown (Mandel 1976).

Pathology

According to Shearn (1971), quoting Morgan and Castleman (1953), the diagnosis of Sjögren's syndrome can be strongly supported, even made with certainty by the demonstration of the characteristic pathologic changes in the salivary and lacrimal glands. Other authors (Katzen and DuPlessis 1964; Evans and Cruickshank 1970; Kelly, Spiegel, and Maves 1975; Batsakis and Sylvest 1977; Konno and Ito 1979) state that these changes in themselves are not specific for the diagnosis of Sjögren's syndrome but may represent a nonspecific reaction of the parotid gland to chronic insult or deficiency of recognized or unrecognized nature.

The histologic findings in the salivary glands in Sjögren's syndrome have been thoroughly described (Godwin 1952; Morgan and Castleman 1953; Patey and Thackray 1955; Bernier and Bhaskar 1958; Hemenway 1960). They consist of (fig. 4.1) (1) dense infiltration of lymphocytes and to a lesser degree by plasma cells and immunoblasts, so that entire lobules may be replaced and there may be organization into germinal follicles; (2) atrophy and disappearance of acini; and (3) proliferation of duct epithelial cells and epimyoepithelial cells, especially in the intercalated and striated ducts (Ericson 1968) to form solid cords, obliterating the duct lumens. Cross sections of these solid cords are the so-called epimyoepithelial islands (Morgan and Castleman 1953), which are seen in biopsy of approximately half of the parotid glands in

Sjögren's syndrome (Shearn 1971). Godwin (1952) suggested the term *benign lymphoepithelial lesion of the parotid gland* for this lesion. In addition to the findings described, cystic structures as large as 1.5 cm have been found in some instances, possibly the result of marked dilatation of larger ducts (Morgan and Castleman 1953) (fig. 4.15).

While these changes may be most marked in the parotid gland (Ericson 1968), they are also present in the submandibular glands, the sublingual glands, and the lacrimal glands (Sjögren 1933; Morgan and Castleman 1953; Waterhouse 1966; Waterhouse and Doniach 1966), and are also found in the minor salivary glands (Cifarelli, Bennett, and Zaino 1966; Bertram 1967; Chisholm and Mason 1968; Talal, Asofsky, and Lightbody 1970; Whaley and Buchanan 1980).

Although a probable diagnosis of Sjögren's syndrome can be made on clinical and serological grounds, the diagnosis can be confirmed by biopsy of a minor salivary gland of the lower lip as recommended by Chisholm and Mason (1968, 1973), Chisholm (1969), and by Chisholm, Waterhouse, and Mason (1970). The dominant histopathologic abnormality in these particular glands is focal lymphocytic sialadenitis, accompanied by acinar atrophy. Marked changes in the ductal epithelium have not been demonstrated, although mild hyperplasia of the intraglandular duct system epithelium may be seen in approximately one third of instances (Chisholm 1969). Epimyoepithelial islands are not seen in the labial glands (Chisholm 1969; Talal, Asofsky, and Lightbody 1970; Shearn 1971), although they have been reported in the glands of the palate (Bertram 1967). According to a survey of the literature by Mason and Chisholm (1975), focal lymphocytic infiltrates in the labial salivary glands have been demonstrated in approximately 70% of patients with Sjögren's syndrome but occur only infrequently in other conditions (Whaley et al. 1973) and are not demonstrable in normal controls (Chisholm and Mason 1968; Talal, Asofsky, and Lightbody 1970; Chisholm, Waterhouse, and Mason 1970; Greenspan et al. 1974). Thus, a definite positive biopsy can be obtained in about 70% of patients with Sjögren's syndrome by performing a biopsy of the labial salivary glands (Chisholm 1969; Whaley and Buchanan 1980).

In order to distinguish between the less severe degrees of lymphoid infiltration that are commonly seen in the salivary glands in the absence of Sjögren's syndrome, and to quantitate the degree of abnormality seen in the salivary glands in the presence of Sjögren's syndrome, it was suggested by several investigators (Waterhouse 1963; Waterhouse and Doniach 1966; Chisholm and Mason 1968; Talal, Asofsky, and Lightbody 1970; Chisholm, Waterhouse, and Mason 1970) that the number of lymphocytic foci present in a given area of salivary gland tissue be counted. A focus is defined as consisting of "an aggregate of 50 or more lymphocytes and histiocytes, usually with a few plasma cells placed peripherally, adjacent to and apparently replacing gland acini" (Waterhouse and Doniach 1966, 54). According to Greenspan and colleagues (1974), the "focus score" thus obtained correlates well with stimulated parotid flow rate and with the uptake and concentration of ^{99m}Tc-pertechnetate and is a valuable index of the severity of salivary gland involvement in Sjögren's syndrome.

A broad spectrum of lymphoproliferation, extending from benign to malignant, is seen in patients with Sjögren's syndrome (Cummings et al. 1971; Hardin and Bloch 1978). The process most commonly manifests as benign lymphoid infiltration of the salivary and lacrimal glands (Whaley and Buchanan 1980), but in about 25% of cases the lymphoproliferative process may extend to extraglandular sites (Moutsopoulos et al. 1980). Progressive intense lymphocytic infiltration may occasionally supervene on a previously stable process (Whaley and Buchanan 1980). The lungs, kidneys, lymph nodes, and salivary glands are characteristically involved by this process, but the lymphoproliferation may become even more widespread. If the histologic appearances are still benign, this process is sometimes referred to as *pseudolymphoma,* a term adopted by Talal, Sokoloff, and Barth (1967).

Pseudolymphoma involving the salivary glands may present with massive salivary gland enlargement and extensive cervical lymphadenopathy (Deutsch 1967; Anderson and Talal 1972).

Less often, the process may take a malignant form such as non-Hodgkin's lymphoma, Hodgkin's disease, or Waldenström's macroglobulinemia (Bunim and Talal 1963; Talal and Bunim 1964; Bloch et al. 1965; Talal, Sokoloff, and Barth 1967; Pinkus and Dekker 1970; Azzopardi and Evans 1971; Anderson and Talal 1972; Thackray and Lucas 1974; Kassan et al. 1977; Hardin and Bloch 1978; Moutsopoulos et al. 1980) (fig. 4.21). The likelihood of developing a lymphoreticular malignancy is greatly increased in patients with Sjögren's syndrome, the incidence of lymphoma in such patients being between 5% and 10% (Whaley and Buchanan 1980). This malignant process may be intrasalivary or extrasalivary, the latter probably being more common according to these authors. It would appear from the data of Hyman and Wolff (1976) that approximately 12% of cases of intraparotid lymphoreticular neoplasms may be associated with the benign lymphoepithelial lesion. Malignancies of epithelial origin have only rarely been reported in Sjögren's syndrome (Hilderman et al. 1962; Delaney and Balogh 1966; Gravnis and Giansanti 1970; Batsakis and Sylvest 1977).

Laboratory Findings

The volume of saliva may be especially diminished during the acute phases of Sjögren's syndrome and also during the late stages, when extensive destruction of the functioning parenchyma may have occurred. During acute attacks, the saliva may be turbid and flocculent (Blatt 1964), possibly owing to associated infection.

According to Whaley and co-workers (1973b) and Whaley and Buchanan (1980), stimulated salivary flow of less than 0.5 ml per minute from a parotid gland is virtually diagnostic of Sjögren's syndrome. The appearances of dryness in the mouth were correlated with salivary flow rates by Bertram (1967). According to Chisholm and Mason (1973), the demonstration of subnormal stimulated parotid salivary flow rate is the most sensitive index of salivary dysfunction in Sjögren's syndrome, occurring in 90% of patients. According to Shearn (1971), however, simple clinical observation usually is adequate to diagnose the presence or absence of salivary insufficiency.

Radionuclide scans using ^{99m}Tc-pertechnetate (Alarcon-Segovia et al. 1974) measure the capacity of the salivary cells to concentrate iodide and transport it into the saliva. The normal gland is able to concentrate the iodide ion 30 to 40 times its original concentration in the blood. In Sjögren's syndrome, there is decreased uptake of the isotope because of the destruction and consequent diminished function of the acinar cells. According to Stephen and colleagues (1971), almost 60% of patients with salivary gland involvement in Sjögren's syndrome had values below those in the control group. The findings, however, are nonspecific since there are many causes for diminished uptake. Schall and associates (1971) and Cummings and co-workers (1971) observed that the findings in sequential salivary scintigraphy paralleled the clinical symptoms, the salivary flow rate, and the sialograhic findings in Sjögren's syndrome. Scintigraphy provides a convenient method of measuring the progress of Sjögren's syndrome.

Anemia and leukopenia occur in less than one third of patients with Sjögren's syndrome (Bloch et al. 1965). Most patients with Sjögren's syndrome have hyperimmunoglobulinemia (Bloch 1983). Serum rheumatoid factor, antisalivary duct antibodies, and antinuclear antibodies can be demonstrated in approximately 75% of patients with Sjögren's syndrome (Whaley and Buchanan 1980; Moutsopolous et al. 1980). The abnormalities found in the serum of patients with Sjögren's syndrome have recently been discussed and summarized by Moutsopolous and colleagues (1980) and Bloch (1983).

The determination of serum protein values and electrophoretic patterns has generally been normal, and antibodies have been absent where sought for in most cases of recurrent parotitis in children (Katzen and DuPlessis 1964), so that participation of the immune system in the development of this disease has not been clarified (Konno and Ito 1979).

Radiologic Findings

Although sialography and CT are not recommended as primary methods to establish the diagnosis of Sjögren's syndrome, these examinations may be requested on the basis of swellings, inflammation, or a mass in the parotid region before the diagnosis of Sjögren's syndrome is suggested.

Sialography   The sialographic abnormalities of the parotid glands in Sjögren's syndrome are usually present bilaterally, though not necessarily in symmetrical fashion, and they may be progressive (Blatt 1964). Some authors (Blatt 1964; Som et al. 1981a,b) state that these changes are pathognomic for Sjögren's syndrome. Others believe them to be a nonspecific reaction of the parotid glands to chronic inflammation from various causes (Patey and Thackray 1955; Ericson 1967; Konno and Ito 1979). A number of characteristic findings have been described. The parotid gland may be enlarged because of swelling of the parenchyma or masses within the gland (figs. 4.2A,B, 4.4, 4.5). There may be failure of many of the duct branches to fill (figs. 4.3, 4.4, 4.7A,B). This may be explained by obliteration of the lumens by piled up epithelial cells as well as by compression by the swollen parenchyma. Acinar opacification is usually deficient, explained by the changes in the ducts as well as by the destruction and replacement of parenchyma by lymphatic cells (figs. 4.2–4.8). There may also be mild to moderate sialectasia with fusiform or tubular dilatation or "clubbing" of the intermediate and smaller duct branches within the gland (Patey and Thackray 1955; MacKenzie, Parker, and Gonzelez 1970; Konno and Ito 1979) (figs. 4.2A, 4.4A, 4.6, 4.7B, 4.8). Strictures may accompany such dilatation.

Perhaps the most characteristic finding is the presence of numerous spherical collections of contrast material distributed throughout the parotid glands (figs. 4.2–4.7, 4.8B,C, and 4.9, 4.18A). These have been shown in histologic sections to be localized to the striated and intercalated ducts; they appear relatively early during the injection when only a moderate degree of duct filling has occurred and before there is acinar filling (Ranger 1957; Katzen and DuPlessis 1964; Ericson 1968). In the early stages of Sjögren's syndrome these appear as myriad tiny punctate collections (fig. 4.5), giving rise to the term *chronic punctate parotitis* (Hemenway 1971). This appearance is also present in the accessory processes along the parotid duct (figs. 4.3, 4.5A, 4.7A, 4.14). As the disease progresses, these tiny collections may become larger (figs. 4.4, 4.6, 4.8) and may subsequently coalesce to form large cavities, ultimately with total destruction of the gland and bizarre pooling and puddling of contrast material (Blatt et al. 1956; Blatt 1964). In a series of 93 patients with Sjögren's syndrome reported by MacKenzie, Parker, and Gonzalez (1970), parotid sialography showed punctate sialectasis to be present in 75% of cases, tubular or cylindrical sialectasis of the interlobular or smaller ducts in 70% (22% had tubular dilatation as the dominant or only abnormality), globular collections in 21%, and cavitary destructive changes in 5%. Gonzalez, MacKenzie, and Tarar (1970) report a somewhat lower incidence of each of these findings: punctate sialectasis in 28% and cylindrical peripheral sialectasis, the most common radiologic finding, in 55% of cases. Any one of these changes may predominate in a gland, but all admixtures of punctate, globular, cavitary, and tubular abnormalities may occur together (MacKenzie, Parker, and Gonzalez 1970).

Postevacuation films have shown much of the contrast material in the spherical, punctate, or globular collections to be retained in the gland (figs. 4.7A, 4.10C, 4.15C, 4.16C). Some of this may persist for months or even years (fig. 4.4B), presumably trapped in the gland because of extravasation or partial duct obstruction and diminished salivary flow.

Although abnormalities of the main parotid duct are not a prevalent feature of Sjögren's syndrome or recurrent parotitis of children (Patey and Thackray 1955; Gonzalez, MacKenzie, and Tarar 1970), irregularities of the wall, sialectasia, and stricture of the main duct may occur, especially late in the disease and in the more severe cases (Katzen and DuPlessis 1964; Ericson 1968; Whaley et al. 1972) (figs. 4.6, 4.7B, 4.8). This could be the result of secondary infection or inflammation of the duct. Calcifications and calculi occasionally occur (Patey and Thackray 1955; Ericson 1968; Shearn 1971) (fig. 4.19A). Cysts (fig. 4.15), which may be lined with hyperplastic or metaplastic epithelium (Godwin 1952; Morgan and Castleman 1953), and abscesses occasionally occur.

Focal masses may be present in the parenchyma because of the lobular character of the process (Patey and Thackray 1955) (figs. 4.4, 4.9) or because a neoplasm has developed.

Even though the submandibular gland may show the same pathologic alterations found in the parotid gland in Sjögren's syndrome (Morgan and Castleman 1953; Bernier and Bhaskar 1958; Waterhouse 1963, 1966; Bloch et al. 1965; Waterhouse and Doniach 1966; Ericson 1968; Shearn 1971), sialographic changes such as have been described in the parotid glands are much less common in the submandibular gland, seen in 8 of 18 adults reported by Blatt (1964), but in none of the cases reported by Patey (1965) and in none of the children reported by Blatt (1966) (fig. 4.20A). Only "fine leakage shadows" were reported by Konno, Kitamura, and Ishikawa (1970), without any of the punctate changes seen typically in the parotid gland.

The sialographic appearances in the parotid gland in recurrent parotitis in children and adults are indistinguishable from those of Sjögren's syndrome (figs. 4.10–4.16). Punctate collections of contrast material were reported by Konno and Ito (1979) to be present in 45 of

52 patients. According to these authors, the clinical course is milder in those patients who do not manifest these punctate sialographic appearances than in those who do.

Although the presence of the collections of contrast material seen in the parotid gland in Sjögren's syndrome and recurrent parotitis and their location near the intercalated ducts is easily demonstrated in pathologic material (fig. 4.17), there is controversy over whether these collections are extravasated contrast material associated with rupture of the weakened duct wall (Patey and Thackray 1955; DuPlessis 1957; Ranger 1957; Katzen and DuPlessis 1964; Patey 1965; Som et al. 1981a), or whether they represent contrast material in actual dilatations of the salivary ducts or cystic cavities connected to these ducts (Ericson 1968). According to Konno and Ito (1979), pathologic examination in recurrent parotitis in children has shown most of these punctate or globular collections of contrast material to be in cystic spaces lined with one to several layers of cells and connected to peripheral ducts, although some do represent actual extravasations. These authors postulate that these dilatations and cystic cavities extending from the peripheral duct system are due to increased ductal pressure and obstruction to outflow of saliva, resulting from proliferation and regeneration of the duct epithelium.

Typical sialographic changes were present in 59%, 80% to 90%, 92%, 97%, and 94% of patients with Sjögren's syndrome (respectively, Whaley et al. 1972; Whaley and Buchanan 1980; MacKenzie, Parker, and Gonzalez 1970; Bloch et al. 1965; Gonzalez, MacKenzie, and Tarar 1970), and in 86% of patients with recurrent parotitis of childhood (Konno and Ito 1979). Possibly the variation in the frequency of involvement may relate to the severity of the disease process in different series. Such findings are commonly demonstrable in the parotid glands of patients with rheumatoid arthritis alone or with Sjögren's syndrome, even in the absence of any history of salivary gland disease (Ericson 1968). Thus, Bloch and colleagues (1965) reported such changes in 20 or 21 of 21 patients with Sjögren's syndrome with no history of salivary gland enlargement but who underwent sialography. In four of these patients the changes were advanced. According to Blatt (1964), Patey (1965), Ericson (1968), and Whaley and co-workers (1972), the punctate sialectatic appearances are usually bilateral even though the clinical symptoms may be unilateral.

Blatt (1966) reported these same sialographic changes also to be present in both parotid glands in patients with recurrent parotitis of childhood who had only unilateral symptoms. Konno and Ito (1979) reported such changes to be present bilaterally in 22 of 27 patients (81%) in whom swelling was unilateral, although the changes were milder on the asymptomatic side. The tendency to develop punctate collections of contrast material during sialography in recurrent parotitis of children may disappear as the child grows older. Among 13 cases of recurrent parotitis in children studied by repeat sialography (Konno and Ito 1979), 9 had such sialangioectatic lesions at the first visit. In two of these patients there was nearly complete disappearance of the tendency to form these punctate collections, while in six there was marked improvement but not complete disappearance. In one case there was progression of the changes so that the second sialogram showed enlargement and fusion of the cystic cavities. According to Konno and Ito (1979), it is very rare for punctate collections of contrast material to appear during repeat sialography in patients with signs and symptoms of recurrent parotitis if they were not present in the initial sialogram. Nevertheless, Katzen and DuPlessis (1964) did report one case in which a sialogram that had been normal initially showed the development of punctate sialectasis three years later.

CT   CT in Sjögren's syndrome reveals the parotid glands to be enlarged, symmetrically or asymmetrically (figs. 4.18B, 4.19B, 4.20B). They are of soft tissue density rather than the density closer to fat often seen in normal patients. Multiple small low density areas are distributed throughout the gland. Calcifications (fig. 4.19A,B) or masses (fig. 4.21) may be present. As further experience accrues, these appearances may prove to be typical of Sjögren's syndrome. The submandibular glands may be enlarged but much less often than the parotid glands. Similar appearances to those in Sjögren's syndrome can be seen in recurrent parotitis as shown in fig. 4.22A,B.

CASES

Benign lymphoepithelial lesion

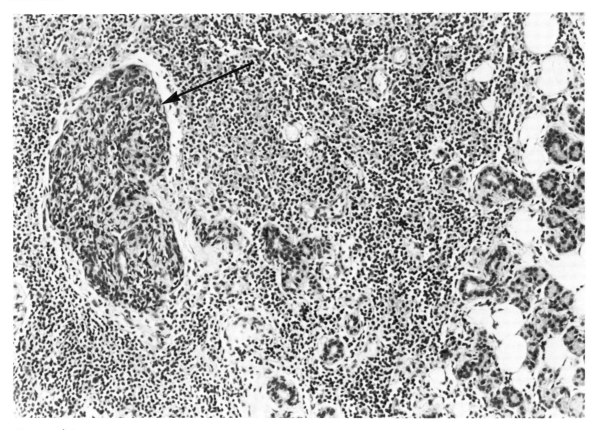

Figure 4.1

Light microscopic examination showing changes consistent with the benign lymphoepithelial lesion. A large epimyoepithelial island is present (*arrow*). Much of the normal parotid acinar tissue has been replaced by lymphoid tissue. (From J. G. Batsakis and V. Sylvest, *Pathology of the Salivary Glands* [Chicago: American Society of Clinical Pathologists, 1977]. Reprinted with permission.)

Sjögren's syndrome, right parotid sialogram

CM = small collections of contrast material
PD = parotid duct
S = strictures
Si = mild sialectasis

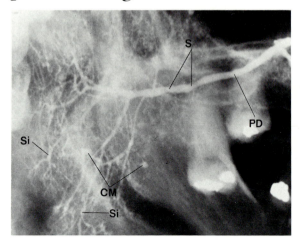

Figure 4.2A

Lateral view.

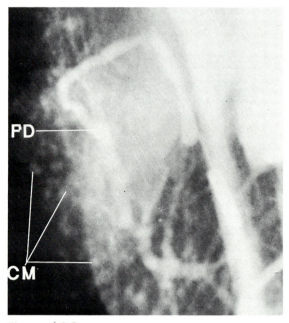

Figure 4.2C

Lupus erythematosus with sicca complex. A different patient. Parotid sialogram, AP view. The contrast material is water soluble (Sinografin). Numerous punctate collections of contrast material are present throughout the gland. The main duct shows minimal sialectasis. There is very poor acinar opacification.

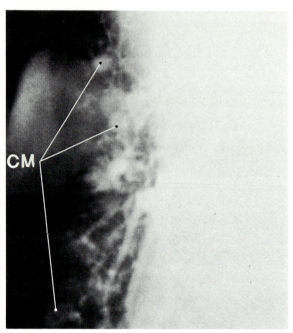

Figure 4.2B

AP view. Contrast material is water soluble (Sinografin). The gland is enlarged and the branches within the gland are spread apart by the swollen parenchyma. Numerous small collections of contrast material are seen, more obvious on the AP projection than on the lateral view. Many are quite faintly visualized, possibly because of the water-soluble nature of the contrast material. The main duct is slightly dilated and several slight strictures are seen. Mild irregularities are also present in some of the intraglandular duct branches, with slight sialectasis and areas of slight narrowing. Acinar opacification is poor.

The patient in figures 4.2A and B is a 56-year-old woman. Both parotid and lacrimal glands have been enlarged for a year. The patient has bilateral pleural effusions, a clinical diagnosis of rheumatoid arthritis, anemia, hyper-gammaglobulinemia and a positive rheumatoid agglutinin factor. Skin biopsy was interpreted as consistent with erythema nodosum. Lower lip biopsy was interpreted as consistent with Sjögren's syndrome.

The patient in figure 4.2C is a 58-year-old woman with history of pain and swelling in the right parotid region during eating, beginning several years ago. There has been recent onset of dryness in the eyes and in the mouth of severe degree. Studies of the serum have shown positive tests for ANA and rheumatoid factor. Biopsy of a minor salivary gland of the lower lip revealed abnormal changes not severe enough to be definitely diagnostic of Sjögren's syndrome but which were considered suggestive of early Sjögren's syndrome. A diagnosis of lupus erythematosus with vasculitis and the sicca complex has been reached.

Sjögren's syndrome, parotid sialogram, lateral view

The patient is a 35-year-old woman in whom a mass was discovered in the right parotid gland 10 years ago. Over the past 10 years it increased and decreased in size without any significant symptoms of pain. Over the past two or three months it increased in size, but it remained nonpainful. For the past seven or eight months the patient has noted dryness in the eyes and in the mouth and a general arthritic condition that began shortly after the birth of her child eight years previously. Laboratory work at the time of admission revealed tests positive for rheumatoid factor and negative for ANA, normal Coombs' test, and serum compliment levels. A Vim-Silverman needle biopsy had been performed, together with a biopsy of the buccal mucosa. Pathologic interpretation of the specimen was Mijulicz's disease. Because a parotid tumor or lymphoma was still suspected, partial parotidectomy was performed. The final diagnosis was Sjögren's syndrome.

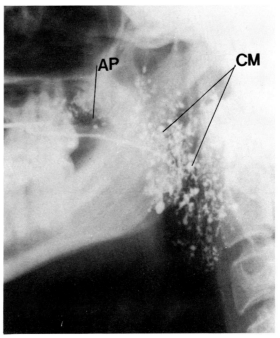

AP = accessory process of the parotid gland
CM = small collections of contrast material distributed throughout the gland as well as in the accessory process of the gland

Figure 4.3

Note the poor filling of the intraglandular branches and numerous small collections of contrast material in the main gland and in the accessory process as well. The main duct is normal. The contrast material is Ethiodol. Acinar opacification is poor.

Sjögren's syndrome, parotid sialogram

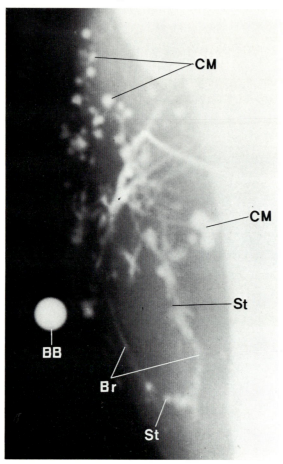

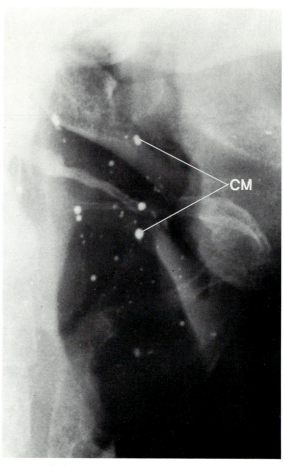

Figure 4.4A

AP view, performed 13 months prior to the current examination. Note the two large branches in the inferior portion of the gland; the medial one of these, moderately dilated, and containing several strictures showed only fragmentary filling on a subsequent sialogram, and apparently has become further obliterated (fig. 4.4D). Note the globular collections of Ethiodol within the gland. Some of these were still present 13 months later (fig. 4.4B). Parenchymal opacification is very poor. The BB indicates a large palpable mass.

Figure 4.4B

Preliminary lateral view of the parotid area taken 13 months after the sialogram shown in figure 4.4A, showing numerous small residual collections of Ethiodol in the parotid gland.

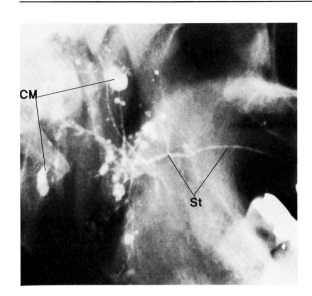

Figure 4.4C

Lateral view. Same examination shown in Fig. 4.4D.

Br = duct branches in the inferior portion of the parotid gland
CM = globules of contrast material
M = mass
St = strictures (mild)

Figure 4.5F

AP view; my
are distribut
accessory pr
glandular br.
larities. Acin
parotid glan
between the
2.0 cm. Com

Figure 4.4D

AP view of parotid sialogram performed 13 months after the sialogram shown in figure 4.4A. Numerous globular collections of contrast material of varying size are present throughout the enlarged gland, gathered mostly about the intra-glandular duct branches. The branches are attenuated and many are not filled. The main duct is not dilated but shows minimal areas of slight narrowing and stricture formation. There is only fragmentary filling of the large medial-inferior duct branch (*arrow*), although it was well filled and moderately dilated on the earlier sialogram (fig. 4.4A). The mass in the inferior part of the gland has enlarged somewhat in the interval. Acinar opacification is very poor. The gland is moderately enlarged.

The patient is a 55-year-old woman with progressively enlarging right parotid mass over the past 12 months. She has noted dryness in the mouth for years, and more recently has noted dryness in both eyes.

At surgery, a large mass was present in the superficial portion of the parotid gland, extending somewhat into the deep portion. This was removed without incident. Pathologic interpretation of the mass was benign lympho-epithelial lesion consistent with Sjögren's syndrome.

Sjögren's syndrome, right parotid sialogram

AP = acces
process of th
parotid glanc
CM = punc
collections of
contrast mate
Ma = manc
PD = parot
duct

CM = collections
of contrast
material in the
parotid gland
PD = main
parotid duct
showing moderate
dilatation

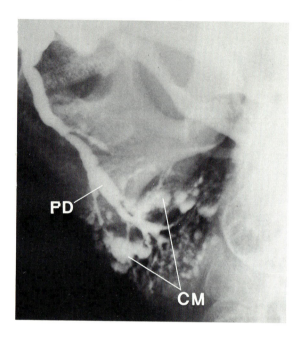

Figure 4.6A

Lateral-oblique view.

Figure 4.6B

AP view. The main duct is moderately dilated and there is mild irregular dilatation of some of the intraglandular branches, many of which are not well filled. Numerous small and larger collections of contrast material are seen throughout the gland. Acinar opacification is poor.

The patient is a 52-year-old woman with a mixed connective tissue disorder who complained of recurrent swelling of the right parotid gland. Superficial parotidectomy had been performed on the opposite (left) side seven years previously for a mass in that gland. Pathologic interpretation of that specimen was benign lymphoepithelial lesion. The diagnosis of Sjögren's syndrome has thus been made on the basis of the clinical and pathologic findings.

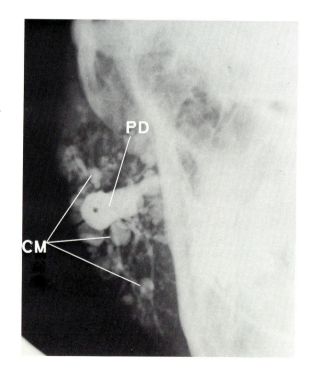

Sjögren's syndrome

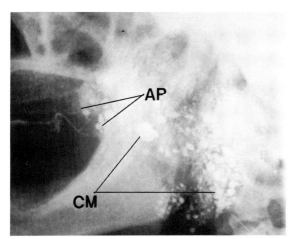

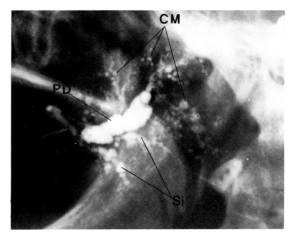

AP = accessory process of the parotid gland
CM = contrast material distributed throughout the gland
PD = parotid duct, markedly dilated
Si = sialectasis and strictures of duct branches

Figure 4.7A

Right parotid sialogram, lateral view, evacuation phase; contrast material is Ethiodol. Note that there is retention of numerous globules of contrast material in the main part of the gland and in the accessory process. Many of the intraglandular duct branches are not filled. Note the poor acinar filling.

Figure 4.7B

Same patient as in figure 4.7A, left parotid sialogram, lateral view, performed four years after the right parotid sialogram shown. Many of the intraductal branches are not filled and those that are opacified show irregular dilatation and stricture formation. The main duct shows marked irregular dilatation. There are numerous small collections of contrast material throughout the gland. Acinar filling is poor.

The patient was a 44-year-old woman who had been in good health until she experienced swelling of the right side of the face of two or three months duration, along with a dull ache in the jaw and ear on the right side. She was admitted to the hospital. There was no fever or chills. The mass increased in size for periods of two or three days and the area became purple but the pain level did not change. Symptoms were unrelated to eating. Saliva expressed from the right parotid duct was normal. The sialogram was performed (fig. 4.7A), and the patient subsequently received radiation to the right parotid area, 600 rad, and the right parotid duct was ligated. Antibiotics were administered, with improvement. Over the next 4 years the patient developed xerostomia and xerophthalmia, and a left parotid sialogram was performed (fig. 4.7B). The patient has Raynaud's phenomenon and fleeting arthralgias, but no definite rheumatoid arthritis. Laboratory analysis revealed tests positive for rheumatoid factor and negative for ANA. Punch biopsy of a rash over the legs and feet revealed allergic cutaneous vasculitis. Schirmer's test was positive. A diagnosis of Sjögren's syndrome was made on clinical grounds.

Sjögren's syndrome, left parotid sialogram

BB = marker

CM = globular collections of contrast material. These became more apparent as the injection continued.

PD = parotid duct

S = strictures of the main duct

Si = sialectasis of the branches which appear somewhat club shaped

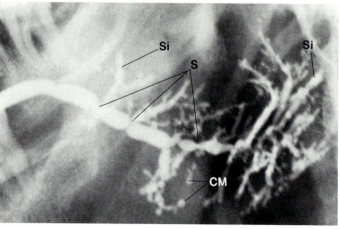

Figure 4.8A

Lateral view; there is sialectasis with multiple strictures in the main duct. A moderate stricture was also present near the duct orifice. There is clubbing and dilatation of many of the duct branches. Globules, which are beginning to become evident in the lower portion of the gland, became more prominent as the injection continued. Contrast material is Ethiodol. The degree of acinar opacification was very poor on this and subsequent pictures.

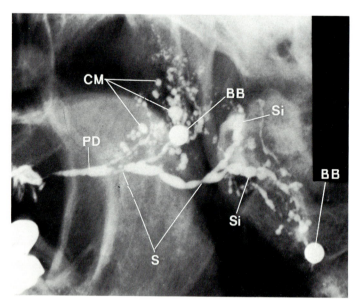

Figure 4.8B

Another patient, lateral view, left parotid sialogram.

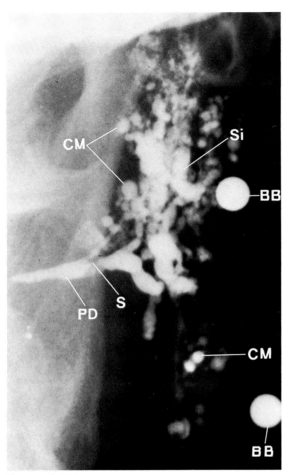

Figure 4.8C

AP view. Multiple strictures are visible in the main duct together with intervening stretches of irregular sialectasis. The duct branches are not as numerous as usual, suggesting that many are not opacified, and others show dilatation. Numerous globular collections of Ethiodol vary considerably in size. Acinar opacification is absent. The BBs indicate small palpable masses in the gland.

The patient in figure 4.8A is a 44-year-old man with a 12-year history of recurrent attacks of swelling and pain of both parotid glands, lasting three to four days at a time. There has been mild to moderate dryness of the mouth and mild dryness of the eyes, and progressive active rheumatoid arthritis. A diagnosis of Sjögren's syndrome has been made on clinical grounds.

The patient in figures 4.8B and C, a 62-year-old woman at the time of the sialogram, complained of swelling of the parotid area for three months. Several small palpable masses were present in the gland, thought possibly to be enlarged lymph nodes. These subsequently disappeared. She had had a mass removed from the tail of the parotid gland 13 years earlier. Histologic examination of the specimen, which included a 1-cm cyst containing yellow tinged fluid, showed changes consistent with Sjögren's syndrome. The patient has recently (six years after the sialogram) complained of increasing dryness of the mouth so that she cannot swallow food alone, and must drink liquids while eating or she is unable to swallow. There has been no dryness of the eyes or rheumatoid arthritis, but a diagnosis (by biopsy) of primary biliary cirrhosis has recently been made. The diagnosis is Sjögren's syndrome with primary biliary cirrhosis.

Sjögren's syndrome

CM = tiny punctate collections of contrast material in the parotid gland
M = mass
PG = parotid gland

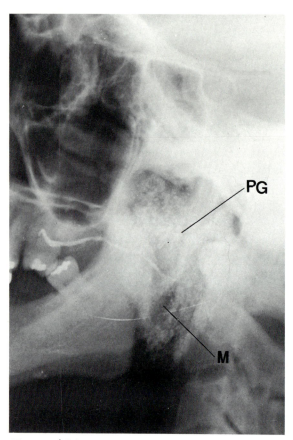

Figure 4.9A

Parotid sialogram, lateral view.

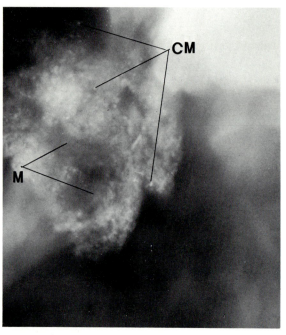

Figure 4.9B

Parotid sialogram, lateral view, laminogram. A mass is present within the gland. Note also tiny punctate collections of contrast material (Ethiodol) throughout the gland. The gland appears rather dense, but most of the contrast material is extravasated.

The patient is a 37-year-old man with a 17-year history of rheumatoid arthritis, and a two-month history of a lump in the right neck. This had fluctuated in size but there had been no pain or swelling with eating. Examination revealed a freely mobile ovoid 2 × 3-cm firm mass in the tail of the parotid gland. Right superficial parotidectomy was performed. Pathologic examination of the specimen revealed dense lymphoid infiltrate and myoepithelial proliferation, and the diagnosis of Mikulicz's disease was made at that time. The patient subsequently developed histiocytic lymphoma.

Recurrent parotitis in childhood, left parotid sialogram

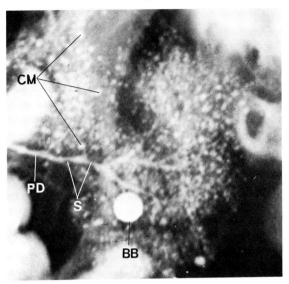

Figure 4.10A

Lateral view.

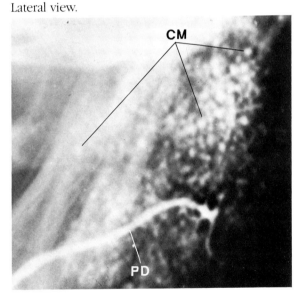

Figure 4.10B

AP view. Tiny punctate collections of Ethiodol are distributed throughout the gland. Some of the intraglandular ducts are poorly filled. There is mild irregularity of the main duct. The gland is moderately enlarged. Acinar opacification is poor. The BB indicates an area of clinically palpable prominence of the gland.

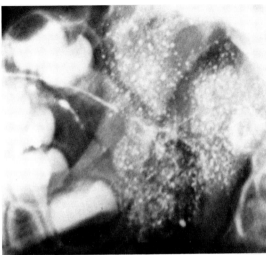

CM = contrast material
S = mild strictures of the parotid duct
PD = parotid duct

Figure 4.10C

Evacuation phase following administration of lemon juice. Much of the Ethiodol remains in the gland and ducts.

The sialogram was performed when the patient was six years old. Up to that time there had been six episodes of recurrent painful swelling of the left parotid gland with some fleeting joint symptoms. There was no evidence of rheumatoid arthritis. Several episodes of ocular irritation occurred but these were thought to be traumatic in nature. The Schirmer's test was normal. Tests including rheumatoid factor and LE cells were negative; the sedimentation rate was normal. There have been no episodes of recurrent parotitis during the eight years following the performance of this sialogram (the patient is now 15 years old), and the patient is now asymptomatic.

Recurrent parotitis in childhood, right parotid sialogram

CM = contrast material distributed throughout the parotid gland
PD = parotid duct
S = stricture (slight)

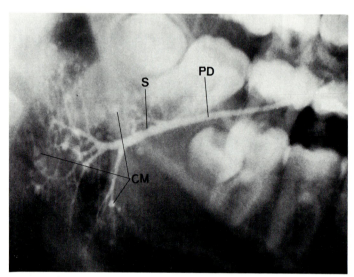

Figure 4.11A

Lateral view.

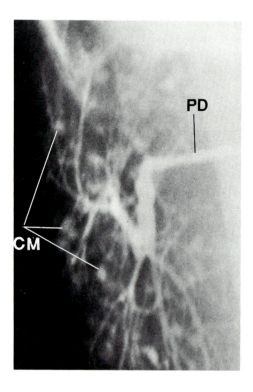

Figure 4.11B

AP view. Water-soluble contrast material is used (Sinografin). There are numerous small globular collections of contrast material throughout the gland. The main duct has a slight stricture. Acinar opacification is poor. The gland is within normal limits of size.

The patient is a 15-year-old boy who had had two episodes of swelling of the right parotid gland. A biopsy of the lower lip was interpreted as mild chronic sialadenitis, not consistent with Sjögren's syndrome. The patient has been asymptomatic during the three years following the sialogram.

Recurrent parotitis in childhood continuing into adulthood

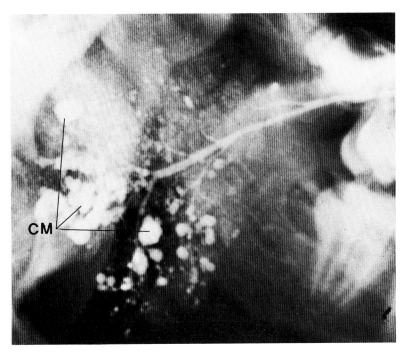

CM = globular and punctate collections of contrast material distributed throughout the gland

Figure 4.12

Left parotid sialogram, lateral view. Larger globular collections of Ethiodol are seen in the posterior and inferior portions of the gland, with smaller punctate collections in the upper anterior portions. There is compression of some of the intra-glandular branches. The main duct is within normal limits. There is rather poor filling of the intraglandular branches, and acinar opacification is very poor.

The patient was an 11-year-old girl at the time of the sialogram with a history of multiple episodes of marked recurrent swelling of the left parotid gland especially during eating. Thirteen years later (the patient is now 24 years old) there is still intermittent swelling and tenderness of the left parotid gland during eating, though less than earlier. The patient complains of dryness of the mouth, but there are no symptoms related to the eyes. Recently a small mass has appeared under the left ear and has since disappeared. There is no evidence of arthritis.

Recurrent parotitis in childhood

CM = collections of contrast material throughout the gland

S = strictures

Si = sialectasis (mild)

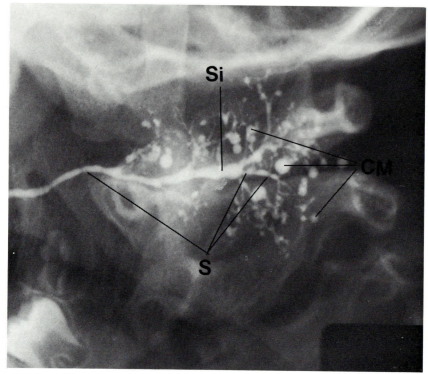

Figure 4.13

Parotid sialogram, lateral view. There are globular and punctate collections of contrast material distributed throughout the gland. The intra-glandular branches show irregular mild dilatation and stricture formation, as does the main duct. There is deficient acinar opacification throughout the gland.

The patient is a 10-year-old boy with a one- to two-year history of recurrent episodes of swelling of the parotid glands, involving both sides, but occurring unilaterally at each episode. The attacks lasted 10 days to three weeks. Sialograms revealed that the changes were bilateral. There was a history of chronic conjunctivitis, and there was some watering of the eyes but no evidence of keratitis. The patient has dysgammaglobulinemia.

Recurrent parotitis in childhood

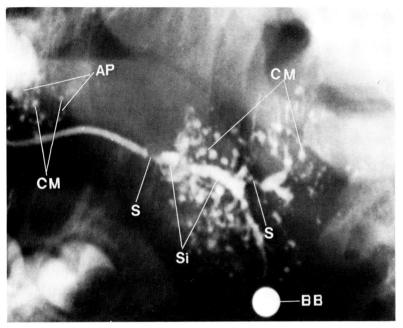

AP = accessory process
CM = globular collections of contrast material throughout the gland, including the accessory process
S = strictures
Si = sialectasis (mild)

Figure 4.14

Left parotid sialogram, lateral view. Punctate-globular collections of Ethiodol are distributed throughout the gland, somewhat unevenly. The accessory process shows similar changes. The main parotid duct anterior to the gland appears normal. There is poor filling of many of the intraglandular ducts, while others show obstruction, stricture formation, and irregular dilatation, including the portion of the main duct within the gland. Acinar opacification is markedly deficient. The BB indicates an area of palpable enlargement of the parotid gland.

At the time of the sialogram, the patient was a two-year-old boy who had had two clinical episodes of left-sided parotitis in recent months, accompanied by fever of 101°F and lasting about a week. There were no abnormal ocular findings and no arthritis or systemic abnormalities. Between episodes, the parotid gland was normal at physical examination. The patient has been asymptomatic during the eight years following the sialogram (he is now 10 years old).

Recurrent parotitis in childhood with cystic structure; progression of disease into adulthood; right parotid sialogram

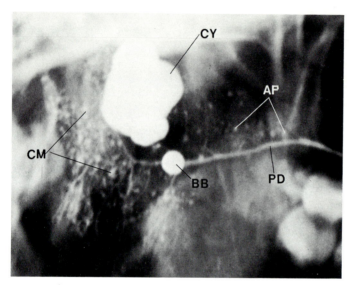

Figure 4.15A

Lateral view.

At surgery the large cystic area was found to contain approximately 5 ml of yellow watery fluid. This was drained surgically. Pathologic examination of several large biopsies of the cyst wall revealed dense fibrous tissue and chronic active inflammation. The adjacent parotid tissue showed mildly inflamed salivary gland lobules and lobules incorporated into an inflammatory mass with dilated ducts, small collection of polymorphonuclear leukocytes, and large germinal centers, findings interpreted as consistent with Mikulicz's disease. Cultures of the cyst contents were sterile.

At the time of the sialogram the patient was a 15-year-old diabetic boy who had developed a tender enlarging mass in the right parotid region. A 3-cm fluctuant mass could be palpated at the angle of the mandible just above the area of palpable firmness. Nine years following the performance of the sialogram (the patient is now 24 years old), the patient has some dryness of the month and eyes and is still having occasional bouts of swelling and tenderness in the right parotid gland. There is no evidence of rheumatoid arthritis. The right parotid gland is moderately enlarged, the left is slightly enlarged. The serum tests for antinuclear antibodies and rheumatoid factor have been negative. The patient has recently developed gluten enteropathy. Figures 4.22A&B show CT examination performed ten years later.

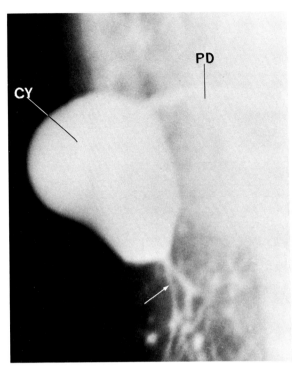

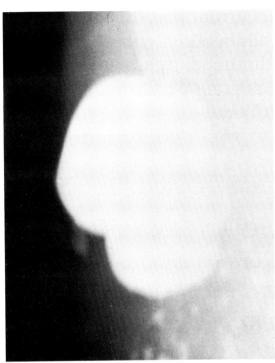

AP = accessory processes

CM = punctate collections of contrast material

Cy = cystic structure in the parotid gland

PD = parotid duct

BB = indicates palpable mass below the cyst

Figure 4.15B

AP view. Numerous punctate collections of Ethiodol are distributed throughout the gland. The main duct appears normal. The intraglandular branches may be slightly compressed. A large lobulated collection of contrast material in the upper anterior portion of the gland could be seen to enlarge progressively during injection, apparently filling from the smaller of two nearby ducts (*arrow*). The BB indicates a clinically palpable enlargement in the parotid gland below the cystic collection. Note the poor acinar opacification.

Figure 4.15C

AP view, evacuation phase; although the ducts have emptied following stimulation of salivary flow with lemon juice, punctate collections and the large pool of contrast material remain in the gland.

Sjögren's syndrome

CM = small collections of contrast material in the parotid gland

LD = low density areas in the enlarged right parotid gland

PD = parotid duct showing mild sialectasis

S = stricture

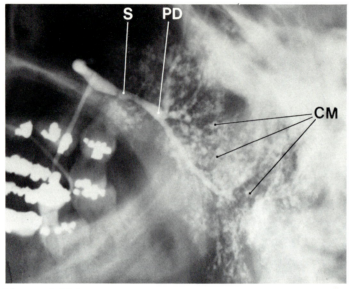

Figure 4.18A

Right parotid sialogram, lateral view. Innumerable small collections of contrast material are distributed throughout the enlarged parotid gland. There is incomplete filling of many of the intraglandular duct branches. The main duct shows mild irregular sialectasis and a short stricture.

Figure 4.18B

Axial CT performed following administration of intravenous contrast material. The right parotid gland is moderately enlarged and its density is in the range of enhanced soft tissue. Multiple small low (near water) density areas are present within the gland. The left parotid gland is only slightly enlarged and contains a few small areas of increased (soft tissue) density.

The patient is a 38-year-old man with a 9-year history of left parotitis treated with antibiotics. Recently the right parotid gland has become enlarged. Biopsy of the right parotid gland showed changes consistent with Sjögren's syndrome.

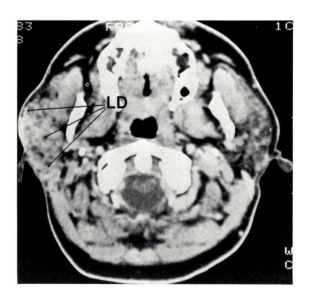

Sjögren's syndrome

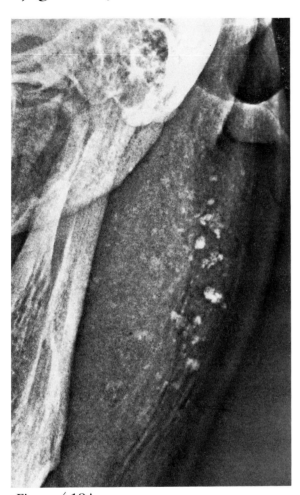

Figure 4.19A

Anterior-posterior view of the right parotid gland. Xerox technique. Multiple small calcifications are present in the enlarged parotid gland.

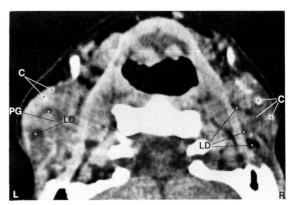

Figure 4.19B

C = calcifications in the parotid gland
LD = low density areas within the parotid glands—these measure 7 to 29 Hounsfield units and may be areas of fluid collection within the glands
PG = moderately enlarged left parotid gland

CT, performed without contrast material, semiaxial view with the chin extended and the gantry angled craniad. The left parotid gland is moderately enlarged. The right is slightly enlarged. Both are of irregular soft tissue density with some focal areas of low density. Calcifications are visible in the right parotid gland and were seen better in the left parotid gland in other sections.

The patient is a 28-year-old woman in first trimester of pregnancy. Painless parotid enlargement was recently first noted by her obstetrician, greater on the left than on the right. Biopsy of a salivary gland of the lower lip showed changes consistent with chronic sialadenitis or Sjögren's syndrome. A diagnosis of primary Sjögren's syndrome has been made on the basis of clinical, serological, and histological findings.

Sjögren's syndrome associated with lupus erythematosus

LD = low density areas within the enlarged right parotid gland

SD = dilated submandibular duct

SG = enlarged left submandibular gland

S = stricture of submandibular duct

Si = sialectasis in submandibular ducts within the gland

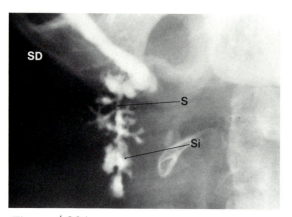

Figure 4.20A

Left submandibular sialogram showing sialectasis in the duct and gland.

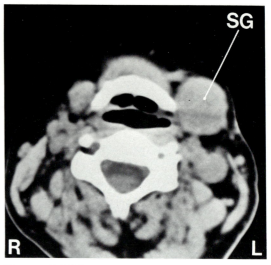

Figure 4.20C

CT of the submandibular glands. The left gland is markedly enlarged and of homogeneous soft tissue density.

The patient is a 45-year-old woman with a 20-year history of lupus erythematosus. The parotid and submandibular glands had been enlarged for two years. Left parotidectomy had been performed. Pathological findings were those of Sjögren's syndrome.

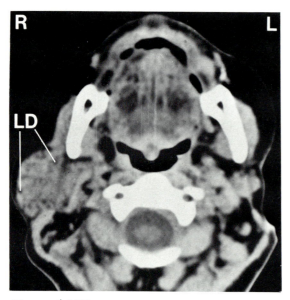

Figure 4.20B

CT of the parotid glands performed without contrast material. The right parotid gland is enlarged and contains numerous tiny low density areas. The left parotid gland has been removed.

Lymphoma in Sjögren's syndrome

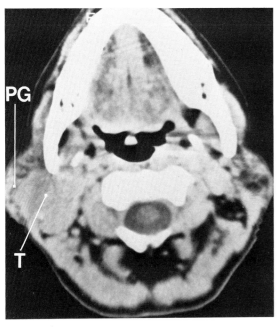

PG = com-
pressed parotid
gland
T   = tumor

Figure 4.21

Axial CT shows a large mass occupying the deep portion of the parotid gland. The parenchyma is compressed outward into a moderately thin layer. Small low density areas are seen within this compressed parotid parenchyma.

The patient is a 75-year-old female with a large growing mass in the right parotid region, first noted four years earlier. Biopsy of this mass was interpreted as lymphoma. Both parotid glands had fluctuated in size over the past four years; biopsy of the parotid gland itself earlier had shown lymphoepithelial tissue consistent with Sjögren's syndrome.

Recurrent parotitis. Same patient as 4.15A,B,C

BA = barium marker on skin indicating mass

CM = contrast material in normally opacifying parotid parenchyma

LD = low density areas in parotid glands

M = mass

PG = enlarged right parotid gland

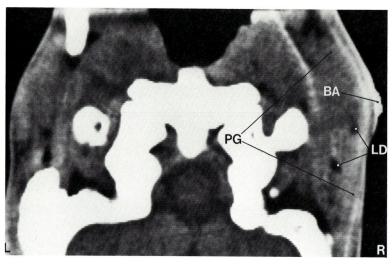

Figure 4.22A

Axial CT performed without contrast material. The parotid glands are of soft tissue density and are enlarged, the right more than the left. Numerous tiny low (near water) density areas are present within the parotid glands.

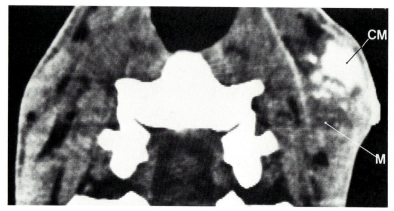

Figure 4.22B

Axial CT performed during injection of 20% Renografin into the duct by hydrostatic method. The parenchyma in the anterior part of the parotid gland opacifies normally. A mass occupies the posterior part of the gland.

The patient was 25 years old at the time of the CT examination. Right superficial parotidectomy was performed because of an enlarging mass in the right parotid gland. Pathology revealed chronic sialadenitis and severe fibrosis.

References

Alarcon-Segovia, D., et al. Salivary gland enlargement in diseases associated with Sjögren's syndrome. Radionuclide and roentgenographic studies. *J. Rheumatol.* 1:159–165, 1974.

Anderson, L. G., and Talal, N. The spectrum of benign to malignant lymphoproliferation in Sjögren's syndrome. *Clin. Exp. Immunol.* 10:199–321, 1972.

Azzopardi, J. G., and Evans, D. J. Malignant lymphoma of parotid associated with Mikulicz disease (benign lymphoepithelial lesion). *J. Clin. Pathol.* 24:744–752, 1971.

Batsakis, J. G., and Sylvest, V. *Pathology of the salivary glands.* Chicago: American Society of Clinical Pathologists, 1977, pp. 22–26.

Bernier, J. L., and Bhaskar, S. N. Lymphoepithelial lesions of salivary glands. Histiogenesis and classification based on 186 cases. *Cancer* 11:1156–1179, 1958.

Bertram, U. Xerostomia. Clinical aspects, pathology, and pathogenesis. *Acta Odontol. Scand.* 25 (Suppl. 49):1–126, 1967.

Blatt, I. M. On sialectasis and benign lympho-sialadenopathy (the pyogenic parotitis, Gougerot-Sjögren's syndrome, Mikulicz's disease complex). A ten-year study. *Laryngoscope* 74:1684–1746, 1964.

Blatt, I. M. Chronic and recurrent inflammations about the salivary glands with special reference to children. A report of 25 cases. *Laryngoscope* 70:917–933, 1966.

Blatt, I. M., et al. Secretory sialography in diseases of the major salivary glands. *Ann. Otol. Rhinol. Laryngol.* 65:295–317, 1956.

Bloch, K. J. Sjögren's syndrome. In *Internal medicine,* ed. J. H. Stein. Little, Brown: Boston, 1983, pp. 1034–1036.

Bloch, K. J., et al. Sjögren's syndrome: a clinical, pathological and serological study of sixty-two cases. *Medicine* 44:187–231, 1965.

Bunim, J. J. A broader spectrum of Sjögren's syndrome and its pathogenetic implications. *Ann. Rheum. Dis.* 20:1–10, 1961.

Bunim, J. J., and Talal, N. The association of malignant lymphoma with Sjögren's syndrome. *Trans. Assoc. Am. Physicians* 76:45–55, 1963.

Chisholm, D. M. Minor salivary gland pathology in Sjögren's syndrome and rheumatoid arthritis. In *Fourth Proceedings of the International Academy of Oral Pathology.* New York: Gordon and Breach, 1969, pp. 44–56.

Chisholm, D. M., and Mason, D. K. Labial salivary gland biopsy in Sjögren's disease. *J. Clin. Pathol.* 21:656–660, 1968.

Chisholm, D. M., and Mason, D. K. Salivary gland function in Sjögren's syndrome. *Br. Dent J.* 135:393–399, 1973.

Chisholm, D. M.; Waterhouse, J. P.; and Mason, D. K. Lymphocytic sialadenitis in the major and minor glands: a correlation in postmortem subjects. *J. Clin. Pathol.* 23:690–694, 1970.

Chused, T. M. Lymphoma and autoantibodies in Sjögren's syndrome. *Ann. Intern. Med.* 92:212–215, 1980.

Cifarelli, P. S.; Bennett, M. J.; and Zaino, E. C. Sjögren's syndrome. A case report with an additional diagnostic aid. *Arch. Intern. Med.* 117:429–431, 1966.

Cummings, N. A., et al. Sjögren's syndrome—newer aspects of research, diagnosis and therapy. *Ann. Intern. Med.* 75:937–950, 1971.

David, R. B., and O'Connell, E. J. Suppurative parotitis in children. *Am. J. Dis. Child.* 119:332–335, 1970.

Delaney, W. E., and Balogh, K., Jr. Carcinoma of the parotid gland associated with benign lympho-epithelial lesion (Mikulicz's disease) in Sjögren's syndrome. *Cancer* 19:853–860, 1966.

Deutsch, H. J. Sjögren's syndrome and pseudolymphoma. *Ann. Otol.* 76: 1075–1084, 1967.

DuPlessis, D. I. Some important features in the development, structure and function of the parotid salivary glands. *South Afr. Med. J.* 31:773–781, 1957.

DuPlessis, D. I. The problem of Mikulicz's disease. *South Afr. Med. J.* 32:264, 1958.

Epstein, O.; Thomas, H. C.; and Sherlock, S. Primary biliary cirrhosis is a dry gland syndrome with features of chronic graft-versus-host disease. *Lancet* 1:1166–1168, 1980.

Ericson, S. Sialographic study of the parotid glands in rheumatoid arthritis. *Odont. Rev.* 18:163–172, 1967.

Ericson, S. The parotid gland in subjects with and without rheumatoid arthritis. *Acta Radiol. [Suppl.]* 275, 1968.

Evans, R. W., and Cruickshank, A. H. Mikulicz-Sjögren syndrome. Solid adenolymphoma, benign lymphoepithelial lesion and lymphatoid adenoma. In *Epithelial tumors of the salivary glands*, ed. R. Winston and A. H. Cruickshank. Philadelphia: W. B. Saunders, 1970, pp. 279–295.

Godwin, J. Benign lymphoepithelial lesion of the parotid gland (adenolymphoma, chronic inflammation, lymphoepithelioma, lymphocytic tumor, Mikulicz disease. Report of eleven cases). *Cancer* 5:1089–1103, 1952.

Gonzalez, L.; MacKenzie, A. H.; and Tarar, R. A. Parotid sialography in Sjögren's syndrome. *Radiology* 97:91–93, 1970.

Gougerot, M. Insuffisance progressive et atrophie des glandes salivaires et muqueuses de la bouche, des conjonctives (et parfois des muqueuses, nasale, laryngée, vulvaire): "Sécheresse" de la bouche, des conjonctives, etc. *Bull. Soc. Franc. Derm. Syph.* 32:376–379, 1925.

Gravnis, M. B., and Giansanti, J. S. Malignant histopathologic counterpart of the benign lympho-epithelial lesion. *Cancer* 26:1332–1342, 1970.

Greenspan, J. S., et al. The histopathology of Sjögren's syndrome in labial salivary gland biopsies. *Oral Surg.* 37:217–229, 1974.

Hadden, W. B. On "dry mouth," or suppression of the salivary and buccal secretions. *Tr. Clin. Soc. Lond.* 21:176–179, 1888.

Hardin, J. A., and Bloch, K. J. Sjögren's syndrome. In *Immunological diseases*, ed. M. Samter. Boston: Little, Brown, 1978, pp. 1151–1157.

Hemenway, W. G. The parotid gland in Mikulicz disease and Sjögren's syndrome. *Ann. Otol. Rhinol. Laryngol.* 69:849–868, 1960.

Hemenway, W. G. *Chronic punctate parotitis.* Boulder, Col.: Colorado Associated University Press, 1971.

Hilderman, W. C., et al. Malignant lymphoepithelial lesion with carcinomatous component apparently arising in parotid gland. A malignant counterpart of benign lymphoepithelial lesion? *Cancer* 15:606–610, 1962.

Houwer, A. W. M. Diseases of the cornea: 1. Keratitis filamentosa and chronic arthritis. *Trans. Ophthalmol. Soc. UK* 47:88–96, 1927.

Hyman, G. A., and Wolff, M. Malignant lymphomas of the salivary glands. Review of the literature and report of 33 new cases, including four cases associated with the lymphoepithelial lesion. *Am. J. Clin. Pathol.* 65:421–438, 1976.

Kassan, S. S., et al. Increased incidence of malignancy in Sjögren's syndrome (abstr.). *Arthritis* Rheum. 20:123, 1977.

Katzen, M., and DuPlessis, D. J. Recurrent parotitis in children. *South Afr. Med. J.* 38:122–128, 1964.

Kelly, D. R.; Spiegel, J. C.; and Maves, M. Benign lymphoepithelial lesions of the salivary glands. *Arch. Otolaryngol.* 101:71–75, 1975.

Konno, A., et al. Clinical study on recurrent swellings of the parotid gland: part I, Sjögren's syndrome. (In Japanese.) *Jpn. J. Otol.* 73:397–408, 1970.

Konno, A., and Ito, E. A study on the pathogenesis of recurrent parotitis in childhood. *Ann. Otol. Rhinol. Laryngol. (Suppl. 63)* 88, part 4: 1979.

Leber, T. Über die Entstehung der Netzhautablösung Klin. Mbl *Augenheilk* 20:165–166, 1882.

MacKenzie, A. H.; Parker, W.; and Gonzalez, L. New sialographic criteria for Sjögren's syndrome. *Arthritis Rheum.* 12:679, 1970.

Mandel, L. Inflammatory disorders. In *Diseases of the Salivary Glands*, ed. I. M. Polayes and R. M. Rankow. Philadelphia: W. B. Saunders, 1976, pp. 202–228.

Mason, D. K., and Chisholm, D. M. *Salivary glands in health and disease.* Philadelphia: W. B. Saunders, 1975, p. 178.

Maynard, J. D. Recurrent parotid enlargement. *Br. J. Surg.* 52:784–789, 1965.

Mikulicz, J. Discussion at Verein fur wissenschaftliche Heilkunde zu Konigsberg January 23, 1888. *Berl. Klin. Wchschr.* 25:759, 1888.

Mikulicz, J. Uber eine eigenartige symmetrische Erkrankung der Thranen—und Mundspeicheldrusen. *Beitr Chir Festschrift fur Billroth* 610–630, 1892.

Mikulicz, J. Concerning a peculiar symmetrical disease of the lacrymal and salivary glands. *Med. classics* 2:137–186, 1937.

Morgan, W. S. The probable systemic nature of Mikulicz's disease and its relation to Sjögren's syndrome. *N. Engl. J. Med.* 251:5–10, 1954.

Morgan, W. S., and Castleman, B. A clinicopathologic study of "Mikulicz's disease." *Am. J. Pathol.* 29:471–503, 1953.

Moutsopoulos, H. M., et al. Sjögren's syndrome (sicca syndrome): current issues. *Ann. Intern. Med.* 92:212–226, 1980.

Patey, D. H. Inflammation of the salivary glands with particular reference to chronic and recurrent parotitis. *Ann. R. Coll. Surg. Engl.* 36:26–46, 1965.

Patey, D. H., and Thackray, A. C. Chronic "sialectatic" parotitis in the light of pathological studies on parotidectomy material. *Br. J. Surg.* 43:43–50. 1955.

Payne, R. T. Recurrent pyogenic parotitis: its pathology, diagnosis and treatment. *Lancet* 1:348–353, 1933.

Pearson, R. S. B. Recurrent swelling of the parotid glands. *Arch. Dis. Child.* 10:363–376, 1935.

Pearson, R. S. B. Recurrent swellings of the parotid gland. *Gut* 2:210–217, 1961.

Pinkus, G. S., and Dekker, A. Benign lymphoepithelial lesion of the parotid glands associated with reticulum cell sarcoma. Report of a case and review of the literature. *Cancer* 25:121–127, 1970.

Ranger, I. An experimental study of sialography, and its correlation with histological appearances, in normal parotid and submandibular glands. *Br. J. Surg.* 44:415–418, 1957.

Schall, G. L. Sjögren's syndrome—newer aspects of research, diagnosis, and therapy. *Ann. Intern. Med.* 75:937–950, 1971.

Schall, G. L., et al. Xerostomia in Sjögren's syndrome. *JAMA* 216:2109–2116, 1971.

Shearn, M. A. Sjögren's syndrome. In *Major problems in internal medicine*, vol. II. Philadelphia: W. B. Saunders, 1971, pp. 1–255.

Sjögren, H. Zur Kenntnis der Keratoconjunctivitis sicca (keratitis filiformis bei hypofunktion der tränendrüsen). *Acta Ophthalmol.* 11 (Suppl. 2):1–151, 1933.

Sjögren, H. Further studies of keratoconjunctivitis sicca. *Acta Ophthalmol.* 15:519–520, 1937.

Sjögren, H. Keratoconjunctivitis sicca and chronic polyarthritis. *Acta Med. Scand.* 130:484–488, 1948.

Sjögren, H. Some problems concerning kerato-conjunctivitis sicca and the sicca syndrome. *Acta Ophthalmol.* 29:33–47, 1951.

Sjögren, H., and Bloch, K. J. Keratoconjunctivitis sicca and the Sjögren's syndrome. *Surv. Ophthalmol.* 16:145–159, 1971.

Som, P., et al. Manifestations of parotid gland enlargement: radiographic, pathologic, and clinical correlations. Part I: The autoimmune pseudo-sialectasias. *Radiology* 141:415–419, 1981a.

Som, P. M., et al. Manifestations of parotid gland enlargement: radiographic, pathologic, and clinical correlations. Part II: The diseases of Mikulicz's syndrome. *Radiology* 141:421–426, 1981b.

Stephen, K. W., et al. Diagnostic value of quantitative scintiscanning of the salivary glands in Sjögren's syndrome and rheumatoid arthritis. *Clin. Sci.* 41:555–61, 1971.

Talal, N.; Asofsky, R.; and Lightbody, P. Immuno-globulin synthesis by salivary gland lymphoid cells in Sjögren's syndrome. *J. Clin. Invest.* 49:49–54, 1970.

Talal, N., and Bunim, J. J. Development of malignant lymphoma in the course of Sjögren's syndrome. *Am. J. Med.* 36:529–540, 1964.

Talal, N.; Sokoloff, L.; Barth, W. F. Extrasalivary lymphoid abnormalities in Sjögren's syndrome (reticulum cell sarcoma, "pseudolymphoma," macro-globulinemia). *Am. J. Med.* 43:50–65, 1967.

Thackray, A. C. Sialectasis. *Archives of the Middlesex Hospital* 5:151–159, 1955.

Thackray, A. C., and Lucas, R. B. Atlas of tumor pathology. Tumors of the major salivary glands. Washington, D.C.: Armed Forces Institute of Pathology, 1974.

Touloukian, R. J. Salivary gland disease in infancy and childhood. In *Diseases of the salivary glands*, ed. R. M. Rankow and I. M. Polayes. Philadelphia: W. B. Saunders, 1976, pp. 284–303.

Waterhouse, J. P. Focal adenitis in salivary and lacrimal glands. *Proc. R. Soc. Med.* 56:911–918, 1963.

Waterhouse, J. P. Inflammation in the salivary glands. *Br. J. Oral Surg.* 3:161–171, 1966.

Waterhouse, J. P., and Doniach, I. Post-mortem prevalance of focal lymphocytic adenitis of the submandibular salivary gland. *J. Pathol. Bacteriol.* 91:53–64, 1966.

Whaley, K., et al. Sialographic abnormalities in Sjögren's syndrome, rheumatoid arthritis, and other arthritides and connective tissue diseases. A clinical and radiological investigation using hydrostatic sialography. *Clin. Radiol.* 23:474–482, 1972.

Whaley, K., et al. Sjögren's syndrome. 2. Clinical associations and immunological phenomena. *Q. J. Med.* 42:513–548, 1973a.

Whaley, K., et al. Sjögren's syndrome. 1. Sicca components. *Q. J. Med.* 42:279–304, 1973b.

Whaley, K., and Buchanan, W. W. Sjögren's syndrome and associated diseases. In *Clinical Immunology*, ed. C. W. Parker. Philadelphia: W. B. Saunders, 1980, pp. 632–666.

Chapter 5   Asymptomatic Enlargement of the Parotid Glands

Clinical Findings

Asymptomatic parotid enlargement, also called asymptomatic parotid hypertrophy, sialosis, and sialadenosis, is characterized by nonneoplastic, noninflammatory chronic or recurrent enlargement of the parotid glands (Rauch 1959; Seifert 1965; Rauch and Seifert 1970; Thackray and Lucas 1974). According to an historical review by Borsanyi (1962), this condition has been recognized since early in this century, when a report described malnourished fellahin in Egypt (Sandwith 1905). The condition involves mainly the parotid glands (Batsakis and McWhirter 1972) and especially the preauricular portions (Davidson, Leibel, and Berris 1969; Rauch and Gorlin 1970; Mason and Chisholm 1975). The submandibular glands may be enlarged as well (Sandstead, Koehn, and Sessions 1955; Wolfe, Summerskill, and Davidson 1957; Banks 1967; Davidson, Leibel, and Berris 1969; Hemenway and Allen 1959), occasionally without parotid enlargement (Barbero and Sibinga 1962; Thomson, McCrossan, and Mason 1974). According to a review by Sandstead, Koehn, and Sessions (1955), all races and all age groups are affected (Kenawy 1937; Hemenway and Allen 1959; Katsilambros 1961). The age incidence parallels the age distribution of the underlying cause. Both sexes may be equally involved (Borsanyi and Blanchard 1961; Davidson, Leibel, and Berris 1969). The onset of the salivary gland enlargement is slow and usually is not accompanied by pain or symptoms of inflammation (Mason and Chisholm 1975). The enlargement is usually bilateral and symmetrical but may be unilateral or asymmetrical (DuPlessis 1956; Duggan and Rothbell 1957; Hemenway and Allen 1959; Batsakis and McWhirter 1972; Conley 1975; Zeit 1981). The enlargement may wax and wane, reflecting worsening or improvement in the underlying condition (Borsanyi and Blanchard 1960, 1961; Batsakis 1979). It may be reversible (DuPlessis 1956; Wolfe, Summerskill, and Davidson 1957;

may be ongoing or may have occurred in the distant past (Sandstead, Koehn, and Sessions 1959; Duggan and Rothbell 1957; Hemenway and Allen 1959). Enlargement of the submandibular glands may accompany the parotid enlargement, as occurred in 2 of 16 patients reported by Wolfe, Summerskill, and Davidson 1957).

A wide variety of drugs have also been implicated as causative agents in this condition. Reviews of this subject can be found in Borsanyi (1962), Rauch and Gorlin (1970), Batsakis and McWhirter (1972), Mason and Chisholm (1975), and Hausler and associates (1977). The findings are summarized here. Phenylbutazone and oxyphenbutazone have been reported to be associated with enlargement of the parotid and submandibular glands, in some instances with pain and tenderness consistent with acute sialadenitis (Murray-Bruce 1966; Banks 1967, 1968; Garfunkel et al. 1974). Iodides (Oppenheimer, Nelson, and Gandhi 1960; Carter 1961; Sussman and Miller 1956; Navani et al. 1972) and sulfisoxazole (Nidus, Field, and Rammelkamp 1965) have also been reported to be associated with the enlargement of the parotid and submandibular glands, sometimes with acute sialadenitis. Despite the term *iodide mumps*, which suggests parotid enlargement (Kohri et al. 1977), the submandibular glands may be more affected than the parotid glands (Harden 1968; Talner et al. 1971; Batsakis and McWhirter 1972). Isoproterenol also has been implicated (Borsanyi 1962). Other drugs listed by Hausler and colleagues (1977) as being associated with asymptomatic parotid enlargement are atropine and its derivatives, imipramine, phenothiazides, benzodiazepines, MAO inhibitors, drugs used in the treatment of Parkinson's disease, and hypotensive agents such as reserpine and guanethidine and their derivatives. Heavy metals such as lead, mercury, and bismuth (Borsanyi and Blanchard 1960; Sprinkle 1968; Batsakis and McWhirter 1972) and drugs used in the treatment of thyroid disease, including methimazole, thiocyanates, and thiourea drugs (Batsakis and McWhirter 1972) such as Thiouracil and Propylthiouracil, have also been reported to cause enlargement of the major salivary glands. In the case of exposure to heavy metals the submandibular glands may be particularly involved and may show signs and symptoms of inflammation. According to Curtis and Swenson (1948), swelling of the submandibular glands is also a frequent development in patients receiving Thiouracil; parotid enlargement also has been reported. Signs and symptoms of acute sialadenitis may accompany administration of Thiouracil.

It would appear from a review of the literature that either the parotid glands or the submandibular glands or both may develop acute or chronic swelling and sometimes pain as adverse reactions to certain drugs. Such swelling and pain and tenderness as a result of drug reactions tend to appear and disappear in shorter intervals—days, or in some instances hours or even minutes—than is the case with sialosis associated with nutritional or hormonal causes, and may also be associated with more local signs and symptoms suggestive of sialadenitis. It apparently is not true, as suggested by Banks (1968), that parotid enlargement secondary to drugs is invariably asymptomatic.

Prolonged starch ingestion (Merkatz 1961; Silverman and Perkins 1966), obesity (Hemenway and Allen 1959; Batsakis and McWhirter 1972), and hyperlipoproteinemia (Kaltreider and Talal 1969; Shanoff 1970) have also been reported to be associated with this condition. Kaltreider and Talal (1969) state that because of the presence of obesity, mild alcoholism, or diabetes in the patients with hyperlipoproteinemia, it is difficult to ascribe an etiologic relationship between the parotid enlargement and the hyperlipoproteinemia. Batsakis (1979, 113) states that "identifiable metabolic disorders such as diabetes mellitus, hypertension, hyperlipidemia, and obesity are often so intermixed that the singling out of one as the underlying cause is impossible."

Sialosis has also been described in uremia (Rauch and Gorlin 1970; Batsakis 1979) and in cystic fibrosis, where the submandibular glands are selectively involved (Barbero and Sibinga 1962).

Various mechanisms by which salivary gland enlargement may be produced have been suggested. Often the pathogenesis is not clear (Wolfe, Summerskill, and Davidson 1957; Brick 1958; Hemenway and Allen 1959; Borsanyi and Blanchard 1960, 1961; Davidson, Leibel, and Berris 1969; Parret et al. 1979). Batsakis and McWhirter (1972) suggest that the viscid saliva produced by atropine and drugs with atropinelike effect finds difficulty exiting the gland, thus producing enlargement of the glands. It is also possible that the xerostomia produced by these and other drugs, including phenylbutazone and phenothiazines, may predispose to ascending infection in the gland (Banks 1967; Batsakis 1979), although enlargement can occur without infection (Worthington 1965). The iodides, which are concentrated by the salivary glands (Harden, Mason, and Alexander 1966), as are the heavy metals, are thought to exert a direct toxic effect on the salivary glands (as is a high local concentration of ammonia in uremia) (Batsakis 1979). Borsanyi (1962) suggested that enlargement may be due to a sialogogic action that may be caused by some drugs. Rothbell and Duggan (1957) and Davidson, Leibel, and Berris (1969) draw attention to the occurrence together of fatty infiltration in the parotid glands and fatty liver in alcoholism, chronic malnutrition, and diabetes, suggesting that a disturbance of nutrition or metabolism underlies the changes in both organs. Duggan and Rothbell (1957) state that asymptomatic parotid enlargement is of unknown pathogenesis but always seems to be associated with disturbed nutrition. These authors and others (Sandstead, Koehn, and Sessions 1955) note that the enlargement may accompany malnutrition or that the glands may enlarge upon the reinstitution of proper nutrition. DuPlessis (1956) (quoting Gillman, Gilbert, and Gilman [1947]) and Gillman and Gillman (1951) note that the serous acini are much more susceptible to malnutrition than the mucous acini, thus explaining why the parotid glands, which are almost entirely serous in nature, are usually more affected in malnutrition than are the submandibular glands with their mixed serous and mucous acini. These authors go on to state that if the submandibular glands are affected, only the serous acini are involved until a later stage, when the mucous acini are also affected.

Prolonged starch ingestion is thought to produce enlargement of the acinar cells by continual stimulation (Merkatz 1961; Silverman and Perkins 1966). Hyperfunction of the parotid gland has also been suggested in cirrhosis of the liver (Borsanyi and Blanchard 1961). Work hypertrophy has also been suggested by DuPlessis (1956). Batsakis and McWhirter (1972) postulate that hypertrophy of the glandular tissue and eventual fatty atrophy may result from some excessive or prolonged stimulation of unknown nature.

Duggan and Rothbell (1957, 1266) state that "it is not clear whether all cases of asymptomatic parotid enlargement, either within this series or globally, should be considered as variants of a single process. Unity among the observed cases is not established. Perhaps no unity should be expected, for one is dealing in a sense with nondescript parotid enlargement, defined only by the absence of inflammatory disease." Merkatz (1961, 1366) states that "it need not be assumed that the etiology of parotid enlargement is invariably the same in cases of starvation, dietary aberrations, obesity, cirrhosis and diabetes mellitus."

Pathology

The pathologic findings have been well described. Autopsy studies have shown that the parotid glands may be two to four times normal weight (Kenawy 1937). Batsakis and Sylvest (1977) point out that fatty replacement of salivary glandular tissue normally increases with age, but that such fatty replacement occurs in an exaggerated form in malnutrition, alcoholism and cirrhosis, diabetes and obesity. According to Thackray and Lucas (1974), the pathologic findings in asymptomatic parotid enlargement consist of increase in the size of acinar cells with loss of their granulation, atrophy of the striated ducts, interstitial edema, and infiltration of fat into the salivary glands. These authors state also that fatty replacement of the gland parenchyma and the enlargement and degranulation of the parenchymal cells may take place together, but either change may take place alone. Thus, two different histologic patterns exist (fig. 5.1, 5.6d). Fibrosis may also be present (Borsanyi 1962). According to Borsanyi and Blanchard (1960, 1961), the acini may be enlarged, reaching almost double normal size in some instances (Hemenway and Allen 1959). The cells themselves may be distended with granules and may be enlarged to 50% of their normal dimension (Batsakis 1979). The pale vacuolated cytoplasm seen in some instances (Bonnin 1954; Bonnin, Moretti and Geyer 1954), with few or no zymogen granules, has been interpreted as possibly caused by fatigue of the cells following prolonged and excessive stimulation (Wolfe, Summerskill, and Davidson 1957; Hemenway and Allen 1959). Silverman and Perkins (1966) also reported depletion of zymogen granules and hydropic swelling of the acinar cells, possibly similar to the appearances of the foamy cytoplasm in the acinar cells described by Hausler and co-workers (1977) (fig. 5.1).

According to Batsakis and McWhirter (1972), the acinar hypertrophy and increased zymogen granulation occurs predominantly in the early stages, while fatty atrophy and fibrosis dominate in the later stages. The fibrosis is of mild to moderate degree and is confined to the interlobular septa. The pathologic appearances are notable for the absence of any inflammatory changes.

The enlargement of the parotid glands noted clinically is due presumably to various combinations of these pathologic changes.

Radiology

Findings on conventional sialography include enlargement of the salivary glands so that the duct branches are separated farther from each other than normal, and compression and narrowing of the intraglandular branches so that some of the smaller peripheral branches may not fill (Nash and Morrison 1949; Borsanyi and Blanchard 1960, 1961; Borsanyi 1962; Mandel and Baurmash 1969; Batsakis and McWhirter 1972) (figs. 5.2, 5.3, 5.4A,B, 5.5B,C, 5.6B,C). These findings appear to be due to compression of the ducts by the increased volume of parenchyma and fat within the gland. Such changes may be reversible, provided that fatty replacement of the gland tissue has not taken place (Batsakis 1979). DuPlessis (1956), for example, reported a case of carcinoma of the esophagus in which these sialographic appearances returned to normal within 23 days following correction of malnutrition by feeding through a gastrostomy.

Very little information has been available on CT examination of sialosis (Zeit 1981). CT, which can be done without contrast material (figs. 5.4C, 5.5D, 5.6E,F, 5.7B,C, 5.8A,B, 5.9, 5.10A,B), shows the parotid glands to be enlarged; they may be of lower density than normal (Zeit 1981) if an increased amount of fat has been deposited in the gland at the expense of the functioning glandular tissue, and provided that a great deal of fibrosis has not occurred. We do not agree with Zeit (1981) that normal parotid tissue has a density equal to that of muscle. According to Sone and co-workers (1982), the density of the parotid gland on CT image varies considerably among normal patients, ranging from a slightly higher density than fatty tissue to a slightly lower density than muscle. It is also known that fatty replacement of salivary tissue is a normal finding with increasing age (Batsakis and Sylvest 1977). Indeed, approximately 25% of the parenchymal cell volume is lost between childhood and old age (Batsakis 1979). Furthermore, according to these authors, such fatty replacement may occur in an exaggerated form in asymptomatic enlargement of the parotid glands, especially in the later stages of this process.

The density of the parotid glands in the cases of asymptomatic parotid enlargement that we have examined have ranged from −100 to +40 Hounsfield units. Thus the density of the glands alone as shown on CT is not necessarily diagnostic of asymptomatic parotid enlargement. If the glands are enlarged, however, and the Hounsfield numbers are lower than the usual range of soft tissue density, suggesting a high fat content, the findings are consistent with this diagnosis (figs. 5.6E, 5.7B,C, 5.8A, 5.9, 5.10A). Hemenway and Allen (1959) reported that parotid biopsies in a series of seven patients with sialosis showed the amount of fat in the involved parotid glands to vary from practically none to over 90% in different instances. On the other hand, if the enlargement of the gland in sialosis were to be due predominantly to enlargement of the acinar cells (Batsakis and McWhirter 1972; Thackray and Lucas 1974), or if a great deal of fibrosis has been laid down, the Hounsfield measure might not approach that of fat, and thus CT examination might be less specific (figs. 5.4C, 5.5D). In either event, the tissue density and texture are either relatively even throughout the gland without any focal areas of increased density, or there may be a more or less regular lobular pattern with fibrous septa between the lower density fattier areas evenly distributed throughout the gland.

The submandibular glands may be normal in size or slightly to moderately enlarged (figs. 5.6F, 5.7C, 5.8B, 5.10B) and may be normal in density (+25 to +50 Hounsfield units) or lower than normal in density (−50 to +15 Hounsfield units). The lobular architecture is preserved.

Differential Diagnosis

There are a number of diseases in addition to asymptomatic parotid enlargement that may be associated with enlargement of the salivary glands and not necessarily accompanied by signs or symptoms of inflammation, such as Sjögren's syndrome, granulomatous diseases such as sarcoid, tuberculosis, and fungus, and bilateral salivary gland tumor such as Warthin's tumor or lymphoma.

The differential diagnosis between Sjögren's syndrome and benign parotid hypertrophy may be difficult on a clinical basis alone since each of these entities may be associated with xerostomia, xerophthalmia, and swelling of the salivary glands (Hausler et al. 1977). According to these authors, this differential diagnosis may be greatly aided by quantitative scintigraphy, since the uptake of the isotope in the salivary glands is markedly diminished in Sjögren's syndrome, while it is elevated in asymptomatic parotid hypertrophy (fig. 5.11).

The diagnosis of asymptomatic parotid enlargement can usually be suspected on the basis of the clinical history and physical findings and may be confirmed by the CT examination if the gland is shown to be enlarged and of relatively fatty density evenly distributed throughout the gland. The differential diagnosis will also be aided by the presence of pertinent clinical, laboratory, radioisotopic, and sialographic findings. It may be necessary in some instances to resort to biopsy of the involved gland.

Asymptomatic parotid enlargement is not of itself a significant condition, and no local treatment is indicated (Hemenway and Allen 1959). Its importance lies in differentiating it from inflammatory or neoplastic enlargements of the gland and in drawing attention to possible serious underlying diseases that may be responsible for the enlargement of the salivary glands. Because its true nature has not always been recognized, surgical excision of such glands has occasionally been performed in the past (Gilman, Schwartz, and Gilman 1956; Davidson, Leibel, and Berris 1969). With the kinds of radiologic examinations available today, it is possible that even such occasional surgery may be avoidable in the future.

CASES

Biopsy of a parotid gland from a patient with sialosis

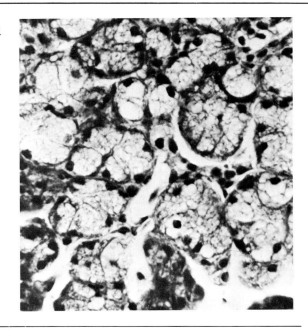

Figure 5.1

Swollen serous acinar cells with foamy cytoplasm (× 512). (Hausler et al. 1977. Reprinted with permission.)

Asymptomatic parotid enlargement. Left parotid sialogram performed with Ethiodol

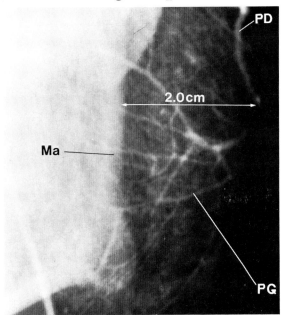

Figure 5.2A

AP view.

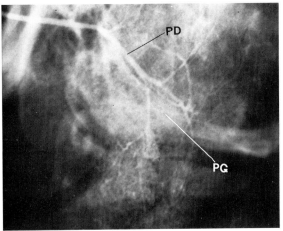

Figure 5.2B

Lateral view. The parotid gland is moderately enlarged; the main duct is displaced moderately laterally at 2 cm from the lateral margin of the mandible. The intraglandular branches are spread apart by the enlarged parenchyma. Only modest acinar opacification could be obtained.

Ma = mandible
PD = parotid duct
PG = parotid gland

The patient is a 42-year-old man with a two-year history of swelling and soreness of both parotid glands. This patient has a long history of severe acute and chronic alcohol abuse and also has diabetes mellitus. The sialogram was performed in 1971. Follow-up in 1977 showed continued severe alcohol abuse; the parotid glands continued to be enlarged.

275

Asymptomatic parotid enlargement

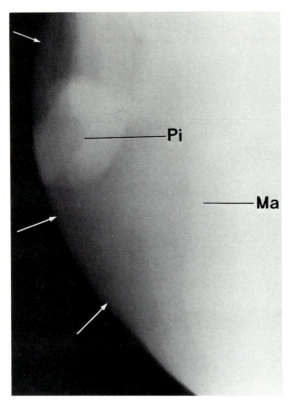

Figure 5.3A

Soft-tissue plain film of the right parotid area without contrast material, AP view. The soft-tissue swelling is due to marked enlargement of the parotid gland (*arrows*).

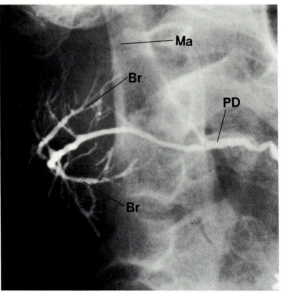

Figure 5.3B

Right parotid sialogram, anterior-oblique view, early duct filling phase, with Ethiodol. The intraglandular duct branches are somewhat spread apart.

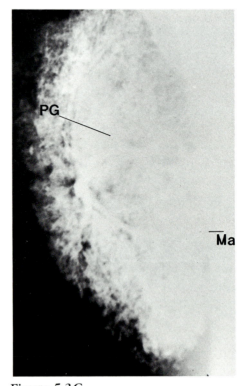

Figure 5.3C

AP view, acinar opacification phase.

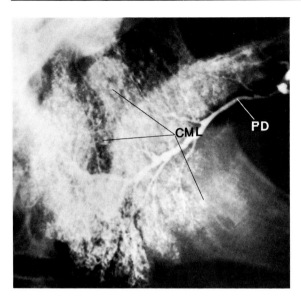

Figure 5.3D

Lateral view, acinar opacification phase. The gland is markedly enlarged, confirming the appearances shown in figure 5.3A. That much of the contrast material is extravasated is suggested by the pattern of multiple small, rather discrete, curvilinear collections of Ethiodol in a lobular distribution throughout the parotid gland.

The patient was 58 years old with chemical diabetes and a history of alcohol abuse at the time the sialogram was performed (1973). At that time there was a two-month history of gradual painless swelling of the parotid glands, the right more than the left. The right parotid gland was enlarged and quite firm.

Follow-up clinical examination 10 years later, with cessation of alcohol abuse in the meantime, shows that the parotid enlargement has disappeared and the parotid glands are normal in size.

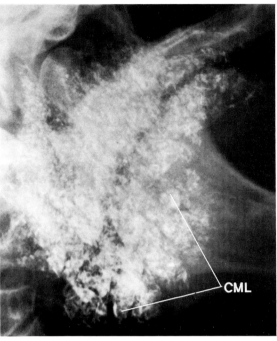

Br = branches of parotid duct
CML = contrast material in lobular pattern
Ma = mandible
PD = parotid duct
PG = parotid gland
Pi = pinna

Figure 5.3E

Postevacuation phase, lateral view, showing much retained contrast material, confirming that there is much extravasated contrast material in the parenchyma. This may be due to overinjection of contrast material or to increased fragility of the epithelium of the ducts, or both, and is not believed to be particularly characteristic of sialosis.

Asymptomatic parotid enlargement, left parotid sialogram

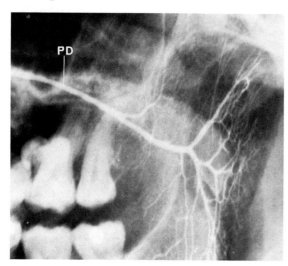

Figure 5.4A

Lateral view, with Ethiodol. This sialogram and that of figure 5.4B were obtained in 1980.

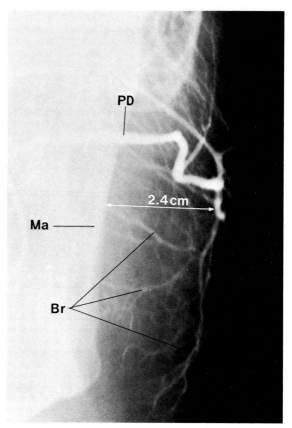

Figure 5.4B

AP view; the parotid gland is moderately enlarged; the main duct is displaced laterally, located approximately 2.4 cm lateral to the lateral margin of the mandible. The branches are moderately spread apart. No acinar filling could be obtained. Compare with figures 2.7B and 2.8A.

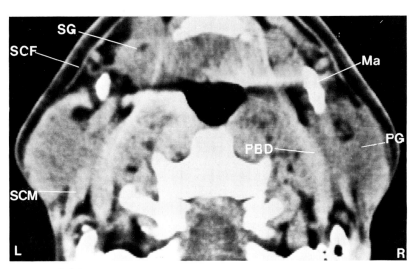

Br = parotid duct branches
Ma = mandible
PBD = posterior belly of digastric muscle
PD = parotid duct
PG = parotid gland
SCF = superficial layer of external cervical fascia
SCM = sternocleidomastoid muscle
SG = submandibular gland
R = right
L = left

Figure 5.4C

CT examination, the head extended and the gantry angled 20 degrees craniad, performed without contrast material in 1983. No basic clinical change had occurred in the parotid glands in the interval since the sialogram. The parotid glands are both enlarged. Density within the parotid glands ranged from 30 to 39 Hounsfield units. Compare with figure 2.21.

The patient was a 49-year-old man at the time of sialography. He was moderately obese but had lost approximately 40 pounds four years previously by dieting. The left parotid gland had been enlarged for many years; the swelling varied at approximately six-month intervals, but the glands had not basically changed in size over many years. During times of increased swelling, the left parotid gland was slightly sensitive but not painful. There was no history of diabetes, alcohol abuse, liver disease, or medication. The cause for the sialosis in this instance is not known.

Physical examination done at follow-up approximately three years after the sialogram, at the time of the CT study, showed the left parotid gland to be moderately enlarged and the right to be slightly enlarged. Both glands were moderately firm, with clearly palpable edges. The submandibular glands were normal clinically and on CT study.

Asymptomatic parotid enlargement

Br = parotid duct branches

Ma = mandible

MM = masseter muscle

MPM = medial pterygoid muscle

PBD = posterior belly of the digastric muscle

PD = parotid duct

PG = parotid gland

PP = posterior process of the parotid gland

SCM = sterno-cleidomastoid muscle

SMP = stylo-mandibular process of the parotid gland

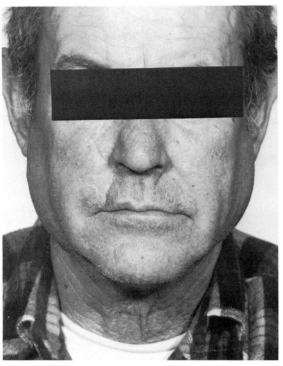

Figure 5.5A

Photograph of the patient taken in 1983 showing markedly enlarged bulging parotid glands bilaterally.

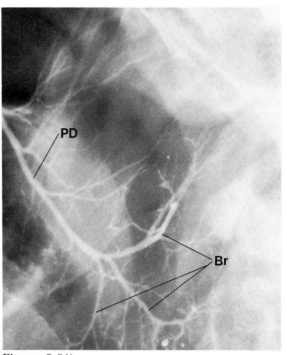

Figure 5.5B

Left parotid sialogram performed in 1979 with injection of Ethiodol; lateral view. Acinar opacification is deficient.

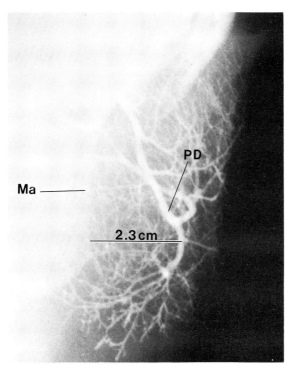

Figure 5.5C

AP view; the parotid gland is moderately enlarged. The main duct is displaced approximately 2.3 cm lateral to the lateral margin of the mandible. The duct branches are all moderately spread apart. Compare with figures 2.7B and 2.8A. (Rabinov 1981. Reprinted with permission.)

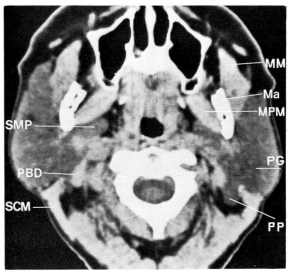

Figure 5.5D

Straight axial CT performed without contrast material in 1983. The parotid glands are markedly enlarged bilaterally but only relatively low in density, measuring + 11 to + 13 Hounsfield units. The tissue density and texture are the same in the various regions of both glands. No focal masses are present. The neck fat measured − 93 Hounsfield units, and the masseter muscle measured + 66 Hounsfield units. Compare with figure 2.20.

The patient was a 50-year-old man at the time of sialography. He had a long history of severe chronic alcohol abuse and cirrhosis of the liver and was diabetic. Both parotid glands had been markedly enlarged for more than eight years, with some variation in size intermittently so that sometimes the right gland would be enlarged, sometimes the left, and sometimes both. The patient noted that when alcohol abuse diminished; the size of the parotid glands also diminished for example, during a recent 18-day hospital stay, the parotid glands had temporarily returned almost to normal size. There was no history of xerostomia or xeropthalmia. The basic condition of the parotid glands had not changed in the interval between sialography and the CT examination. Physical examination revealed both parotid glands to be markedly enlarged, to three to four times normal size, and quite firm but not tender.

Asymptomatic parotid enlargement

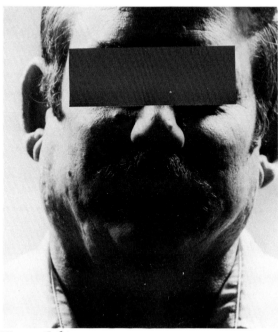

Figure 5.6A

Recent photograph of the patient (1983); marked enlargement of both parotid glands is evident.

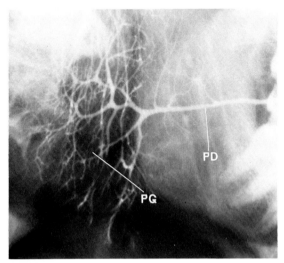

Figure 5.6B

Right parotid sialogram performed in 1981; the contrast material is Ethiodol; lateral view.

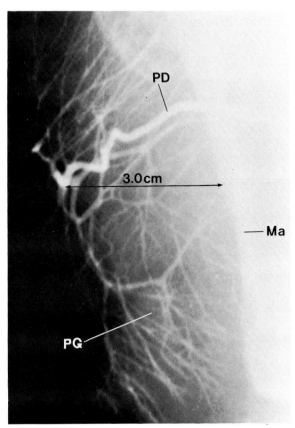

Figure 5.6C

AP view; the parotid gland is enlarged and the duct branches are spread apart. The distance between the main duct and the lateral margin of the mandible measures 3 cm. Compare with figures 2.7B, 2.8A. Acinar filling could not be easily obtained without causing discomfort and was not accomplished. The appearances of the sialogram performed at the same time on the left parotid gland were similar.

The patient was a 41-year-old moderately obese man at the time of performance of the sialography, with a three- to four-year history of gradual enlargement of both parotid glands. There has been occasional "aching" sensation in the left parotid gland. There is no history of diabetes, alcohol abuse, or medication, and the

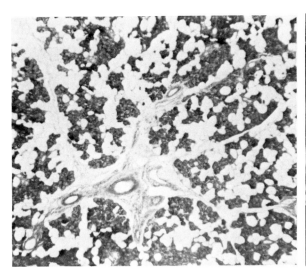

Figure 5.6D

Biopsy of the right parotid gland performed in 1981 showing "considerable fatty infiltration, minimal chronic inflammation around rare ducts and slight fibrosis of the stroma."

While moderate amounts of fat are commonly present in the normal parotid gland, the amounts shown in this specimen are unusually large.

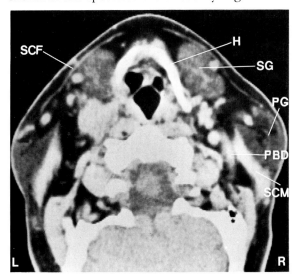

Figure 5.6F

CT of the submandibular glands, same position as in figure 5.6E; the submandibular glands are normal in size but lower in density than usually seen, measuring + 7 to + 11 Hounsfield units. The right one is best shown in this particular image. The left one was better seen in an adjacent image. Compare with figure 2.30.

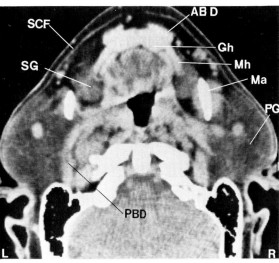

Figure 5.6E

Semiaxial CT of the parotid glands, performed in 1983; no contrast material was used. The head is extended and the gantry is angled 17 degrees craniad. The parotid glands are markedly enlarged bilaterally and measured − 7 to − 20 Hounsfield units. The density and tissue architecture are the same in various regions of both glands. Note preservation of lobular pattern. Compare with figure 2.21.

ABD = anterior belly of digastric muscle
GH = genio-hyoid muscle
H = hyoid bone
Ma = mandible
MH = mylo-hyoid muscle
PBD = posterior belly of digastric muscle
PD = parotid duct
PG = parotid gland
SCF = super-ficial layer of external cervical fascia
SCM = sterno-cleidomastoid muscle
SG = subman-dibular gland

cause of the sialosis in this patient has not been determined. The enlargement was first noted by the patient's friends approximately three years earlier, when he was on a strict diet and had lost approximately 30 pounds. Physical examination at the time of the sialogram revealed that the parotid glands were soft in consistency, approximately two to three times normal size, and not tender. Two years later, at the time of performance of the CT examination done in follow-up, the degree of enlargement of the parotid glands and the intermittent aching sensation were unaltered, with the glands still moderately severely enlarged, the right slightly more than the left, and soft in consistency.

Asymptomatic parotid enlargement, CT of the salivary glands without contrast material

ABD = anterior belly of the digastric muscle
ECA = external carotid artery
Ma = mandible
PBD = posterior belly of digastric muscle
PG = parotid gland
PFV = posterior facial vein
SCF = superficial layer of the external cervical fascia
SCM = sternocleidomastoid muscle
SG = submandibular gland

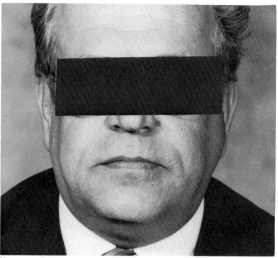

Figure 5.7A

Recent photograph of the patient; both parotid glands are enlarged, the left more than the right. A large lipoma is present in the left parotid gland.

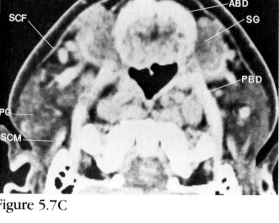

Figure 5.7C

Lower CT section through the parotid and submandibular glands, same projection as in figure 5.7B. The submandibular glands are within normal limits of size but measure + 8 to + 16 Hounsfield units, somewhat lower than is normally seen.

The patient is a 48-year-old man with a five- to six-month history of enlargement of both parotid glands, the left more than the right. There is no history of alcoholism, diabetes, or medication, and the cause for the sialosis in this patient is undetermined.

Physical examination showed both parotid glands to be moderately enlarged, soft in consistency; the left was enlarged two to three times normal, the right, one and a half times normal size. There was no tenderness. The submandibular glands were not clinically enlarged. A 2.5-cm lipoma (not shown) was also present in the left parotid gland, shown by CT in other sections.

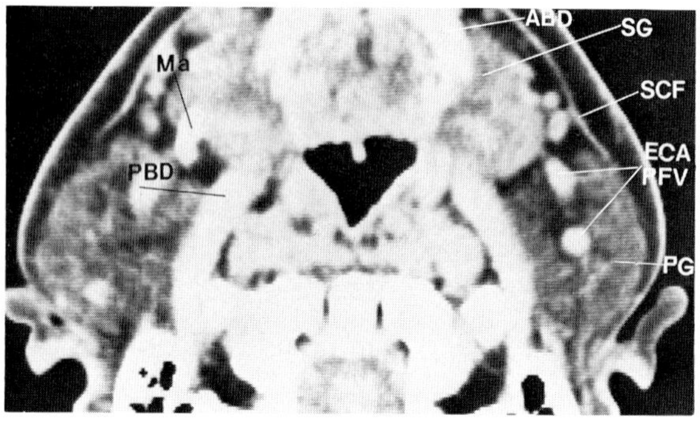

Figure 5.7B

CT performed through the midportion of the parotid glands; the head is extended and the gantry is angled 20 degrees craniad. Both parotid glands are moderately enlarged. The CT measurement of the parotid parenchyma ranged from − 9 Hounsfield units to − 27 Hounsfield units. Subcutaneous fat measured − 76 Hounsfield units. The lobular architecture of the glands is preserved.

Asymptomatic parotid enlargement, CT of the salivary glands without contrast material

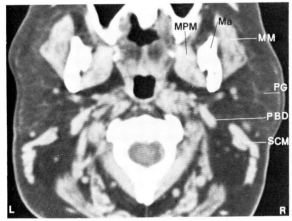

Figure 5.8A

Near axial CT through the parotid glands with the head flexed and the gantry angled 6° degrees caudad. The glands are both enlarged, the right more than the left; the left parotid gland is flattened by the positioning cushion. The density of the parotid glands is less than usual measuring − 66 to − 100 Hounsfield units. A regular pattern of lobules and interlobular septa is demonstrated throughout the glands.

The patient was a 47-year-old obese woman at the time of the CT, complaining of recurrent fluctuating swelling of the parotid glands, more on the right than on the left and of the submandibular glands, also more on the right than on the left. The patient has a history of chronic alcohol abuse. The parotid glands were bilaterally diffusely enlarged, the right larger than the left, and there was bilateral enlargement of the submandibular glands, also more on the right than on the left. The glands were not tender. Six months later, with cessation of alcohol abuse, the right parotid gland has become considerably smaller and appears almost normal when clinically examined.

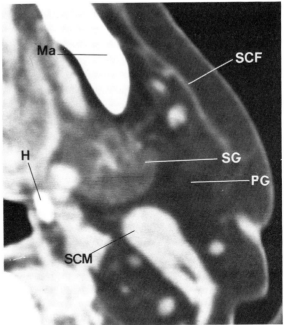

H	= hyoid bone
Ma	= mandible
MM	= masseter muscle
MPM	= medial pterygoid muscle
PBD	= posterior belly of the digastric muscle
PG	= parotid gland
SCF	= superficial layer of external cervical fascia
SCM	= sternocleidomastoid muscle
SG	= submandibular gland

Figure 5.8B

Lower CT section through the right submandibular gland, same patient and position as in figure 5.8A. This gland is possibly slightly enlarged and is lower in density than is usually seen in the normal, measuring in this instance − 20 to − 51 Hounsfield units. Cervical fat measured − 102 to − 118 Hounsfield units. The lobular pattern within the gland is visible because of the increased fat content in the parenchyma.

Asymptomatic parotid enlargement

Ma = mandible
PBD = posterior belly of digastric muscle
PG = parotid gland
SCM = sterno-cleidomastoid muscle
SG = submandibular gland

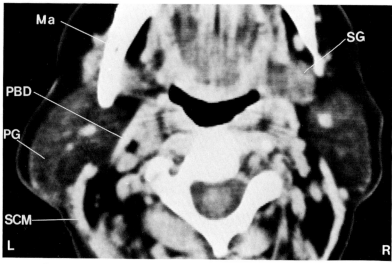

Figure 5.9

Straight axial plain CT of the parotid glands. The parotid glands are both moderately enlarged, the left more than the right, and both are low in density, measuring −34 to −57 Hounsfield units. The lobular architecture is preserved in both glands.

The patient was a 76-year-old woman who was referred to CT for evaluation of a mass in the neck on the right side; this was shown by CT to be due to enlargement of the right submandibular gland of undetermined cause. The parotid glands were also noted clinically to be enlarged bilaterally, the left more than the right. No specific etiology could be found for this enlargement. The glands were soft to slightly firm to palpation.

Asymptomatic parotid enlargement, CT examination without contrast material

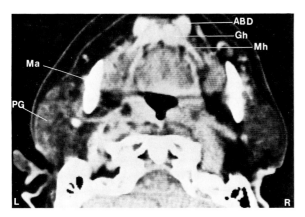

ABD = anterior belly of digastric muscle
GH = genio-hyoid muscle
H = hyoid bone
Ma = mandible
MH = mylo-hyoid muscle
PBD = posterior belly of the digastric muscle
PG = parotid gland

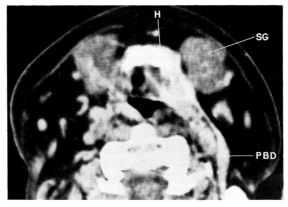

Figure 5.10A

Semiaxial projection with the head extended and the gantry angled 20 degrees craniad; section through the mid portion of the parotid glands showing these glands to be enlarged bilaterally, the left more than the right. The glands are moderately low in density, the parenchyma ranging from − 10 to − 41 Hounsfield units. The tissue architecture is the same throughout both glands. No masses are seen.

The patient is a 53-year-old woman with a history of enlargement of the left parotid gland for 25 years and of the right parotid gland for three or four years. The glands have sometimes been larger than at present and occasionally have been tender. There is a probable history of alcohol abuse. On physical examination both parotid glands were enlarged two to three times normal size, the left was somewhat larger than the right, and both were firm in consistency but not tender.

Figure 5.10B

Section through the submandibular glands, showing these to be possibly slightly larger than average; the submandibular gland parenchyma ranged from + 15 to + 30 Hounsfield units.

Salivary gland scintigraphy, right lateral views

BP = bucco-
pharyngeal region
P = parotid
gland
S = subman-
dibular gland
T = thyroid
gland

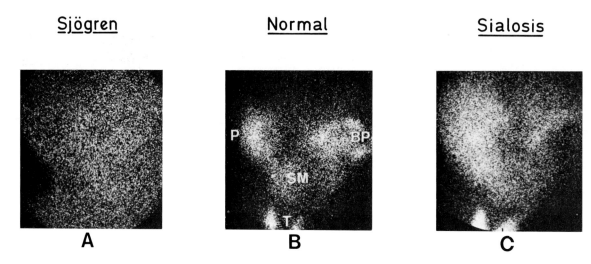

Sjögren

Normal

Sialosis

A

B

C

Figure 5.11A

Lack of glandular uptake in a woman with xerostomia from Sjögren's syndrome.

Figure 5.11B

Normal uptake of parotid, submandibular gland, and buccopharyngeal region in a man with normal salivation.

Figure 5.11C

Increased uptake and hypertrophy of the parotid gland in a woman with xerostomia caused by sialosis. (Hausler et al. 1977. Reprinted with permission.)

References

Banks, P. Hypersensitivity and drug reactions involving the parotid gland. *Br. J. Oral Surg.* 5:60–67, 1967.

Banks, P. Non-neoplastic parotid swellings: a review. *Oral Surg.* 25:732–745, 1968.

Barbero, G. J., and Sibinga, M. S. Enlargement of the submaxillary glands in cystic fibrosis. *Pediatrics* 29:788–793, 1962.

Batsakis, J. G. *Tumors of the head and neck. Clinical and pathological considerations.* Baltimore: Williams & Wilkins, 1979.

Batsakis, J. G., and McWhirter, J. D. Non-neoplastic diseases of the salivary glands. *Am. J. Gastroenterol.* 57:226–247, 1972.

Batsakis, J. G., and Sylvest, V. *Pathology of the salivary glands.* Chicago: American Society of Clinical Pathologists, 1977.

Bonnin, M. La parotidose des cirrhoses alcooliques. *Bull. Acad. Natl. Med. (Paris)* 138:322–324, 1954.

Bonnin, M.; Moretti, G.; and Geyer, A. Les grosses parotides des cirrhoses alcooliques. *Le Presse Med.* 62:1449–1451, 1954.

Borsanyi, S. J. Chronic asymptomatic enlargement of the parotid glands. *Ann. Otol. Rhinol. Laryngol.* 71:857–867, 1962.

Borsanyi, S. J., and Blanchard, C. L. Asymptomatic enlargement of the parotid glands. Its diagnostic significance and particular relation to Laennec's cirrhosis. *JAMA* 174:102–105, 1960.

Borsanyi, S. J., and Blanchard, C. L. Asymptomatic enlargement of the parotid glands in alcoholic cirrhosis. *South. Med. J.* 54:678–682, 1961.

Brick, I. B. Parotid enlargement in cirrhosis of the liver. *Ann. Intern. Med.* 49:438–451, 1958.

Carter, J. E. Iodide "mumps." *N. Engl. J. Med.* 264:987–988, 1961.

Conley, J. *Salivary glands and the facial nerve.* New York: Grune & Stratton, 1975.

Conner, S.; Iranpour, B.; and Mills, J. Alteration in parotid salivary flow in diabetes mellitus. *Oral Surg.* 30:55–59, 1970.

Curtis, G. M., and Swenson, R. E. Thiouracil and its allies in the treatment of hyperthyroidism. An experimental and clinical survey. *Int. Abstr. Surg.* 86:105–123, 1948.

Davidson, D.; Leibel, B. S.; and Berris, B. Asymptomatic parotid gland enlargement in diabetes mellitus. *Ann. Intern. Med.* 70:31–38, 1969.

Diamont, H. Enlargement of the parotid gland. *Acta Otolaryngol. (Stockh.)* 52:299–310, 1960.

Duggan, J. J., and Rothbell, E. N. Asymptomatic enlargement of the parotid glands. *N. Engl. J. Med.* 257:1262–1267, 1957.

DuPlessis, D. J. Parotid enlargement in malnutrition. *S. Afr. Med. J.* 30:700–703, 1956.

Garfunkel, A. A., et al. Phenylbutazone-induced sialadenitis. *Oral Surg.* 38:223–226, 1974.

Gillman, J.; Gilbert, C.; and Gillman, T. The Bantu salivary gland in chronic malnutrition, with a brief consideration of the parenchyma-interstitial tissue relationship. *S. Afr. J. Med. Sci.* 12:99–109, 1947.

Gillman, J., and Gillman, T. *Perspectives in human malnutrition.* New York: Grune & Stratton, 1951.

Gilman, R. A.; Schwartz, M.; and Gilman, J. S. Fatty infiltration of the parotid gland. Report of a case simulating a tumor. *JAMA* 160:48–49, 1956.

Harden, R. McG. Submandibular adenitis due to iodide administration. *Br. Med. J.* 1:160–161, 1968.

Harden, R. McG.; Mason, D. K.; and Alexander, W. D. The relation between salivary iodide excretion and the plasma inorganic iodine concentration. *Q. J. Exp. Physiol.* 51:130–135, 1966.

Hausler, R. J., et al. Differential diagnosis of xerostomia by quantitative salivary gland scintigraphy. *Ann. Otol. Rhinol. Laryngol.* 86:333–341, 1977.

Hemenway, W. G., and Allen, G. W. Chronic enlargement of the parotid gland: hypertrophy and fatty infiltration. *Laryngoscope* 69:1508–1523, 1959.

John, H. J. Mikulicz's disease and diabetes. *JAMA* 101:184–187, 1933.

Kaltreider, H. B., and Talal, N. Bilateral parotid gland enlargement and hyperlipoproteinemia. *JAMA* 210:2067–2070, 1969.

Katsilambros, L. Asymptomatic enlargement of the parotid glands. *JAMA* 178:513–514, 1961.

Kenawy, M. R. Endemic enlargement of the parotid gland in Egypt. *Trans. R. Soc. Trop. Med. Hyg.* 31:339–350, 1937.

Kohri, K., et al. Bilateral parotid enlargement ("iodide mumps") following excretory urography. *Radiology* 122:654, 1977.

Mandel, L., and Baurmash, H. D. Asymptomatic parotid hypertrophy. In *Diagnosis of diseases of the mouth and jaws*, ed. E. V. Zegarelli; A. H. Kutscher; and G. A. Hyman. Philadelphia: Lea & Febiger, 1969, pp. 384–385.

Mason, D. K., and Chisholm, D. M. *Salivary glands in health and disease.* Philadelphia: W. B. Saunders, 1975.

Merkatz, I. R. Parotid enlargement resulting from excessive ingestion of starch. *N. Engl. J. Med.* 265:1304–1306, 1961.

Murray-Bruce, D. J. Salivary gland enlargement and phenylbutazone. *Br. Med. J.* 2:1599–1600, 1966.

Nash, L., and Morrison, L. F. Asymptomatic chronic enlargement of the parotid glands—review and report of a case. *Ann. Otol. Rhinol. Laryngol.* 58:646–664, 1949a.

Nash, L., and Morrison, L. F. Functions of the parotid gland. *Ann. Otol. Rhinol. Laryngol.* 58:976–987, 1949b.

Navani, S., et al. Evanescent enlargement of the salivary glands following tri-iodinated contrast media. *Br. J. Radiol.* 45:19, 1972.

Nidus, B. D.; Field, M.; and Rammelkamp, C. H. Salivary gland enlargement caused by sulfisoxazole. *Ann. Intern. Med.* 63:663–665, 1965.

O'Hara, A. E. Sialography: past, present, and future. *CRC Crt. Rev. Radiol. Sci.* 4:87–139, 1973.

Oppenheimer, P.; Nelson, K.; and Gandhi, K. Bilateral parotid enlargement due to iodides. *Quart. Bull. North-Western Univ. Med. School* 34:299–301, 1960.

Parret, J., et al. Sialoses hypertrophiques—reflexions sur 13 observations. *Rev. Stomatol. Chir. Maxillofac.* 80:329–333, 1979.

Phillips, L. G. Parotid swelling associated with lactation, with the report of a case. *Am. J. Obstet. Gynecol.* 22:434–435, 1931.

Rauch, S. *Die speicheldrusen des menschen. Anatomic, physiologie und klinische pathologie.* Stuttgart: Georg Thieme, 1959.

Rauch, S., and Gorlin, R. J. Diseases of the salivary glands. In *Thoma's Oral Pathology*, ed. R. J. Gorlin and H. M. Goldman. St. Louis: C. V. Mosby, 1970, pp. 962–1070.

Rauch, S., and Seifert, G. Sialadenoses (sialoses). *Encycl. Med. Chir., Paris*, Stomatol 3 B10 22057:4–10, 1970.

Rothbell, E. N., and Duggan, J. J. Enlargement of the parotid gland in diseases of the liver. *Am. J. Med.* 22:367–372, 1957.

Sandstead, H. R.; Koehn, C. J.; and Sessions, S. M. Enlargement of the parotid gland in malnutrition. *Am. J. Clin. Nutr.* 3:198–214, 1955.

Sandwith, F. M. Medical diseases in Egypt, part 1. London: Henry Kimpton, 1905, p. 295.

Seifert, G. Die pathologische anatomie der speicheldrusen-erkrankungen (sialadenitis, sialadenose, sialome syndrome). *HNO* 13:1–11, 1965.

Shanoff, H. M. Parotid enlargement and hyperlipoproteinemia. *JAMA* 211:2016, 1970.

Shearn, M. A. *Sjögren's syndrome. Major problems in internal medicine*, vol. II. ed. Lloyd H. Smith. Philadelphia: W. B. Saunders, 1971.

Silverman, M., and Perkins, R. L. Bilateral parotid enlargement and starch ingestion. *Ann. Intern. Med.* 64:842–846, 1966.

Sone, S., et al. CT of parotid tumors. *AJR* 3:143–147, 1982.

Sprinkle, P. M. Recurrent salivary gland disease. *Laryngoscope* 78:654–661, 1968.

Sussman, R. M., and Miller, J. Iodide "mumps" after intravenous urography. *N. Engl. J. Med.* 255:433–434, 1956.

Talner, L. B., et al. Elevated salivary iodine and salivary gland enlargement due to iodinated contrast media. *Am. J. Roentgenol.* 112:380–382, 1971.

Thackray, A. C., and Lucas, R. B. *Tumors of the major salivary glands. Atlas of tumor pathology.* Second series, Fascicle 10. Washington D.C.: Armed Forces Institute of Pathology, 1974.

Thomson, J. A.; McCrossan, J.; and Mason, D. K. Salivary gland enlargement in acromegaly. *Clin. Endocrinol.* 3:1–4, 1974.

Wolfe, S. J.; Summerskill, W. H. J.; and Davidson, C. S. Parotid swelling, alcoholism and cirrhosis. *N. Engl. J. Med.* 256:491–495, 1957.

Worthington, J. J. Parotid enlargement bilaterally in a patient on thioridazine. *Am. J. Psychiatry* 121:813–814, 1965.

Zeit, R. M. Hypertrophy of the parotid gland: computed tomographic findings. *AJR* 136:199–200, 1981.

Chapter 6   Benign and Malignant Salivary Gland Lesions

Introduction

Salivary gland neoplasms occur in less than 3 persons per 100,000 population (Eneroth 1964), although an increased incidence has been reported in Eskimos (Wallace et al. 1963). and survivors of exposure to high doses of radiation from atomic bombs (Belsky et al. 1972). Benign and malignant tumors and miscellaneous lesions can be classified as follows (Thackray and Sobin 1972):

I. Epithelial Tumors
   A. Adenomas
      1. Pleomorphic adenoma (mixed tumor)
      2. Monomorphic adenoma
         a. adenolymphoma
         b. oxyphilic adenoma
         c. other types
   B. Mucoepidermoid tumors
   C. Acinic cell tumors
   D. Carcinomas
      1. Adenoid cystic carcinoma
      2. Adenocarcinoma
      3. Epidermoid carcinoma
      4. Undifferentiated carcinoma
      5. Carcinoma in pleomorphic adenoma (malignant mixed tumor)
      6. Metastatic carcinoma
II. Nonepithelial tumors
   A. Lymphomas
   B. Neurogenic tumors
      1. Neurolemmoma
      2. Neurofibroma
   C. Hemangioma

In most reported series there has been an equal sex incidence or a slight predominance for females. Approximately 80% of all salivary gland tumors occur in the parotid gland, 5% in the submandibular gland, 1% in the sublingual gland, and 10% to 15% in the minor salivary glands (Eneroth 1971). Benign tumors comprise 65% to 80% of parotid tumors, 50% to 60% of submandibular tumors, and 25% to 40% of minor salivary gland neoplasms (Batsakis 1979). From these figures, it is evident that the incidence of malignancy increases in inverse proportion to the size of the gland. Adenolymphoma (Warthin's tumor), oncocytoma, and acinic cell tumor are usually confined to the parotid gland. The acinic cell tumor is the second most frequent tumor after Warthin's tumor to occur bilaterally and multicentrically (Chong, Beahrs, and Woolner 1974). Table 6.1 summarizes the incidence of the various benign and malignant epithelial tumors (Eneroth 1971). In the benign group, the most common lesions are pleomorphic adenoma and adenolymphoma. Mucoepidermoid tumors, adenoid cystic carcinoma, undifferentiated carcinoma, acinic cell tumors, and carcinoma in pleomorphic adenoma are the most common malignancies.

Staging of parotid cancers has been published by the American Joint Committee for Cancer Staging and End Results Reporting (1978). The size of the mass is a prominent factor in the staging of parotid gland cancers, and four classes are defined: T1 (0–2 cm), T2 (2–4 cm), T3 (4–6 cm), and T4 (>6 cm) lesions. The stage of the disease correlates with the recurrence rate, incidence of lymph node and distant metastases, and overall survival rate. The incidence of cervical lymph node metastasis present at the time of initial presentation in all parotid cancers is said to be 13% (Spiro, Huvos, and Strong 1975). An increased rate of local metastasis has been reported in squamous cell carcinoma, T3 parotid cancer, and carcinoma associated with facial nerve paralysis (Johns 1980).

Many factors influence survival of patients with malignant tumors of the salivary glands. Cure rates reported three or five years postdiagnosis are inadequate because recurrence is reported as late as 10 to 25 years after the initial diagnosis (Conley 1975). A prime

Table 6.1.
Percentage distribution of different epithelial tumor types in the parotid and submandibular glands

	Parotid Gland		Submandibular Glands	
	Middlesex Hospital (651 cases)	Karolinska Sjukhuset (2158 cases)*	Middlesex Hospital (60 cases)	Karolinska Sjukhuset (170 cases)*
Adenomas				
Pleomorphic adenoma	72.0	76.2	68.0	60.0
Monomorphic adenoma				
Adenolymphoma	9.0	4.7	1.7	2.4
Oxyphilic adenoma	0.6	1.0	0	0.6
Other types of adenoma	1.8		0	
Mucoepidermoid tumors	2.3	4.1	0	3.6
Acinic cell tumors	1.2	3.0	0	0.6
Carcinomas				
Adenoid cystic carcinoma	3.3	2.3	17.0	15.0
Adenocarcinoma	1.0	2.4	1.7	0
Epidermoid carcinoma	1.0	0.3	3.3	7.0
Undifferentiated carcinoma	3.7	3.9	6.6	9.0
Carcinoma in pleomorphic adenoma	4.1	1.5	1.7	1.8

*Eneroth, C-M. Salivary gland tumors in the parotid gland, submandibular gland, and the palate region. *Cancer* 27:1415–1418, 1971.

example is the adenoid cystic carcinoma, which may recur many years after the initial diagnosis. The prognosis is adversely affected by the following factors: (1) facial nerve paresis, (2) pain, (3) fixation to skin and deep structures, (4) extension of tumor outside the parotid gland, (5) neck or distant metastases, and (6) histologic grade of tumor. Low-grade mucoepidermoid and acinic cell carcinomas have a good long-term survival while malignant mixed tumors, adenoid cystic carcinoma, undifferentiated carcinoma, and high-grade mucoepidermoid carcinoma carry a poor prognosis.

A host of lesions and abnormalities arising in structures adjacent to the salivary glands have to be differentiated from primary benign and malignant salivary tumors. Tumors or cysts originating from the mandible or temporomandibular joint may extend into the parotid and be mistaken for a primary parotid lesion (Kinkead, Bennett, and Tomich 1981; Janecka and Conley 1978; Heydt 1977; Ethell 1979). Large sebaceous or dermoid cysts overlying the salivary glands can simulate intraglandular pathology. A prominent transverse process of the atlas in a thin patient may create the false impression of a parotid lesion. Masseter muscle hypertrophy (detailed in chapter 7) is another condition not to be confused with parotid tumor.

Epithelial Tumors

Adenomas

Pleomorphic Adenoma

(Figs. 6.1–6.11)

Pleomorphic adenoma is the most common tumor of the major salivary glands. In a review of 4245 cases of pleomorphic adenoma by Rauch (1959), 92.5% were seen in the major salivary glands (84% in the parotid gland, 8% in the submandibular gland, and 0.5% in the sublingual glands), 6.5% in the minor salivary glands, and 1% outside the head and neck region. Sites of involvement other than the major salivary glands include the nasopharynx, hard and soft palates, lips, buccal mucosa, tongue, oropharynx, mandible, thyroglossal duct, temporal bone, and hypophyseal duct.

There is a slight preponderance in women with a ratio of about 4:3 (Thackray and Lucas 1974). The majority of patients are between 30 and 50 years of age with a peak incidence around the age of 40. Tumors in children are rare but have been reported in infants (Howard et al. 1950).

Most pleomorphic adenomas develop in the superficial portion of the parotid gland; only about 10% of these tumors are situated in the deep portion (Thackray and Lucas 1974). Tumors may arise from the accessory portions of the parotid gland tissue and may be located far forward on the cheek. Initially the tumor is within the substance of the gland, but subsequently, in large lesions, it protrudes and reduces the gland to a rimlike cap of tissue.

Characterized by slow, intermittent growth, pleomorphic adenomas are smooth, encapsulated, and often lobulated with bosselated surfaces. The majority range in size from approximately 2 to 6 cm (Thackray and Lucas 1974). Mixed tumors grow by expansion and form small excrescences, which arise from the surface of the tumor and penetrate through the shell of fibrous tissue into the adjacent gland. Cyst formation and hemorrhage do occur, especially when the tumor is large. The tumor usually presents as a single lesion and is rarely multifocal or bilateral. There is no exact correlation between the various histologic subtypes and the biological behavior of the tumor. The majority of these adenomas are made up of epithelial and myoepithelial cells with a mesenchymal component, composed of mucoid, myxomatous, cartilaginous, and hyaline elements, spindle cells, and less frequently bone. The lesion is easily movable, round, smooth, and moderately firm and presents as a swelling behind the angle of the mandible or below and in front of the ear. Most often patients complain of a pressure sensation in the region of the parotid gland. Pain is not a common feature and, when present, suggests malignancy.

Recurrences are most often multiple and arranged in nodular

clusters, which are usually mobile and asymptomatic. The clusters may contain 5 to 15 tumor foci dispersed throughout the area of the original surgical field; they also may be diffuse within the residual parotid gland (Conley 1975). The recurrences usually grow very slowly, over a period of 1 to 10 years. Occasionally the rate of growth is more aggressive. Second, third, or fourth recurrences may present as a conglomerate, fixed, bulky mass occupying the entire parotid area and comprising the facial nerve. The recurrence of pleomorphic adenomas has decreased from the rate of 30% to 50% (noted about 30 to 40 years ago, when enucleation was practiced) to approximately 0.5% with the introduction of the removal of the superficial portion of the parotid gland (Conley 1975). Recurrences are usually secondary to rupture of the capsule during surgery, with spillage of primary tumor leading to seeding, failure to remove multiple projections of tumor at the periphery (when enucleation and inadequate excision are carried out), or detachment of tumor projections during enucleation.

Tumors of the deep lobe of the parotid gland are rarely diagnosed in the early stages (Conley 1975). When the tumor is small, the patient usually has no symptoms. Sufficient growth has to occur for the lateral lobe to be displaced outward, thereby simulating a tumor of the superficial portion of the gland, or the tumor has to extend, with its bulk, into the region of the pharynx, which causes a bulging of the palate and tonsils. These deep lobe tumors are difficult to differentiate from minor salivary gland tumors, which present in the region of the soft palate, retropharynx, lateral pharynx, and nasopharynx. Minor salivary gland tumors occur more within the substance of the soft palate rather than in the retropharyngeal or pharyngeal areas and are somewhat mobile. The deep lobe tumors are more pharyngeal in position and usually more fixed. Malignant tumors of the deep lobe appear somewhat earlier, because the patients frequently present with pain and facial nerve paresis. The facial nerve is involved relatively early by these tumors, because it is part of the lateral boundary of the deep extension of the parotid gland. Paresis frequently occurs before there is either any gross visual or palpable abnormality of the gland. The initial presentation of the tumor may be that of a generalized weakness of the face. The development of facial nerve paralysis is gradual and relentless in its course without change or alteration. This paralysis needs to be differentiated from Bell's palsy, which has a rather precipitous type of onset.

Monomorphic Adenoma

Adenolymphoma (Warthin's Tumor, Papillary Cystadenoma Lymphomatosum)
(Figs. 6.12–6.16)
Adenolymphoma is a tumor composed of acinophilic epithelium forming glandular and cystic structures, sometimes with a papillary

cystic arrangement. A variable amount of lymphoid tissue with follicles is contained in the stroma. The Warthin's tumor constitutes approximately 5% to 10% of parotid gland neoplasms (Thackray and Lucas 1974). This tumor occurs primarily in the parotid gland and is rarely encountered in the submandibular gland or minor salivary glands. The majority of these masses occur within the substance of the parotid gland and usually arise from the superficial portion and tail of the gland. A few lesions are situated in the upper part of the neck close, but not continuous, to the gland. These tumors are bilateral in about 5% of cases, with the opposite gland developing a tumor at the same time or up to 15 years later (Thackray and Lucas 1974; Hales and Hansen 1977). There is also a tendency for this tumor to occur in multiple areas within the gland. Adenolymphomas are much more common in men than in women; the incidence ratio of males to females is about 5:1 (Chaudhry and Gorlin 1958). The age range is approximately 20 to 90 years with an average age of 55 years. The tumor may contain a unilocular cyst or may be multicystic. These tumors may become secondarily infected. Adenolymphomas are slow-growing, completely encapsulated lesions and range in size from about 2 to 6 cm with an average of 3 cm (Foote and Frazell 1953). Usually ovoid, the tumor has a smooth surface and varies in consistency from moderately firm to cystic. Cysts contain fluid that is thin, yellow, cloudy—and more often, brown, and tenacious. Up to six separate and distinct tumors in one parotid gland have been reported. The adenolymphoma concentrates technetium 99m pertechnetate, which shows up as a hot spot on the nuclear medicine scan (Thackray and Lucas 1974; Stebner et al. 1968). The tumor has a benign course and recurrences are rare and usually attributed to inadequate local excision particularly if there is multifocal occurrence.

Oxyphilic Adenoma
(Fig. 6.17)
Oxyphilic adenoma (oncocytoma) is a benign tumor (although a few examples of malignant oncocytomas have been reported) consisting of large cells with granular eosinophilic cytoplasm (oncocytes) (Blanck, Eneroth, and Jakobsson 1970; Christopherson 1949). The tumors are circumscribed, round or ovoid, smooth surfaced or slightly lobulated, and moderately firm. Uncommon, they account for less than 1% of parotid tumors. The submandibular gland is rarely involved. These lesions are slightly more common in females and occur predominantly between the ages of 55 and 70 years. Both parotid glands may be involved by this tumor.

Other Types of Adenoma
Other types of adenoma constitute approximately 2% of salivary gland tumors (Batsakis 1979; Thackray and Lucas 1974), and include

sebaceous adenoma, lymphadenoma, basal cell adenoma, and clear cell adenoma. They occur predominantly in the older age groups with a peak incidence in the sixth and seventh decades. These benign tumors are round to oval and are well encapsulated in the salivary glands. Monomorphic adenomas are not uncommon (Thackray and Lucas 1974; Eneroth, Hjertman, and Moberger 1972) in the minor salivary glands.

Mucoepidermoid Tumors

(Figs. 6.18 and 6.19)

Mucoepidermoid carcinomas account for approximately 4% to 9% of salivary gland tumors and nearly one third of all malignant tumors (Patey, Thackray, and Keeling 1965; Morgan and MacKenzie 1968; Eversole 1970). In a review of 550 cases of mucoepidermoid carcinomas of the major salivary glands, 89% involved the parotid gland, 8.4% the submaxillary gland, and 0.4% the sublingual gland (Eversole 1970). In the same review, the minor salivary glands were involved in 265 cases of which 41.1% occurred in the palate and 14% in the buccal mucosa. In adults, the mucoepidermoid tumor is the most common malignancy in the parotid and second only to adenoid cystic carcinoma in the submandibular gland. It represents the most common malignant salivary gland tumor in children (Krolls, Trodahl, and Boyers 1972). This tumor occurs in all age groups, but is most frequent in the fourth and fifth decades of life, with a slight female preponderance.

Low-grade and high-grade malignancies are differentiated; the low-grade malignant group follows a course clinically similar to that of benign mixed tumors of the salivary gland, which are characterized by slow growth, a painless lump, frequent recurrences, and rare metastasis. The tumors are usually circumscribed but poorly encapsulated and may adhere to surrounding structures. They may vary in size from 2 to 6 cm with an average diameter of 2 to 3 cm. The neoplasm occurs most frequently in the superficial lobe of the parotid gland. These tumors contain squamous cells and glandular mucous-secreting cells with a proportion of less differentiated cells usually designated as intermediate. The predominant cell group encountered is the epidermoid cell and intermediate tumor cell, which produces mucus. In the more malignant type of tumors, the epidermoid and intermediate cells dominate the histologic picture. Prognosis seems to be related to histologic differentiation of these lesions and when no tumor is found at the resection margins.

Acinic Cell Tumors

Acinic cell tumors arise from serous acinar cells. Encountered almost exclusively in the parotid gland, they account for 2.5% to 4% of all parotid tumors and 15% to 17% of all malignant tumors of the parotid (Levin, Robinson, and Lin 1975). Bilateral parotid gland involvement occurs in approximately 3% of cases (Levin, Robinson, Lin 1975).

Submandibular and sublingual gland involvement are rare and minor salivary gland involvement is unusual. Acinic cell tumors have been reported in all age groups, including children as young as 4 years old, but occur predominantly in patients in their fifth and sixth decades. Acinic cell tumors occur two to three times more frequently in women.

The acinic cell adenocarcinomas manifest as single, round, lobulated, circumscribed encapsulated masses that may contain areas of necrosis, hemorrhage, or both. The tumor may also be multifocal, as exemplified by Warthin's tumor (Thackray and Lucas 1974; Clarke, Hentz, and Mahoney 1969), and has been found in both parotid glands. Recurrent lesions tend to be multinodular and less well defined and are not limited to the gland, but can occur anywhere in the surgical field.

Clinical presentation consists of a painless slow-growing mass. In some cases, however, pain, rapid growth, and facial nerve involvement have been described.

Five-year survival figures of more than 80% have been recorded (Frazell 1968), but after 20 years' followup reported survival rates fell to 56% (Eneroth, Jakobsson, and Blanck 1966). Some patients need repeated excisions of tumor nodules over a period of many years. Regional lymph node metastases occur in approximately 10% of patients. Distant metastases to the lung and bones develop in 15% of cases (Spiro, Huvos, and Strong 1975).

Carcinomas

Adenoid Cystic Carcinoma

(Fig. 6.20)

Adenoid cystic carcinoma constitutes 4% to 8% of all salivary gland tumors, 2% to 6% of parotid gland tumors, approximately 15% of submandibular gland tumors, and 14.6% to 25% of all minor salivary gland tumors (Foote and Frazell 1954; Fine, Marshall, and Horn 1960). It occurs more often in the minor salivary glands and has a predilection for the hard palate. While the tumor may appear in any age group, it is distinctly rare in patients under the age of 20 and occurs most frequently in patients in the late fifth and early sixth decades of life. The most common initial presentation is the appearance of a mass. Lesions in general are firm with no tendency toward cystic degeneration or hemorrhage. Adenoid cystic carcinomas measure, on the average, from 0.5 to 6 cm (Foote and Frazell 1953). Although some tumors appear encapsulated, most show incomplete encapsulation with regions of infiltrative growth and attachment to adjacent structures. Adenoid cystic carcinomas have a relatively low incidence of lymph node metastases, but have a propensity to cause distant metastases, particularly to the lung. The incidence of metastasis varies from 20% to 50% in various studies, and increases with time following the initial diagnosis (Moran et al. 1961; Spiro, Huvos, and Strong 1975). Invasion

The appearance of hemangiomas on CT is a reflection of their macroscopic distribution within the parotid gland. There is ill-defined enlargement of the gland in the capillary type and a well-defined mass in the cavernous type. Enhancement following contrast media administration is a predominant feature of these vascular tumors.

Lymphangioma

(Figs. 6.41 and 6.42)

Lymphangiomas have been divided into three histologic groupings based on the size of the lymph channels. The classification includes simple or capillary, cavernous, and cystic lymphangiomas (hygromas). All three elements may coexist in the same lesion (Karmody, Fortson, and Calcaterra 1982). Cystic hygromas are most commonly seen shortly after birth and 90% occur prior to the end of the second year of life. They may, however, occur as late as the fourth or fifth decades of life (less than 10% of all lymphangiomas). In 80% of patients, a cystic hygroma involves the neck. Situated in the posterior triangle and extending into adjoining anatomic areas, these cysts are soft, painless compressible masses, which are asymptomatic and have only cosmetic deformity. On CT scan, lymphangiomas display water density (Silverman, Korobkin, and Moore 1983). Enhancing septa may be seen following infusion or bolus injection of contrast material. The parotid or submandibular glands are usually secondarily involved from a lymphangioma in the neck, which may take the form of an indentation of the gland contour or invasion of the parenchyma.

Lipoma

(Figs. 6.43–6.45)

Lipomas, which occur in approximately 1% of parotid tumors, are round to spheroid and soft in consistency (Thackray and Lucas 1974; Seldin et al. 1967). The tumor may be well circumscribed within or diffusely infiltrating the gland. A lipoma may be intraglandular and manifest as a solitary mass or indent or invade the gland from the surrounding periglandular tissue. On CT, the lesion is characterized by low attenuation coefficients (Carter et al. 1981; Som and Sanders 1984).

Miscellaneous Lesions

Cysts

Branchial Cleft Cysts

(Figs. 6.46–6.48)

The typical branchial cleft cyst is a smooth, round nontender mass located between the external auditory canal and the clavicle anterior to and beneath the sternocleidomastoid muscle (Moran and Buchanan 1978; Simpson 1967). The cyst may be situated within the parotid gland simulating a parotid tumor; cysts adjacent to the parotid or submandibular glands cause indentation of the gland. These cysts are lined by epithelial cells and contain lymphoid elements in the wall. They range in size from 1 to 10 cm in diameter. Although congenital in origin, branchial cleft cysts usually present clinically in the third decade of life.

Branchial cleft cysts are usually nontender, but can become painful when inflamed. The cysts enlarge when infection occurs and decrease in size when the infection resolves. An infected branchial cleft cyst may develop into an abscess and rupture to form a sinus tract.

On CT, the cyst cavity is reflected by a water density mass circumscribed by a well-delimited wall. Enhancement of the wall may occur if infection supervenes.

Epidermoid Cysts

(Figs. 6.49 and 6.50)

Cysts in the parotid are rare and may arise from the parotid duct or represent simple cysts lined by epithelial cells and filled with clear fluid (Moore 1950). These cysts cause a well-defined filling defect in the parenchyma after acinar opacification. On CT scans the cyst may be either isodense or of low density depending on the cyst contents.

Ranula

Ranula is a cyst in the floor of the mouth of variable size and shape, caused by obstruction of the sublingual ducts. The cyst appears as a well-circumscribed, water density mass on the CT scan.

Minor Salivary Gland Tumors

(Figs. 6.51–6.54)

Minor salivary gland tumors occur in many different anatomic areas in the head and neck region. They are situated in the hard and soft palate, lips, cheek, floor of the mouth, posterior tongue, retromolar area, tonsil, pharynx, jaw, and outside the vicinity of the major salivary glands (i.e., nasal cavity, paranasal sinuses, lacrimal gland, larynx, trachea, skin, and breast). This wide distribution is responsible for the many diverse tumors encountered in the upper aerodigestive system. Minor salivary gland tumors comprise the same histopathologic types that are seen in the major salivary glands, except for the adenolymphoma, which has been reported to occur only in the major salivary glands. These tumors differ, however, in cell type, incidence, and growth characteristics.

The patients range in age from the first to the ninth decades with a median age of 50 to 60 years for malignant lesions and 40 to 50 years for benign lesions (Spiro, Koss, and Hajdu 1973). There is a slight preponderance of females in the benign group. Benign tumors most frequently produce asymptomatic swelling that has been present for many months and sometimes years before diagnosis. In the vast majority of cases, the mass is mobile, nontender, and nonulcerated. Pain, ulceration, bleeding, anesthesia, and fixation suggest malignancy.

In one large series these neoplasms accounted for 23% of all salivary gland tumors (Spiro, Koss, and Hajdu 1973). Among the benign lesions, pleomorphic adenoma constitutes the most common lesion (60–92%) (Conley 1975). Minor salivary gland tumors tend to be malignant in 60% to 80% of cases (Spiro, Koss, and Hajdu 1973; Crocker, Calalaris, and Finch 1970; Bergman 1966). Adenoid cystic carcinoma, adenocarcinoma, mucoepidermoid carcinoma, and malignant mixed tumor, in that order, represent the most common malignant lesions (Spiro, Koss, and Hajdu 1973). The most frequent location for benign and malignant tumors is the hard and soft palate with adenoid cystic carcinoma the predominant tumor. The size of the primary tumor varies from a few millimeters to more than 6 cm (median 3–4 cm) (Spiro, Koss, and Hajdu 1973).

The overall rate of cervical lymph node metastases reported in one series was 23% (Spiro, Koss, and Hajdu 1973). Most likely to show metastases were those patients with oat cell carcinoma (50%), malignant mixed tumor (38%), mucoepidermoid carcinoma (30%), adenocarcinoma (25%), and adenoid cystic carcinoma (13.8%) (Spiro, Koss, and Hajdu 1973).

Sublingual Gland Tumors

Approximately 90% of sublingual gland tumors are malignant and account for 0.5% to 4.5% of all salivary gland malignancies (Foote and Frazell 1953). Half of these tumors are adenoid cystic carcinomas and the remainder mucoepidermoid carcinomas. There is a small percentage of squamous cell cancers.

Sublingual tumors should be differentiated from lesions in the anterior floor of the mouth or submandibular gland tumors that have extended anteriorly.

Parapharyngeal Space Lesions

(Figs. 6.55–6.58)

Anatomy

The parapharyngeal space is cone shaped and extends from the base of the skull to the greater cornu of the hyoid bone. The greatest transverse diameter is found superiorly at the skull base and the greater cornu of the hyoid bone is the apex. The medial border consists of the lateral pharyngeal wall (superior constrictor muscles) and tonsillar area. The lateral boundary is defined by the ascending ramus of the mandible, medial pterygoid muscle, medial portion of the parotid gland, posterior belly of the digastric muscle, and sternocleidomastoid muscle. Below the level of the mandible, the lateral wall is formed by muscles and soft tissues of the neck. The anterior limit is represented by the pterygomandibular raphe. The posterior boundary is delimited by the carotid artery, jugular vein, and the prevertebral fascia and muscles. The styloid process and its muscles divide the parapharyngeal space into an anterior and posterior compartment or pre- and poststyloid space. The prestyloid space is adjacent to the palatine tonsil and the poststyloid space contains the internal jugular vein, the internal carotid artery, cranial nerves IX through XII, the cervical sympathetic chain, and lymph nodes. The parapharyngeal space communicates posteromedially with the retropharyngeal space and anteriorly with the submandibular space.

Fascia extends as a broad sheath from the entire length of the styloid process to the posterior edge of the ascending ramus of the mandible. Inferiorly, condensation of the fascia forms the stylomandibular ligament. Tumors with their medial extension from the deep portion of the parotid gland protrude above the stylomandibular ligament through a tunnel into the lateral parapharyngeal space.

Masses within the parapharyngeal space are delimited on three sides by bone and thick fascia: superiorly by the skull base, posteriorly by the cervical spine, carotid, and prevertebral fascia, and laterally by the mandible and the fascia of the parotid gland and pterygoid muscles. Masses within this space will extend medially into the tonsillar area, soft palate, and the nasopharyngeal space. Inferior growth proceeds into the retromandibular area producing a mass at the angle of the mandible. Tumors that extend from the parotid gland into the parapharyngeal space through the stylomandibular tunnel are dumbbell shaped with wide medial and lateral portions and a narrowed neck. Tumors in the deep portion of the gland that grow medially into the parapharyngeal space are round to spherical.

Symptoms of parapharyngeal masses are usually minimal and consist of a sore throat, nonspecific discomfort, dysphagia, and otalgia. A bulge in the lateral pharyngeal wall and tonsillar area, displacement of the soft palate, a mass at the angle of the mandible, or external swelling anterior and inferior to the tragus of the ear is found on physical examination.

Tumors of the parapharyngeal space constitute a wide spectrum of benign and malignant neoplasms as outlined in the following list:

1. Tumors from deep lobe of parotid gland
2. Minor salivary gland tumors
3. Neurogenic tumor
4. Paraganglioma
5. Metastatic tumor
6. Lymphoma
7. Sarcoma
8. Extension of tumors from
   a. base of skull
   b. nasopharynx
9. Branchial cleft cyst

10. Hemangioma and lymphangioma

11. Lipoma

The majority of these lesions are benign and arise from the deep portion of the parotid gland (Work and Hybels 1974). Of these deep lobe parotid tumors, 80% to 90% are benign mixed tumors. Less than 10% of all parotid tumors of the parotid gland are located in the deep lobe (Som, Biller, and Lawson 1981). The second largest variety of tumors comprise neurogenic lesions (Work and Hybels 1974; Gore, Rankow, Hanford 1956), of which the schwannoma predominates.

Most of the minor salivary gland lesions are benign mixed tumors and occur in either the palate or the lateral pharyngeal wall. The lesions are separated from the deep portion of the parotid gland by a fibrofatty plane, which can be delineated by CT. Lipomas, liposarcomas, and hibernomas rarely involve the parapharyngeal space and because of their fat content show low attenuation coefficients on the CT scan. Dermoids and teratomas also reveal low-density areas on the CT scan interspersed with isodense or calcified areas.

Paragangliomas (chemodectomas) of the parapharyngeal space arise from the carotid body or the ganglion nodosum of the vagus nerve. Only 8% of carotid body lesions located in the lower neck extend into the parapharyngeal space; however, two thirds of the glomus vagale tumors are parapharyngeal in position. These lesions uniformly enhance and show a characteristic pattern of vascularity on carotid angiography. Meningioma and chordomas may rarely extend inferiorly into the parapharyngeal space from the skull base. Meningiomas have high absorption values and are enhanced significantly following infusion of contrast media.

In some cases CT is capable of differentiating between parotid and extraparotid masses and determining the vascularity of the lesion, which is a reflection of the degree of enhancement following infusion of contrast material. If a lucent line is seen on the CT scan between the posterolateral margin of the parapharyngeal mass and the contrast-filled parotid gland, then the mass is extraparotid in origin. This line represents the fibrofatty supporting matrix of the parapharyngeal space as it is compressed between the mass and the deep lobe of the parotid gland. If no line is seen on the midtumor scans, then the mass is a deep lobe parotid tumor (Som and Biller 1979). The CT scan also allows assessment of the extent of the tumor into the base of the skull or the pterygopalatine space. Chemodectomas and hemangiomas are characterized by marked enhancement, which is a reflection of their hypervascularity.

Pediatric Salivary Gland Tumors

The overall incidence of noninflammatory tumors of the salivary glands in children is low constituting less than 5% of all salivary gland tumors in all age groups (Reiquam 1963; Castro et al. 1972; Kauffman and Stout 1963). More than one-half of benign tumors of the salivary glands in children are vascular in origin (Goldman and Perzik 1969; Wowro, Fredrickson, and Tennant 1955).

The parotid gland is the most common site for neoplastic lesions in children. Schuller and McCabe (1977) reviewed 428 salivary gland neoplasms in children; 392 cases were reported in the literature and 36 cases were from the University of Iowa. Of 428 neoplasms, 149 (35%) were malignant. The most common benign tumor was a hemangioma; the most common malignant tumor was a mucoepidermoid carcinoma, followed by adenocarcinoma. Of the benign epithelial tumors in children, the pleomorphic adenoma was the most common. Table 6.2 enumerates salivary gland neoplasms in children among the 428 collected cases.

Table 6.2.
Salivary gland neoplasms in children (total 428)

Benign		Malignant	
Hemangioma	111	Mucoepidermoid carcinoma	73
Mixed tumor	94	Acinous cell carcinoma	18
"Vascular proliferative"	40	Undifferentiated carcinoma	14
Lymphangioma	18	Undifferentiated sarcoma	9
Lymphoepithelial tumor	3	Carcinoma ex-mixed tumor	9
Cystadenoma	3	Adenocarcinoma	11
Warthin's tumor	3	Adenoid cystic carcinoma	6
Plexiform neurofibroma	2	Squamous cell carcinoma	3
Xanthoma	2	Mesenchymal sarcoma	2
Neurilemmoma	1	Rhabdomyosarcoma	2
Adenoma	1	Malignant epithelial tumor	1
Lipoma	1	Ganglioneuroblastoma	1
Total	279	Total	149

Adapted from Schuller, D. E., and McCabe, B. F., Salivary gland neoplasms in children. *Otolaryngol. Clin. North Am.* 1977.

Evaluation of Salivary Gland Masses by Sialography with Conventional Tomography

Plain sialography with conventional overhead or spot films is unsatisfactory for use in the diagnosis of salivary gland masses in more than 50% of cases. Only large masses cause enough ductal displacement or a parenchymal defect to allow a tumor diagnosis. The addition of conventional tomography, performed when optimal parenchymal opacification has been achieved with an oily contrast medium (Ethiodol), accomplishes delineation of small masses within the parotid and submandibular glands (Weber and Kushner 1977). These masses cause well or poorly defined lucent defects of the opacified glandular parenchyma. Indentation of glandular margins can also be demonstrated by conventional tomography after opacification of the parenchyma. These conventional tomographic methods, however, do not disclose the extraglandular soft tissue component; they also fail to differentiate the various type of lesions (i.e., benign and malignant tumors, enlarged lymph nodes, and cysts).

Benign lesions including enlarged lymph nodes and cysts displace and stretch the intraglandular ducts, if of sufficient size. Lesions totally within the gland are completely surrounded by these ducts. Masses at the peripheral portion of the gland are only partially encircled by duct branches depending on the size of the intra- and extraglandular component. Acinar opacification, preferably with Ethiodol and tomographic sectioning, is capable of demonstrating masses under 1 cm in diameter. CT sialography with water-soluble contrast material may be substituted for conventional tomography.

Invasive malignant lesions cause ductal cutoff, irregular ductal narrowing and stretching, pooling of contrast media within necrotic areas, and an irregular tumor–parenchymal interface. The majority of malignant tumors including lymphoma, however, do not display invasive characteristics and therefore cannot be differentiated from benign tumors by conventional methods or CT.

Normal CT Anatomy

Parotid Gland

The parotid gland is the largest of the major salivary glands and has a triangular configuration in the lateral and axial projections (Karmody, Fortson, Calcaterra 1982; Bryan et al. 1982; Rabinov, Kell, and Gordon 1984; Golding 1982). The parotid gland on CT is more lucent than the surrounding muscles and is also more radiodense than the adjacent fat in the subcutaneous tissues, infratemporal fossa, and lateral pharyngeal space. The low attenuation values are a reflection of the fatty glandular tissue that is encased in a dense capsule. The gland is subdivided into a medial and lateral portion using the facial nerve as a dividing line. The facial nerve exits from the stylomastoid foramen, enters the gland posteriorly, and passes through the gland lateral to the styloid process, external carotid artery, and retromandibular vein. The facial nerve breaks up into five major trunks within the parotid gland, lateral to the mandible. The facial nerve cannot be demonstrated by CT but the styloid process and retromandibular vein, seen on CT, can be used as anatomic landmarks. The main portion of the parotid gland, which is situated on the outer surface of the mandibular ramus and the masseter muscle, extends superiorly to slightly below the zygomatic arch and inferiorly to the level of the angle of the mandible. The parotid gland extends behind the mandible to fill the retromandibular space and abuts more medially the pterygoid muscles anteriorly and projects over a variable distance into the lateral pharyngeal space. The deep portion of the gland is separated posterolaterally from the major neurovascular sheath by the styloid diaphragm and stylopharyngeous ligament. Lesions of the parotid gland tend to remain localized within the gland because of the tough fascial ligamentous and membranous capsule. The parotid gland has two groups of lymph nodes: a superficial group, which lies on the surface of the gland, and deep nodes, which are located within the gland itself. The parotid duct cannot be demonstrated on CT without the introduction of contrast material into the lumen.

Submandibular Gland

The submandibular gland is half the size of the parotid gland. It is composed of a larger superficial part of the gland, which is covered by the platysma muscle and lies inferior to the myelohyoid muscle. The gland extends to the posterior margin of the myelohyoid muscle and lies with its deep portion superior to the myelohyoid muscle. The submandibular duct passes forward from this deep part beneath and adjacent to the sublingual gland to its opening in the papilla in the anterior floor of the mouth. The submandibular gland has no lymph nodes within its parenchyma, but is surrounded by lymph nodes with additional lymph nodes adjacent to the course of the duct. The superficial part of the gland represents a globular soft tissue structure along the superolateral aspect of the hyoid bone. The deeper parts, including the ducts of the submandibular glands, are best seen on coronal scans. The gland is more radiodense than the parotid gland and has about the same density as the adjacent muscle. For masses adjacent to or within the submandibular gland, it may be necessary to use intraductal contrast material.

Sublingual Glands

The sublingual glands are the smallest of the major salivary glands and lie immediately below the lateral mucosa of the floor of the mouth. The glands are relatively lucent, fatty structures superior to the myelohyoid muscle and lateral to the geniohyoid muscles.

CT Findings in Parotid Lesions

CT is an efficient modality to define the intraglandular location of tumors and the presence or absence of spread beyond the gland capsule (Carter et al. 1981; Bryan et al. 1982; Rabinov, Kell, and Gordon 1984; Golding 1982; Rice, Mancuso, and Hanafee 1980; Sone et al. 1982; Stone et al. 1981). Benign tumors appear as discrete, sharply marginated, high-density masses embedded in a normal gland. The CT density of these tumors is about the same as that of muscle, and the degree of enhancement following intravenous infusion of contrast material also is in the same density range. In contrast, invasive malignant tumors are poorly defined and marginated radiodense lesions, which may extend beyond the gland into the fat and fascial planes. These tumors may transgress adjacent anatomic structures and extend into the skull base, lateral pharyngeal space, and neurovascular bundle. In some cases, malignant lesions may simulate benign lesions, in that they are sharply marginated, well defined, and contained within an otherwise normal parotid gland. CT is useful for separating lesions that arise from the deep portion of the gland from lateral pharyngeal tumors. Axial CT sections allow localization into the deep or superficial portion and relate them to the imagined location of the facial nerve; however, in some lesions that straddle the deep and superficial portion of the parotid, relation to the facial nerve—whether medial or lateral—is difficult to determine.

Localized inflammatory lesions within the salivary glands may mimic mass lesions. Inflammatory disease, in general, produces a relatively diffuse, irregular, radiodense lesion in an enlarged gland. If the inflammatory process is well defined and localized, it may simulate a benign tumor and in cases with poorly defined borders, a malignant lesion may be postulated. Inflammatory processes may extend into the adjacent soft tissues.

CT attenuation values of tumors are variable and it is not possible to determine the histologic nature of the lesion. Cysts may have attenuation values similar to water or soft tissue tumors depending on the amount of mucus and other contents within the cyst. Lipomas characteristically present as low-density lesions identical to those observed in other parts of the body. They may be well circumscribed or they may diffusely infiltrate the salivary gland and adjacent structures. Cavernous hemangiomas, encountered in the pediatric age group and in adults, are displayed as lesions that are enhanced strikingly following infusion or bolus injection of contrast material. In suspected vascular lesions a precontrast scan should be used as a baseline study to discern the degree of enhancement following introduction of contrast material. Lymphangiomas present as low or isodense cystic spaces that demonstrate enhancing postcontrast septa.

Masses arising from outside the salivary glands may invade or be adherent to the gland. In these instances a primary intraglandular mass cannot be distinguished from extraglandular masses. A positive diagnosis of an extraglandular lesion can only be made if a fat plane is situated between the lesion and the normal salivary gland. The most common extraglandular lesions represent enlarged lymph nodes of variable etiology (e.g., metastatic disease, lymphoma, inflammatory nodes, and so on).

CASES

Mixed tumor of the left parotid gland

This 57-year-old man noted a mass in the superficial portion of the left parotid gland. There was no pain or tenderness.

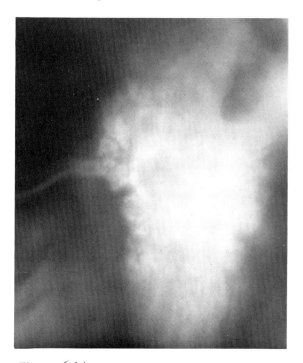

Figure 6.1A

Lateral tomographic section of the opacified parotid gland reveals a sharply marginated lucent defect in the anterior superficial portion of the parotid gland.

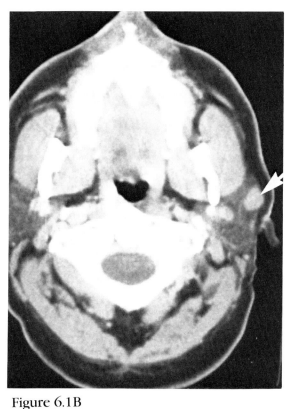

Figure 6.1B

An axial contrast CT section reveals a hyperdense nodule within the superficial anterior portion of the left parotid gland (*arrow*).

Pleomorphic adenoma of the superficial right parotid gland

This 34-year-old woman had had a mass in the right parotid for approximately 10 years. During the last six months, she noted further enlargement of this mass. Examination on admission revealed a firm mass, approximately 5 cm in diameter. She underwent a right superficial parotidectomy with complete excision of the tumor.

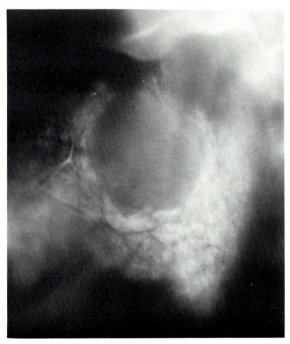

Figure 6.2A

A lateral tomographic section of the parotid sialogram shows a sharply marginated, homogeneous filling defect in the central, anterior, and superior portion of the right parotid gland.

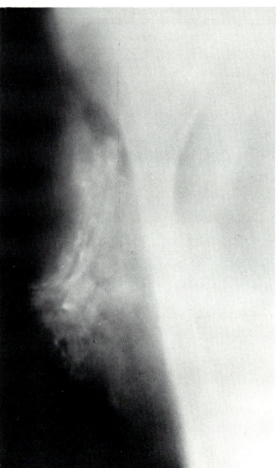

Figure 6.2B

AP tomographic section shows the defect to be in the superficial portion of the gland laterally and superiorly.

Mixed tumor of the superficial lobe of the right parotid gland

A 28-year-old woman had noted a mass in the right parotid gland five years previously. The mass was never painful and remained relatively stable in size. She had no infection or fever. Examination revealed a 4- × 3-cm, oval, smooth parotid mass in the superficial lobe anterior to the tragus. The mass was mobile and nontender. Facial nerve function was intact. She underwent a right superficial parotidectomy. A small portion of tumor extended between the buccal and cervical branch of the facial nerve to the medial part of the gland.

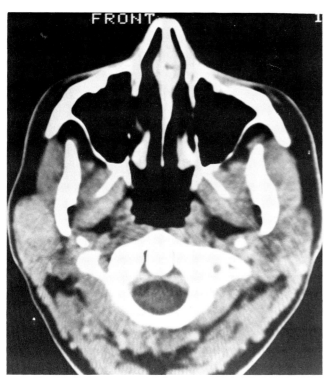

Figure 6.3

Axial contrast CT scan reveals an oval, well-defined mass in the superficial portion of the right parotid gland.

Pleomorphic adenoma of the right parotid gland

The patient was a 76-year-old woman with a large palpable mass in the region of the right parotid gland.

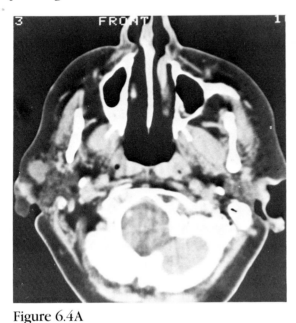

Figure 6.4A

Axial CT study of the region of the parotid gland superiorly reveals a sharply marginated nodule in the superficial portion of the gland.

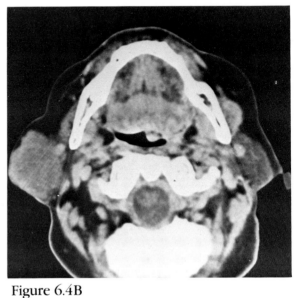

Figure 6.4B

Axial CT study at the angle of the mandible shows the inferior portion of the mass, which is homogeneous and sharply marginated in the superficial portion of the right parotid gland with bulging, but no thickening of the adjacent skin. Note normal left parotid gland for comparison.

Pleomorphic adenoma of the deep portion of the right parotid gland

This 29-year-old woman had a two-month history of a slowly enlarging, nontender right parotid mass. The mass measured 4 cm and was overlying the ramus of the mandible. A right parotidectomy was done for removal of this mass. At surgery, the tumor was found medial to the facial nerve, which was displaced laterally.

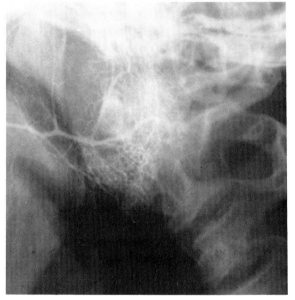

Figure 6.5A

Lateral sialogram suggests a filling defect in the central to anterior portion of the parotid gland.

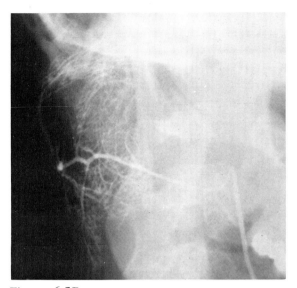

Figure 6.5B

AP view of the conventional sialogram suggests a large defect with lateral displacement of the intraparotid branches.

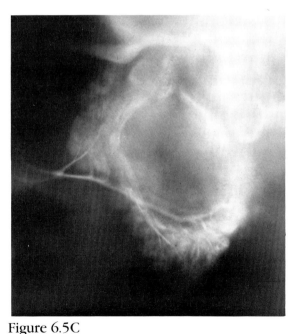

Figure 6.5C

Lateral tomographic section of the parenchymal phase shows a large, homogeneous, well-defined mass in the deep portion of the gland with inferior displacement of the major ducts.

Pleomorphic adenoma of the deep portion of the left parotid gland

This 63-year-old woman noted a feeling of fullness of the left side of her throat and increased sensitivity along with swelling of the soft palate. A biopsy of the tumor from the oral cavity demonstrated a pleomorphic adenoma.

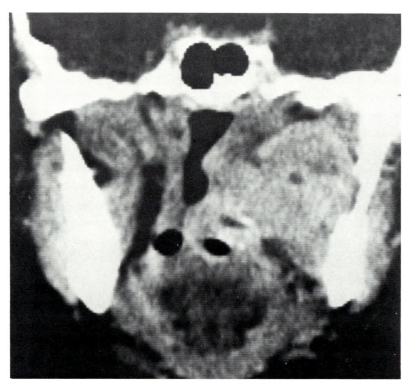

Figure 6.6

Coronal CT section at the level of the oropharynx demonstrates a homogeneous mass arising from the deep portion of the left parotid gland with extension into the parapharyngeal space. Note medial displacement of the lateral oropharyngeal wall secondary to the adjacent tumor, which also obliterates the parapharyngeal fat plane.

Pleomorphic adenoma of the deep portion of the left parotid gland

This 52-year-old woman complained of recurrent serous otitis media of at least five-years' duration. Physical examination showed a retracted tympanic membrane and slight fullness in the lateral aspect of the left anterior tonsillar pillar. A left parotid and cervical operative approach was used and a large pleomorphic adenoma of the deep portion of the parotid gland was excised. There was no facial nerve paralysis.

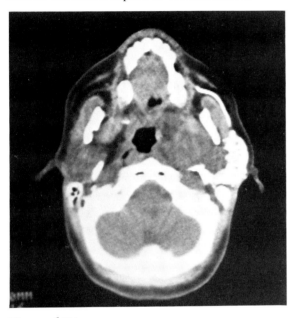

Figure 6.7A

Axial CT sialogram reveals a deep mass of the parotid gland extending into the parapharyngeal space. The interface between the mass and opacified parotid gland is sharply defined. The mass extends medially to the lateral wall of the oropharynx. (Photo courtesy of Hugh D. Curtin, M.D., Eye and Ear Hospital, Pittsburgh, Pennsylvania.)

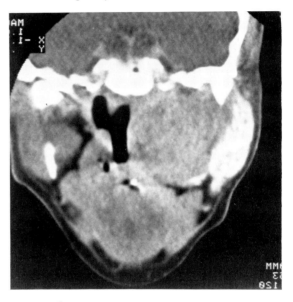

Figure 6.7B

Coronal CT sialogram shows the bulk of the mass within the parapharyngeal space arising from the deep portion of the parotid gland. The lateral wall of the oropharynx is displaced medially by the adjacent tumor. Note the slight inferior displacement of the soft palate on the left. The superficial opacified portion of the left parotid gland is slightly displaced laterally. (Photo courtesy of Hugh D. Curtin, M.D., Eye and Ear Hospital, Pittsburgh, Pennsylvania.)

Two pleomorphic adenomas of the right parotid gland with branchial cleft cyst at the inferior margin of the gland

This 39-year-old woman had a history of asymptomatic bilateral masses in front of both ears. The supraparotid mass on the left was excised and pathologic examination revealed a dermoid.

She subsequently underwent a right sub-total parotidectomy. Two separate spherical, firm, and slightly lobulated tumor masses were found. One mass was found in the body of the parotid superficially; the other was located in the deep portion just medial to the facial nerve. On pathologic examination, these masses proved to be pleomorphic adenomas. A third mass, found in the infraparotid region, was removed and on pathologic examination was classified as a branchial cleft cyst.

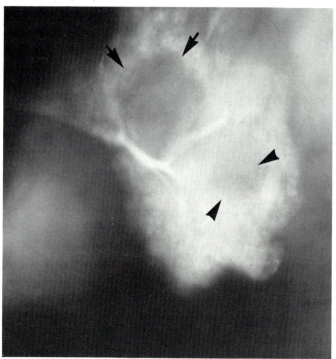

Figure 6.8

Lateral tomographic section of the right parotid gland reveals an oval, sharply marginated defect in the anterior portion of the parotid gland above the main duct (*arrows*). A second, slightly less well-defined mass is seen in the posterior central portion of the gland (*arrowheads*). An indentation of the inferior pole of the parotid gland is secondary to the branchial cleft cyst.

Recurrent mixed tumor of the right parotid gland

This 47-year-old woman had complained of right parotid swelling for several months. Over the past two years, three excisions for a mixed tumor had been performed at other hospitals. Each excision was followed by recurrence. The pathology of each excision was benign mixed tumor. She underwent a total parotidectomy with facial nerve dissection and she subsequently received radiation therapy. Her facial nerve function was returning to normal within two months after surgery.

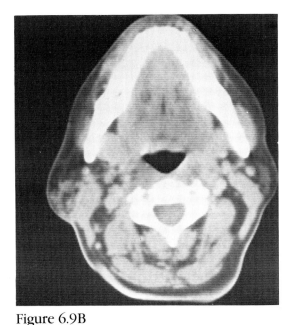

Figure 6.9B

CT scan at mid-parotid gland demonstrates multiple nodules secondary to recurrent tumor in the superficial and deep portion of the gland.

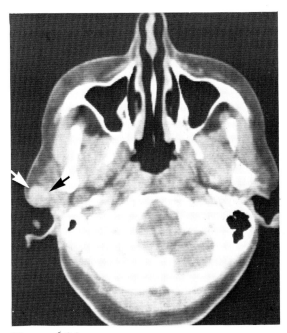

Figure 6.9A

Axial CT section slightly below the external auditory canal shows a nodular density anterior to the tragus (*arrows*).

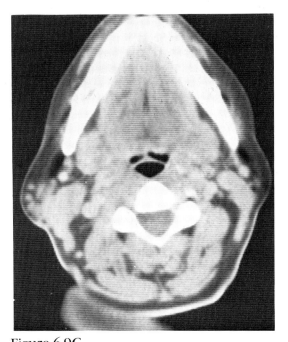

Figure 6.9C

CT section at angle of mandible again shows multiple tumor nodules in the remaining superficial posterior parotid gland.

Ectopic pleomorphic adenoma of the left side of the upper neck area with calcification

This 50-year-old woman had had a mass in the submandibular area for 20 years. It was never painful. On palpation, the mass was firm and sharply defined. At surgery, the mass was separated from the parotid and submandibular gland and represented an ectopic pleomorphic adenoma in the upper neck area.

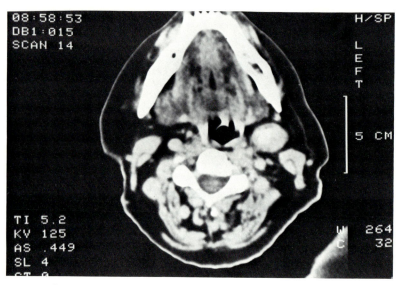

Figure 6.10

Axial CT study of the upper neck area following infusion of contrast material demonstrates a homogeneous, well-defined mass anterior to the sternocleidomastoid muscle and posterior to the left submandibular gland. Note the presence of mottled calcification within the tumor mass.

Pleomorphic adenoma of the right submandibular gland with calcification

This 23-year-old man had complained of a slowly growing right-sided neck mass for five years. The mass recently had increased in size, but no pain or other symptoms were present. On physical examination, a golfball-sized mass was palpated in the right submandibular gland area. It was firm, hard, and nontender. The mass was excised and on pathologic examination was 5 × 3 cm in diameter and encapsulated.

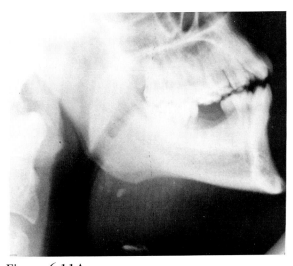

Figure 6.11A

Lateral film of the mandible and upper neck area reveals mottled calcification in the soft tissue below the angle of the mandible.

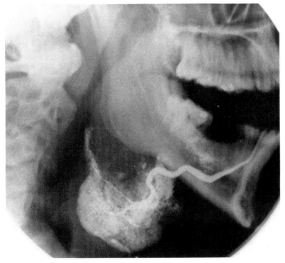

Figure 6.11B

Lateral right submandibular sialogram demonstrates a filling defect in the upper half of the right submandibular gland with irregular interface between the mass and gland. Note the calcification within the mass below the angle of the mandible.

Warthin's tumor of the left parotid gland

This 58-year-old man had a history of swelling of the tail of the left parotid gland.

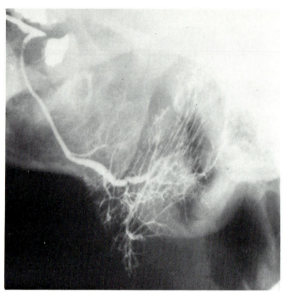

Figure 6.12A

Lateral view of the parotid sialogram reveals a questionable defect in the posterior inferior portion of the parotid gland.

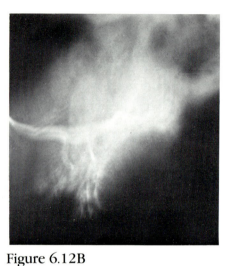

Figure 6.12B

Lateral tomographic study of the opacified parotid gland reveals a sharply marginated, hemispherical shaped defect in the lower posterior portion of the gland.

Warthin's tumor of the left parotid gland

This 62-year-old man gave a history of a slowly enlarging, painless mass of one month's duration on the left side at the angle of the mandible. There was no facial weakness or spasm. On 2/17/78, he underwent a left total parotidectomy with facial nerve dissection and preservation. At surgery, the mass measured 6 × 5 × 3 cm and was located in the superficial and deep lobe of the parotid gland. On pathologic examination, an adenolymphoma (Warthin's tumor) was diagnosed along with chronic sialadenitis.

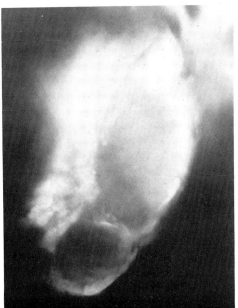

Figure 6.13B

Lateral tomographic section reveals a large lobulated mass reflected by sharply defined filling defects.

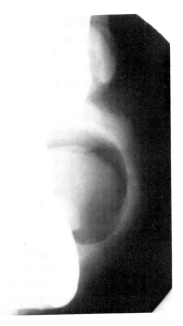

Figure 6.13A

AP puffed-cheek view demonstrates a large round mass projecting into the air-filled, puffed-out cheek.

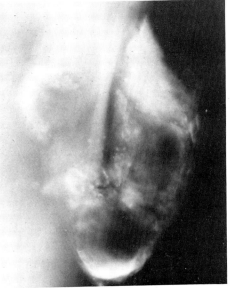

Figure 6.13C

AP tomographic section demonstrates a multi-lobulated lesion in the deep and superficial portion of the parotid gland. Linear, vertical bony density represents the ascending ramus of the mandible.

Warthin's tumor of the left parotid gland

This 95-year-old woman had an asymptomatic mass in her left parotid gland. A superficial parotidectomy was carried out and the histologic diagnosis of a Warthin's tumor was made.

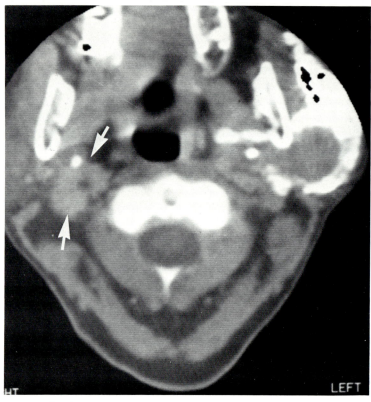

Figure 6.14

Axial CT sialogram shows a sharply defined tumor in the superficial portion of the opacified parotid gland bulging into the deep portion behind the mandible. Note a second lesion in the right parotid gland adjacent to the deep portion posteriorly (*arrows*), which may represent a second Warthin's tumor. The patient's right side has not been explored.

Adenolymphoma (Warthin's tumor) of the left and right parotid glands

This 63-year-old man had a five-year history of bilateral parotid neck masses. Three months ago he noted enlargement of the left parotid mass; however, the gland itself was reduced in size. On PE, a 6- × 4-cm, slightly lobulated mass was felt at the angle of the left mandible. The right parotid mass measured 2 × 3 cm and was soft on palpation. On 11/29/83, he underwent a left parotidectomy with preservation of the facial nerve.

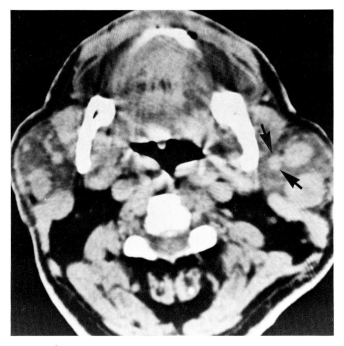

Figure 6.15

Axial CT study of both parotid glands following infusion of contrast material reveals two homogeneous masses in the superficial portion of the left parotid gland. A small rounded density medial to the anterior mass represents the retromandibular facial vein (*arrows*).

On the right, a single round to oval mass is demonstrated in the posterior portion of the right parotid gland, which is consistent with a Warthin's tumor.

Bilateral Warthin's tumors

The patient was a 53-year-old man with a three-year history of mass in the neck. He had no other symptoms. Examination revealed two masses in the left side of the neck in the parotid area. The first mass measured 2 cm and was located anterior to the sternocleidomastoid muscle; the second mass was immediately inferior to the first. These two masses were nontender, slightly mobile, and cystic. There were similar mobile masses posterior and inferior to the mandible on the right. Surgery of the left parotid revealed adenolymphoma.

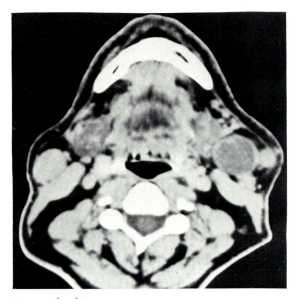

Figure 6.16A

Axial CT study through the lower portion of the parotid glands and submandibular glands after infusion of contrast material reveals two homogeneous, sharply defined masses in the inferior portion of the left parotid gland. The anterior mass contains a water density component that represents a cyst within the tumor. There is some bulging of the adjacent skin as well as indentation of the left submandibular gland by the mass. Note the normal right submandibular gland. On the right, there is an oval homogeneous mass within the inferior portion of the parotid gland anterior and lateral to the sternocleidomastoid muscles.

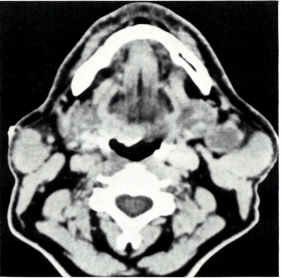

Figure 6.16B

CT scan below the section included in figure 6.16A again demonstrates the masses in both parotid glands with a slightly different configuration at this lower section.

Two oxyphilic adenomas (oncocytomas) of the left parotid gland

This 59-year-old woman had a two-month history of a mass in the left cheek. Physical examination revealed a 1.5-cm, well-demarcated mass in the region of the ramus of the mandible. She underwent a superficial parotidectomy with resection of the anterior portion of the parotid gland. At surgery, two separate masses were found in the anterior-superior portion of the gland.

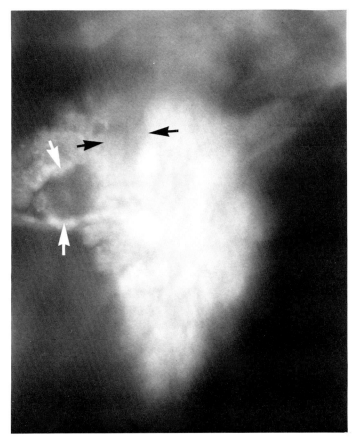

Figure 6.17

Lateral tomographic section of the opacified parenchyma reveals a sharply marginated, round defect in the anterior accessory portion of the parotid gland above the main duct (*white arrows*). A second, less well-defined defect is demonstrated more superiorly (*black arrows*).

Adenoid cystic carcinoma of the left parotid gland

This 66-year-old woman had a history of left-sided otalgia and left-sided facial nerve paralysis of several months' duration. A mass was palpated in the region of the ascending ramus of the mandible. The patient underwent a left superficial and deep parotidectomy.

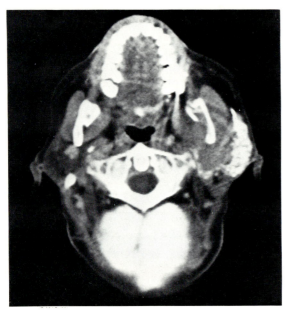

Figure 6.20A

Axial CT sialogram reveals a mass in the superficial and deep portion of the parotid gland. (Photo courtesy of Hugh D. Curtin, M. D., Eye and Ear Hospital, Pittsburgh, Pennsylvania.)

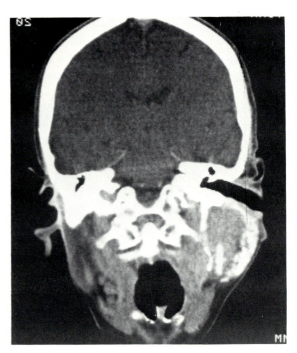

Figure 6.20B

Coronal sections of the CT scan reveal a homogeneous mass in the deep and superficial portion. Normal parotid tissue from the superficial portion caps the mass laterally. Note the normal external ear canal. (Photo courtesy of Hugh D. Curtin, M.D., Eye and Ear Hospital, Pittsburgh, Pennsylvania.)

Adenocarcinoma of the parotid gland

This 71-year-old woman had had a mass beneath the left ear for some time. The mass increased in size, was very hard and semi-fixed, and measured approximately 1 × 2 cm in diameter. She underwent a left parotidectomy. Pathologic examination revealed an adenocarcinoma most likely developing from a pleomorphic adenoma. She received 4400 rad of radiation postsurgery.

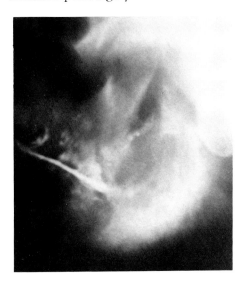

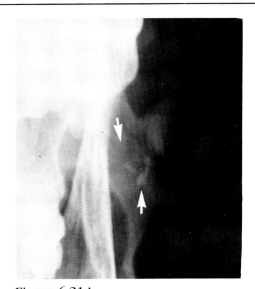

Figure 6.21A

AP view of the left parotid gland reveals mottled, irregular calcifications within the tumor mass (*arrows*).

Figure 6.21B

Lateral tomographic section of the opacified gland reveals an ill-defined, irregular filling defect in the central and anterior portion of the parotid gland, secondary to the malignant tumor. The tumor extends anteriorly into aberrant glandular tissue about the main duct.

Adenocarcinoma of the right parotid gland

This 74-year-old man demonstrated a tumor mass in the right parotid gland for which a total parotidectomy was done. The histologic examination demonstrated an adenocarcinoma of the right parotid gland with extension into the deep lobe and pterygopalatine space.

Figure 6.22

Oblique view of a right parotid sialogram reveals slight dilatation of several ducts in the right parotid gland interspersed with areas of narrowing with fixation.

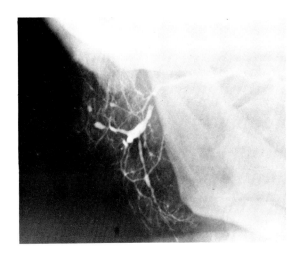

Poorly differentiated adenocarcinoma of the right parotid gland

This 70-year-old man had an eight-week history of a slowly enlarging mass. On physical examination, the mass was approximately 4 cm in diameter. There was slight weakness of the facial nerve, and slight bulging of the pharyngeal wall was noted on oral examination. The patient had a total parotidectomy with sacrifice of the facial nerve, hemimandibulectomy, and right-sided radical neck dissection.

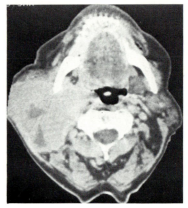

Figure 6.23

Axial contrast CT section at the level of the angle of the mandible reveals a large mass that extends into the parapharyngeal space with obliteration of the space. The mass extends to the skin and bulges laterally. The mass involves the carotid sheath and extends into the posterior triangle. The two lucent areas within the tumor probably represent necrosis. (Photo courtesy of Anton Hasso, M.D., Loma Linda University Medical Center.)

Clear cell carcinoma of the left parotid gland

This 64-year-old woman had a four-year history of a mass in her cheek. She had had facial nerve paralysis for six to seven months. The patient underwent a radical parotidectomy and infratemporal fossa exploration with radical neck dissection and partial temporal bone resection. The tumor extended into the base of the skull at the level of the stylomastoid foramen.

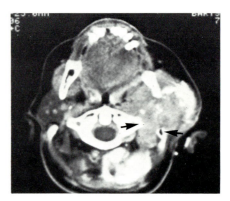

Figure 6.24

Axial CT sialogram reveals a large mass involving the deep portion of the parotid with extension into the parapharyngeal space. The tumor extends posteriorly into the posterior triangle between the mastoid process and the cervical spine (*arrows*). The interface beteen the tumor and the opacified superficial portion of the parotid gland is irregular. Multiple small densities are present within the center of the tumor mass; these represent extravasated contrast material. (Photo courtesy o' Hugh D. Curtin, M.D., Eye and Ear Hospital, Pittsburgh, Pennsylvania.)

Clear cell carcinoma of the right parotid gland

This 23-year-old woman had a two-year history of right-sided mandibular pain. She saw an oral surgeon for this problem and had her wisdom teeth removed. Examination revealed a node in her right neck. She experienced no physical symptoms (e.g., weight loss, fever, sweats, and so on). She had noted paresthesias of the right cheek over the last few months and a twitching of the corner of her mouth. She underwent a needle biopsy on 5/20/83 and on 8/9/83 she underwent a total parotidectomy with resection of the facial nerve and dissection of tumor in the infratemporal and pterygoid fossas.

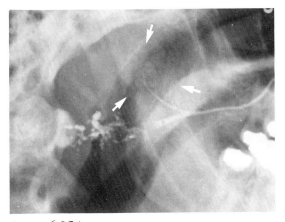

Figure 6.25A

Right parotid sialogram reveals infiltration by the tumor, which is reflected by distortion and narrowing of the intraglandular ducts. The smaller ducts and parenchyma could not be filled. Note normal aberrant glandular tissue superior to the mid-third of the normal parotid gland (*arrows*).

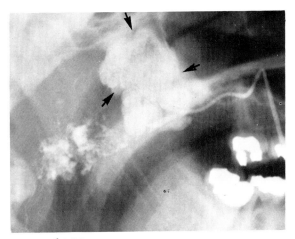

Figure 6.25B

Injection of contrast material under pressure reveals diffuse opacification of the aberrant glandular tissue (*arrows*). There is complete destruction of the gland architecture, which is characterized by ill-defined puddling of contrast material.

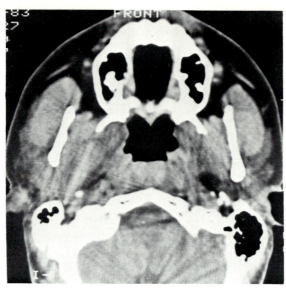

Figure 6.25C

Axial contrast CT scan reveals a diffuse, ill-defined tumor mass in the right parotid gland with extension into the deep portion.

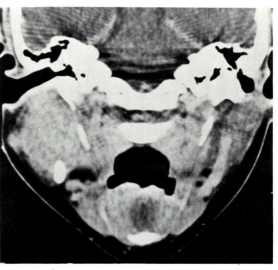

Figure 6.25E

Coronal CT section at the level of the styloid process and external auditory canal shows the tumor in the superficial and deep portion of the parotid gland with extension into the para-pharyngeal space.

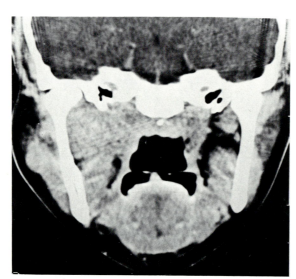

Figure 6.25D

Coronal CT section at the level of the mandible shows the mass in the deep portion of the gland and parapharyngeal space with obliteration of lateral pterygoid muscle and fat plane. (See normal left side for comparison.)

Adenocarcinoma of the right submandibular gland

This 55-year-old woman noted tenderness of the right submandibular gland for three weeks. She also noted twitching of her right eye and the right corner of her mouth. A nodule also was palpated. At surgery and pathologic examination, the tumor was localized within the gland and corresponds to the demonstrated low-density area.

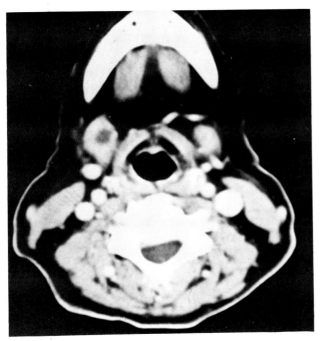

Figure 6.26

Axial CT section through the submandibular glands reveals a round, sharply marginated, low-density area within the right submandibular gland. The gland is sharply marginated and not enlarged.

Squamous cell carcinoma of the right parotid gland

This 50-year-old man was observed for recurrent bilateral parotid swelling with pain. A lip biopsy confirmed the presence of Sjögren's syndrome. He developed a right-sided upper neck mass that biopsy results proved to be squamous cell carcinoma.

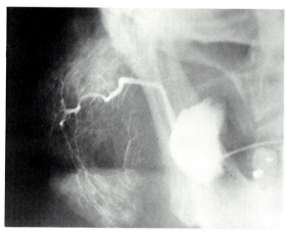

Figure 6.27A

AP film of the parotid sialogram reveals a defect in the central and deep portion of the parotid gland with elevation of the main duct.

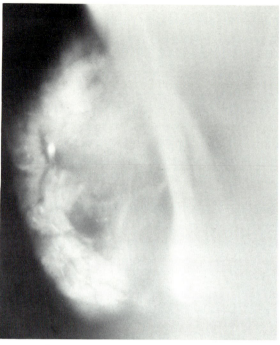

Figure 6.27B

AP tomographic section of the parenchymogram reveals multiple ill-defined defects in the central and deep portion of the right parotid gland.

Figure 6.27C

Axial CT section through the oropharynx demonstrates a large, irregular, homogeneous mass involving the deep portion of the right parotid gland with extension medially into the parapharyngeal space and posteriorly into the vascular sheath and posterior triangle. There is also some extension of this mass anteriorly into soft tissues adjacent to the medial border of the right mandible and base of the tongue. An area of increased density adjacent to the lateral border of the right mandible at the masseter muscle may represent tumor in the anterior-superficial portion of the parotid gland.

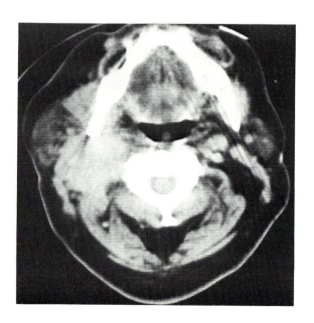

Squamous cell carcinoma of the right parotid gland

A 70-year-old woman with a right-sided upper neck area and cheek mass of 5-weeks' duration complained of slight trismus, but experienced no pain. A biopsy of the mass revealed squamous cell carcinoma.

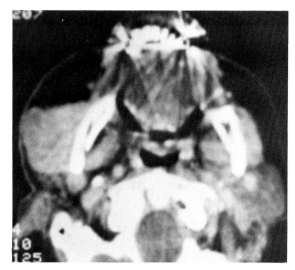

Figure 6.28

Axial contrast CT scan shows a large, homogeneous, sharply defined mass adjacent to the right ascending ramus of the mandible. The right masseter muscle is obliterated. The anterior portion of the parotid gland is involved by tumor.

Undifferentiated carcinoma of the right submandibular gland

This 70-year-old woman had had swelling of the right submandibular gland for several months. Examination revealed a 3- × 4-cm mass; a biopsy revealed undifferentiated carcinoma. She underwent a total excision of the tumor with a right-sided radical neck dissection.

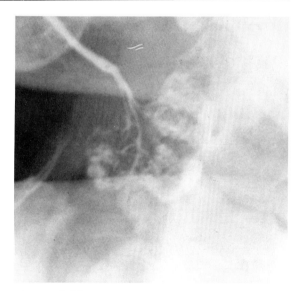

Figure 6.29

An oblique view of a right-sided submandibular sialogram reveals complete destruction of the submandibular gland as reflected by multiple, irregular filling defects within the opacified gland.

Recurrent malignant mixed tumor of the left submandibular gland

A malignant mixed tumor of the left submandibular gland was excised in this 67-year-old woman. Several months following surgery she developed a recurrent mass in the submandibular region, which was mobile and measured 8 cm in diameter. She underwent total excision of this recurrent tumor; pathologic examination revealed malignancy in a recurrent pleomorphic adenoma. On gross examination, the tumor was pink to red with cystic cavities filled with hemorrhagic fluid. The cysts were approximately 5 cm in diameter.

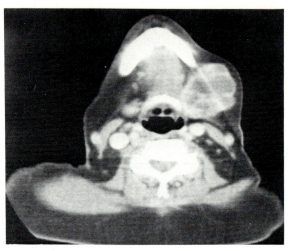

Figure 6.30B

Axial CT section at the level of the hyoid bone reveals extension of the lobulated mass, which contains low-density areas consistent with cavities within the tumor. In between the low-density areas are strands of enhancing tumor tissue. Note the bulging of the adjacent skin.

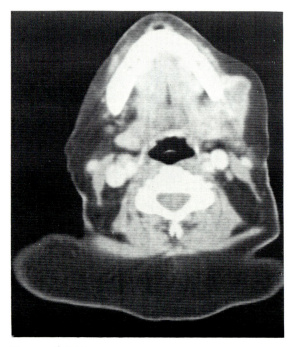

Figure 6.30A

Axial contrast CT scan reveals a large, in-homogeneous tumor mass with low-density areas in the left submandibular region extending laterally to the skin, which bulges. There is no extension posteriorly into the vascular sheath.

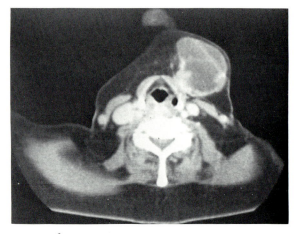

Figure 6.30C

Axial CT section at the level of the thyroid cartilage shows the low-density, septated, and sharply marginated malignant mixed tumor.

Poorly differentiated adenocarcinoma of the lung metastatic to the mandible with extension into the parotid gland

This 56-year-old man had a previous history of a right-sided upper lobectomy for a poorly differentiated adenocarcinoma. He developed right-sided jaw pain and a palpable mass, which was thought to be a tumor of the parotid. Biopsy showed this mass to be metastatic adenocarcinoma from the lung.

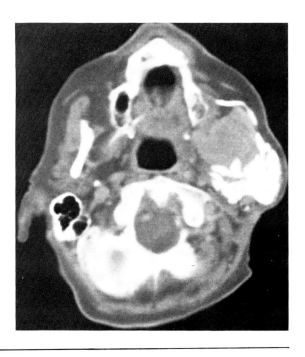

Figure 6.31

Axial CT sialogram shows a homogeneous, fairly well-defined mass invading the anterior portion of the left parotid gland. The mass is adjacent to the main duct, which is slightly displaced laterally. The ascending ramus of the mandible has been destroyed by this tumor. (Note the normal mandible on the opposite side). (Photo courtesy of Hugh D. Curtin, M.D., Eye and Ear Hospital, Pittsburgh, Pennsylvania.)

Squamous cell carcinoma of the right external auditory canal and middle ear cavity with invasion of the right parotid gland

This 84-year-old man had a mass in the right bony external auditory canal and right seventh nerve paresis.

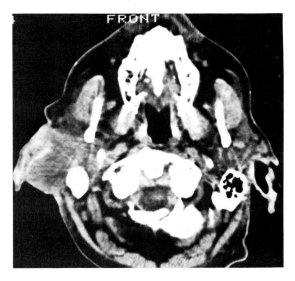

Figure 6.32

Axial CT section reveals a large mass in the right parotid gland that represents extension from a carcinoma of the ear. There is invasion of the skin that bulges laterally. The tumor extends medially to the styloid process.

Malignant lymphoma of the left periparotid lymph nodes

This 52-year-old woman had a six-month history of a progressively enlarging mass in the left side of the upper neck area posterior to the angle of the mandible. PE revealed a 4- × 3-cm, firm, and mobile mass. She underwent a left superficial parotidectomy with excision of the mass. Pathologic examination revealed a malignant lymphoma (nodular, poorly differentiated lymphocytic type) in a lymph node adjacent to the posterior portion of the parotid gland.

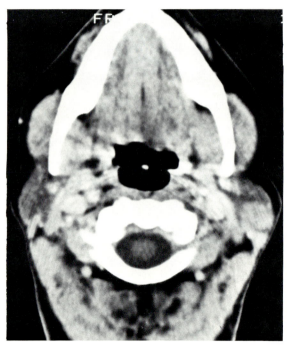

Figure 6.36A

Axial CT study reveals an oval, homogeneous mass in the posterior portion of the left parotid gland. On CT, this lymphomatous lymph node appears intraparotid, but it was in the periparotid lymph node at surgery.

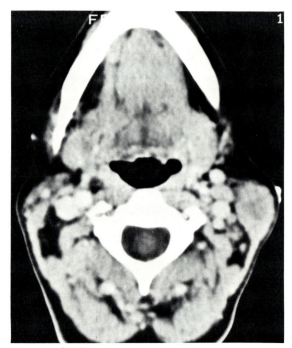

Figure 6.36B

Axial CT section below that covered in figure 6.36A reveals the same enlarged lymph nodes below the left parotid gland with a slight bulge of the skin. There is a low-density area within the otherwise homogeneous, sharply defined lymph node.

Lymphoma in left parapharyngeal space adjacent to the submandibular and parotid glands

This patient was a 49-year-old man with palpable lymph nodes in the left side of the neck.

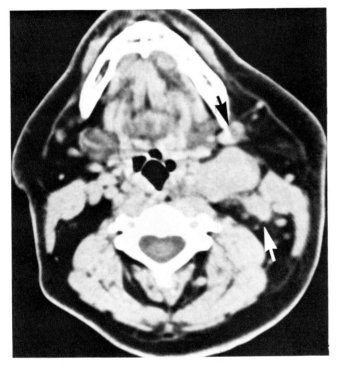

Figure 6.37

Axial CT section at and slightly below the angle of the mandible reveals a sharply marginated, homogeneous mass in the left parapharyngeal space anterior to the left sternocleidomastoid muscle. Two enlarged nodes are noted anterior to the described large mass behind the angle of the mandible (*black arrow*) and posterior to the main mass, medial to the sternocleidomastoid muscle (*white arrow*).

Neurilemmoma from the facial nerve in the right parotid gland

This 55-year-old woman had a four-year history of intermittent pain and swelling in the right parotid region lasting usually one to two days and occurring two to three times a week. The swelling was associated with auricular paresthesia. On physical examination, a firm, nontender mass 5 × 4 cm was palpated in the tail of the right parotid gland. She underwent a right total parotidectomy; pathologic examination revealed a schwannoma with focal necrosis and cystic degeneration.

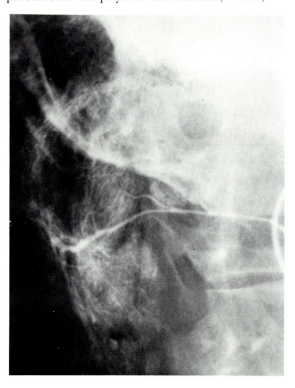

Figure 6.38A

An oblique sialographic spot film reveals a filling defect in the superior half of the gland with stretching of intraglandular branches and displacement of the parenchyma externally. The main duct within the gland is slightly displaced inferiorly.

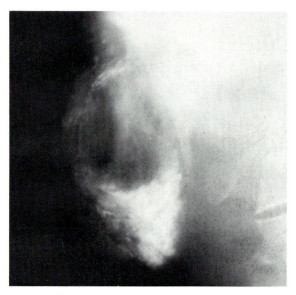

Figure 6.38B

AP tomographic section in the parenchymal phase reveals an oval, sharply marginated defect in the middle and superior portion of the parotid gland. The superficial portion of the gland is draped laterally over the mass.

Cavernous hemangioma of the deep portion of the right parotid gland

This 49-year-old man had a long history of an asymptomatic right parotid mass. Surgery was performed and a cavernous hemangioma was removed from the deep portion of the parotid gland.

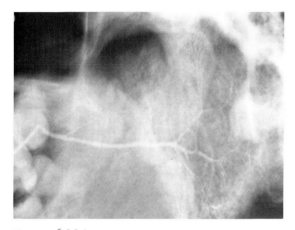

Figure 6.39A

Lateral parotid sialogram demonstrates an ill-defined lucent area in the central portion of the parotid gland.

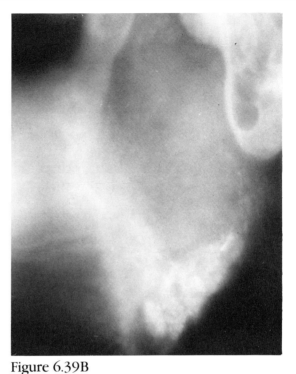

Figure 6.39B

Lateral tomographic section reveals a large, sharply marginated mass in the deep portion of the right parotid gland.

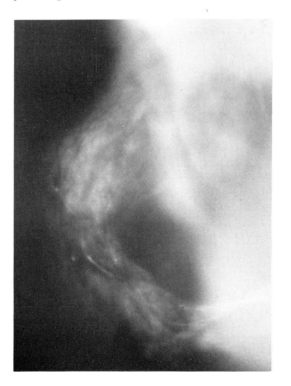

Figure 6.39C

AP tomographic section of the parotid gland demonstrates a mass in the deep portion of the parotid gland laterally displacing the superficial portion.

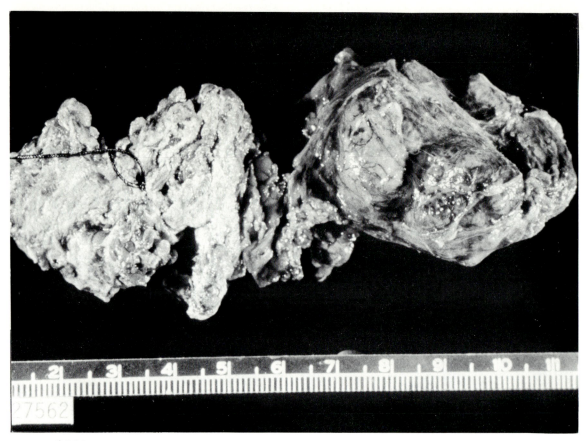

Figure 6.39D

The gross specimen reveals a bosselated
hemangioma. A cross section on the left side of
the figure shows white, glistening tissue.

Capillary hemangioma of the right side of the neck and skull with invasion of the salivary glands

A 9-month-old boy was noted at birth to have a large, cystic-feeling structure on the lateral aspect of his head and neck, which was believed to be a cystic hygroma. He was referred for surgical therapy. At surgery, the lesion was found to be a capillary hemangioma invading the bone. A large segment of skull had to be removed to control the bleeding during the procedure. Postoperatively, he had a brief course of steroids, which were not effective in shrinking the lesion. The lesion increased in size over the next year. He received another course of steroids in November 1982 at 6½ months of age. In January 1983, extremely rapid development of a large posterior occipital mass was noted, which was believed to be an extension of his hemangioma.

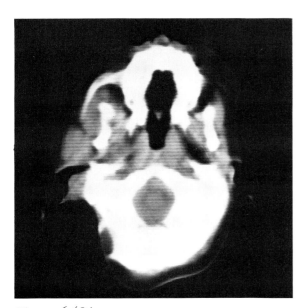

Figure 6.40A

Axial CT study of the parotid glands reveals a homogeneous, enhancing mass in the superficial portion of the right parotid gland. There is associated loss of bone in the right occipital region.

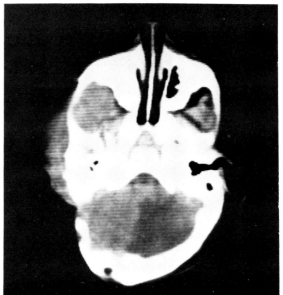

Figure 6.40B

Axial CT section above the parotid gland reveals a mass adjacent to the squamosal portion of the right temporal bone, sphenoid bone with extension into the temporal fossa. Note enhancing areas within the hemangioma. There is loss of bone in the region of the right occipital bone.

Lymphangioma of the right side of the neck with involvement of the right submandibular gland

This 18-year-old woman had had swelling in the right side of her neck, which waxed and waned for several years. Recently, she had complained of pain and tenderness in the region of the neck as well as of some difficulty swallowing. On physical examination, there was a 9- × 5-cm, firm, nontender, and slightly mobile mass in the right submandibular region. This mass was surgically removed and on pathologic examination was diagnosed as a cystic lymphangioma with hemorrhage and mural fibrosis.

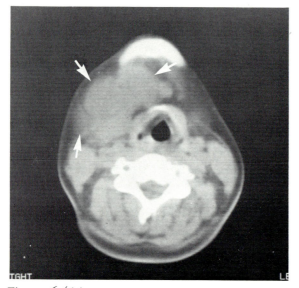

Figure 6.41A

Axial precontrast CT section at the level of the upper margin of the thyroid cartilage reveals a lobulated, homogeneous right-sided neck mass, which extends from the anterior border of the sternocleidomastoid muscle to the midsagittal plane of the thyroid cartilage (*arrows*).

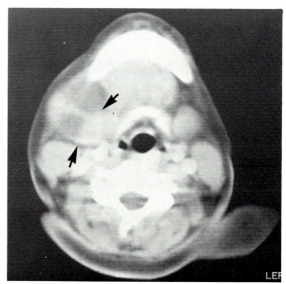

Figure 6.41B

Axial contrast CT section at the level of the hyoid bone demonstrates enhancing tissue outlining cystic areas. Note invasion of the right submandibular gland (*arrows*).

Cystic lymphangioma invading the left submandibular gland

This 27-year-old woman had a cyst (lymphangioma) removed from the left side of the neck on 7/30/81. In August 1982, she noted recurrent swelling after the removal of a tooth. The swelling persisted for six months. On 2/4/83, she underwent excision of a recurrent lymphangioma. At surgery, a 7- × 3-4 cm, multilobulated, cystic mass was removed. The lymphangioma involved the left submandibular gland and periglandular structures of the neck and adjacent floor of mouth.

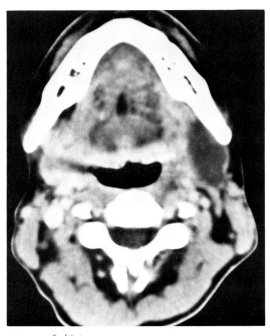

Figure 6.42A

Axial CT section following infusion of contrast material reveals a low-density, sharply defined, oval mass in the floor of the mouth and adjacent submandibular gland on the left.

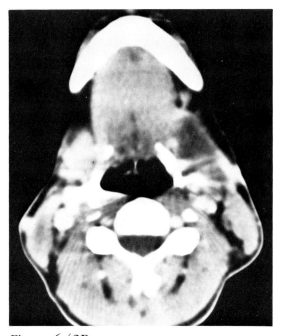

Figure 6.42B

Axial CT section at the level of the posterior tongue and hyoid bone demonstrates extension of the lymphangioma into the left submandibular gland.

Lipoma of the right parotid gland

This 29-year-old man developed an asymp-tomatic mass in the right angle of the mandible 10 months prior to admission. Preoperative examination revealed a 4-cm, smooth, non-tender, cystic-feeling mass in the region of the tail of the parotid. The patient underwent a superficial parotidectomy; pathologic examina-tion revealed a lipoma with fatty infiltration of the right parotid gland.

Figure 6.43

Lateral tomographic section of the parenchymal phase of the sialogram reveals a sharply mar-ginated, cone-shaped mass in the inferior parotid gland.

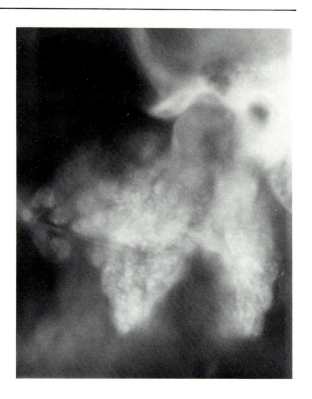

Lipoma of the left parotid gland

A 51-year-old man with a four- to five-year history of a slowly progressive left parotid mass.

Figure 6.44

Axial CT section through the midportion of the parotid glands reveals a lipoma in the left parotid gland. Note septation within the mass.

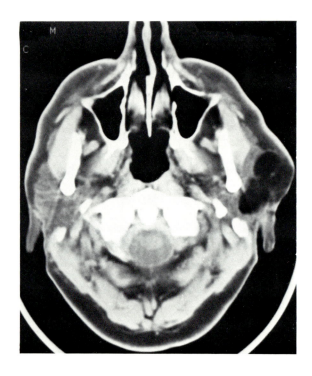

Lipoma in the floor of the mouth indenting and displacing the submandibular gland (not proved surgically)

This 72-year-old man had had a painless swelling in his left submandibular gland for three months. Examination revealed fullness in the region of the left submandibular gland.

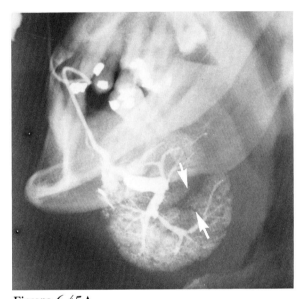

Figure 6.45A

Lateral view of a left submandibular sialogram reveals an ill-defined low-density area posteriorly and superiorly. Note slight spreading of adjacent glandular lobules (*arrow*).

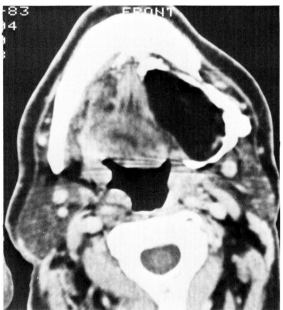

Figure 6.45B

Axial CT sialogram shows indentation and lateral displacement of the submandibular gland caused by a well-defined oval lipoma.

Branchial cleft cyst, type 1, and sinus tract in the left superficial parotid gland

This 24-year-old woman had had a left-sided retromandibular mass for approximately three years. This mass was painless and nontender. Approximately one year ago, the mass became large and was incised; however, the incision revealed only degenerative tissue. One year later she was admitted to the hospital and examination demonstrated a 2- × 3-cm mass, which was mobile and nontender. Superficial parotidectomy was done along with removal of a branchial cleft cyst and sinus tract. The pathologic examination showed a cyst with columnar epithelial lining, fibrosis, and lymphoid tissue with an adjacent amputation-type neuroma. The final diagnosis was branchial cleft cyst, type 1.

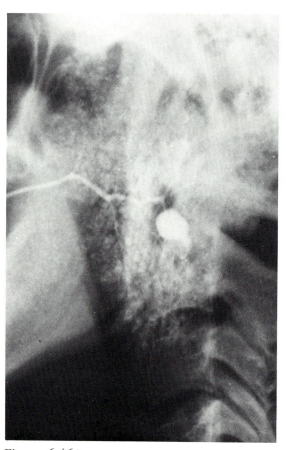

Figure 6.46A

Left parotid sialogram reveals a collection of contrast material in a saccular structure in the midportion of the gland and in a surrounding filling defect.

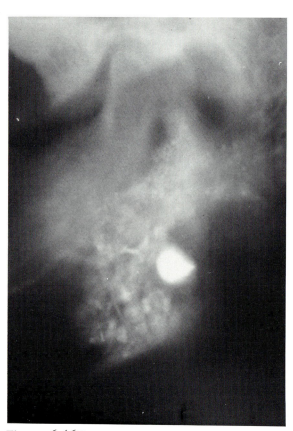

Figure 6.46B

Lateral tomographic cut shows a small cavity filled with contrast material within a large, well-defined hemispherical mass.

Left branchial cleft cyst, type II

This 27-year-old man had a three-year history of a left-sided neck mass that was slowly growing, but which markedly increased in size—doubling over a period of one month. He had no pain or tenderness. He eventually developed fever of 102 degrees and was admitted to the hospital. Examination revealed a 5- × 4-cm, firm, fixed, immobile mass. He underwent excision of this branchial cleft cyst. An angiogram performed prior to the excision revealed an avascular mass.

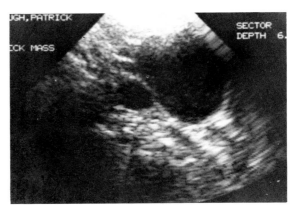

Figure 6.47B

Axial ultrasonic section reveals a hypoechoic mass lateral to the vascular sheath. Some ultrasonic tissue reflections indicate debris within this cyst.

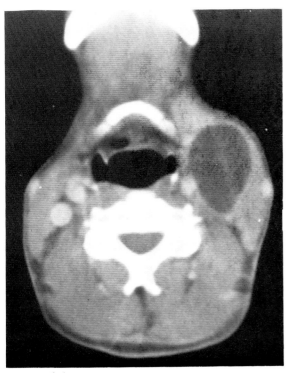

Figure 6.47A

Axial contrast CT study of the neck at the level of the hyoid bone demonstrates an oval, sharply defined, water density mass with no enhancement. The vascular structures are displaced medially. The mass is located in the anterior triangle medial to the left sternocleidomastoid muscle.

Left branchial cleft cyst, type II, in the left parotid gland

This 42-year-old man had a mass removed from the left angle of the mandible four years ago. The mass recurred and has grown steadily larger since then. The mass is painless and measures approximately 4 to 5 cm in diameter. At surgery, the cyst was filled with grayish, slightly turbid fluid.

Figure 6.48

Axial CT study through the level of the mid parotid gland reveals a sharply marginated low density mass within the left parotid. There is slight compression and posterior displacement of the left sternocleidomastoid muscle. There is slight anterior displacement of the retromandibular vein.

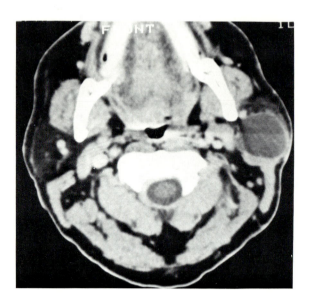

Epidermoid cyst of the left parotid gland

This 39-year-old woman revealed a two-year history of a mass in the left parotid area, which recently had been enlarging. On physical examination, a mass 4 × 6 cm was palpated inferior to the left earlobe. A cyst located in the deep and superficial portion of the parotid gland was excised. On pathologic examination, the cyst contained cheesy white material with an epidermal lining.

Figure 6.49

Lateral tomographic study in the parenchymal phase of the sialogram reveals a sharply defined, round filling defect in the superior deep portion of the parotid gland.

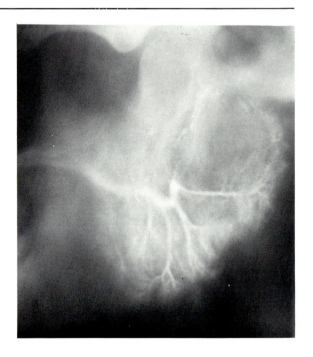

Epidermoid cyst in the left submandibular fossa causing a filling defect in the anterior portion of the submandibular gland

This 24-year-old man had a mass in the left submandibular fossa of two months' duration. Onset was quite sudden and associated with some pain, which subsequently disappeared. Physical examination revealed a 3- × 3-cm mass, nontender and mobile, with a cystic consistency anterior to the submandibular gland. The cyst including a normal submandibular gland was excised. The cyst contained cheesy white material.

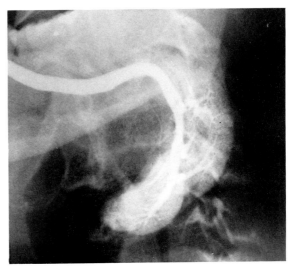

Figure 6.50

Lateral spot film of the left submandibular sialogram reveals a mass indenting the anterior portion of the gland. There is posterior displacement of the main duct and major branches.

Pleomorphic adenoma of the soft palate

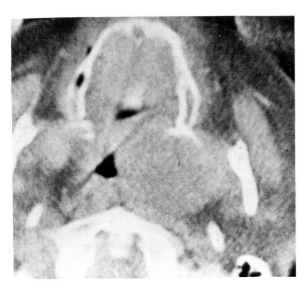

This 61-year-old woman had had a mass in the right soft palate for one year, which increased in size in the six weeks prior to admission.

Figure 6.51

A transverse scan at the level of the maxillary alveolar ridge demonstrates a soft tissue mass involving the right side of the soft palate. It extends posteriorly along the lateral wall of the oropharynx to the left retropharyngeal space. Laterally, the mass blends in with the medial pterygoid muscle. No bone destruction is evident and the lesion is homogeneous with smooth margins. (From Hesselink, J. R., et al. Computed tomography of the paranasal sinuses and face: Part II. Pathological anatomy. *J. Comput. Assist. Tomogr.* 2:568–576, November 1978. Reprinted by permission.)

Pleomorphic adenoma of the hard palate

This 61-year-old man complained of an enlarging palatal mass of several years' duration, which had been causing his dentures to fit poorly. On examination, a firm, centrally ulcerated mass 3 cm in diameter was noted on the left side of the hard palate.

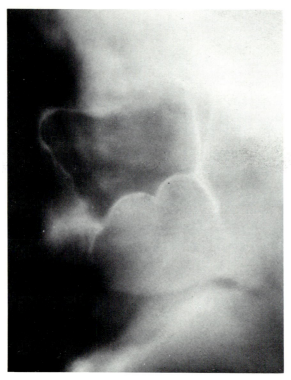

Figure 6.52A

Lateral tomographic study of the hard palate shows a mass arising from the hard palate and causing biconcave, cortical, bony displacement. (From Weber, A. L. Pleomorphic adenoma of the hard palate. *Annals of Otology, Rhinology and Laryngology* 90(2):192–193, March–April 1981. Reprinted by permission).

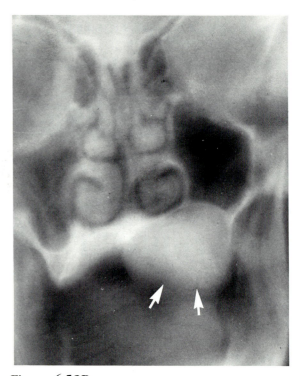

Figure 6.52B

AP tomographic section reveals thinning and superior displacement of bone in the region of the left alveolar ridge, floor of the antrum and adjacent hard palate. A mass projects below the left alveolar portion of the maxilla into the adjacent oral cavity (*arrows*). (From Weber, A. L. Pleomorphic adenoma of the hard palate. *Annals of Otology, Rhinology and Laryngology* 90(2):192–193, March–April 1981. Reprinted by permission).

Adenocarcinoma of the palate

A 60-year-old woman with a six-month history of adenocarcinoma of the hard palate was treated with two courses of chemotherapy without success. She was admitted for palatectomy.

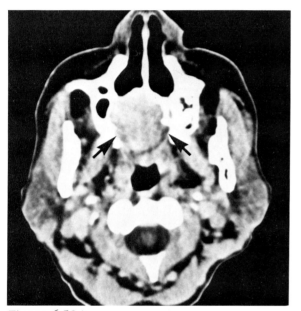

Figure 6.53A

Axial contrast CT scan at the level of the palate reveals a homogeneous mass projecting into the upper portion of the oral cavity (*arrows*).

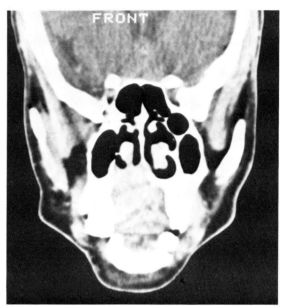

Figure 6.53B

Coronal CT scan shows the same mass in the oral cavity arising from the hard palate with extension into the lower portion of the right nasal cavity. There is destruction of the central and right portion of the hard palate.

Mucoepidermoid carcinoma in a thyroglossal duct cyst

This 58-year-old woman had noted a slowly enlarging midline neck mass with occasional discomfort, but no acute pain. A thyroid scan was normal Physical examination revealed a 7- × 7-cm, anterior, firm neck mass extending from the cricoid cartilage to the submentum. There was no adenopathy. The mass was completely resected and there was no invasion of intralaryngeal structures.

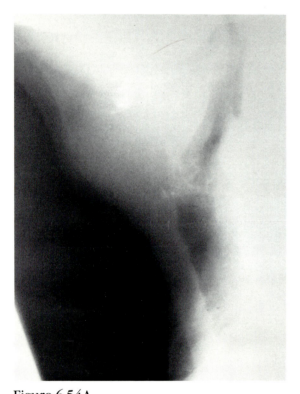

Figure 6.54A

Lateral view of the neck reveals a homogeneous mass anterior to the larynx and below the hyoid bone. The epiglottis is slightly displaced posteriorly.

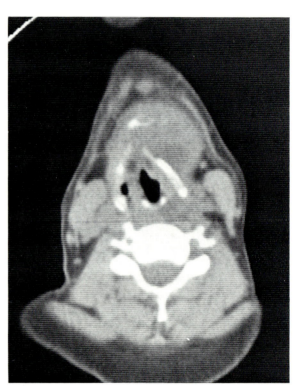

Figure 6.54B

Axial noncontrast CT section at the level of the thyroid cartilage shows a sharply marginated mass anterior to the thyroid cartilage, predominantly on the left. There are some speckled calcifications in the anterior portion of this mass.

Pleomorphic adenoma arising in the deep portion of the left parotid gland with parapharyngeal extension

This 75-year-old woman was noted to have an asymptomatic mass in the left oropharynx during hospitalization for pneumonia. Physical examination demonstrated a mass in the peritonsillar region and adjacent soft palate extending into the nasopharynx. Through an external approach after a superficial parotidectomy, the parapharyngeal tumor was removed.

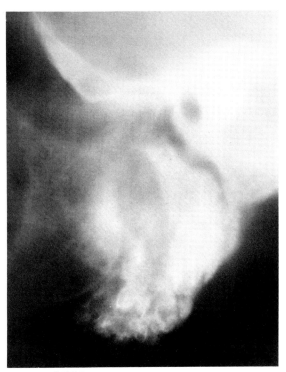

Figure 6.55B

Lateral tomographic section in the parenchymal phase of the parotid sialogram reveals an ill-defined defect in the deep portion of the left parotid gland.

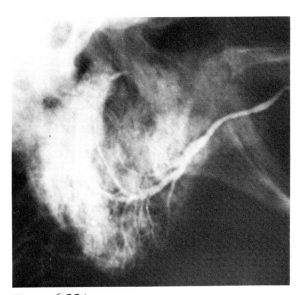

Figure 6.55A

Lateral view of a left parotid sialogram reveals an ill-defined defect in the anterior superior portion of the parotid gland. Note stretching of intraparotid branches around this tumor mass. The main duct is displaced inferiorly.

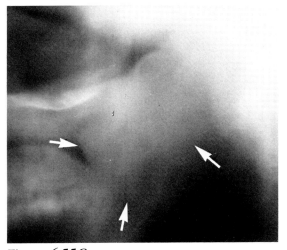

Figure 6.55C

Lateral tomographic section through the oronasopharynx reveals a homogeneous, sharply marginated mass in the region of the oropharynx and nasopharynx (*arrows*).

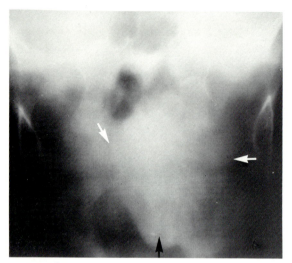

Figure 6.55D

AP tomographic section of the oronasopharynx demonstrates a left-sided, oval, homogeneous mass that is sharply marginated superiorly, medially, and inferiorly (*arrows*). The lateral component of this mass arising from the deep portion of the parotid cannot be discerned on this conventional tomographic study.

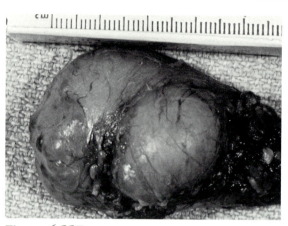

Figure 6.55E

Photograph of specimen shows an encapsulated slightly lobulated mass.

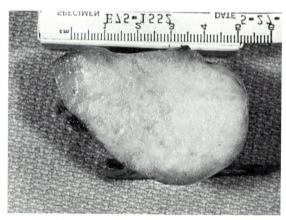

Figure 6.55F

Cut section through the mass shows a glistening grayish white surface with a well-defined capsule.

Pleomorphic adenoma with calcification of the left side of the parapharyngeal space arising from the minor salivary glands

This 40-year-old woman noted a painless lump in the back of her throat. Physical examination revealed a 3- × 3-cm mass displacing the soft palate medially and inferiorly.

The patient underwent an excision of the left parapharyngeal mass via a cervical approach. The pathologic examination revealed a pleomorphic adenoma.

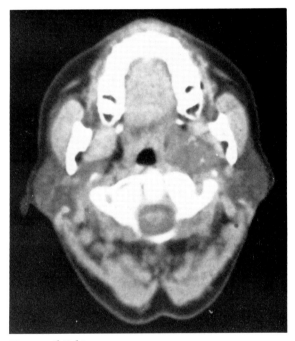

Figure 6.56A

Axial contrast CT study reveals a low-density lesion in the left parapharyngeal space adjacent to the deep portion of the parotid gland. Note punctate calcifications within the homogeneous, sharply defined mass. There is slight medial displacement of the oropharyngeal wall.

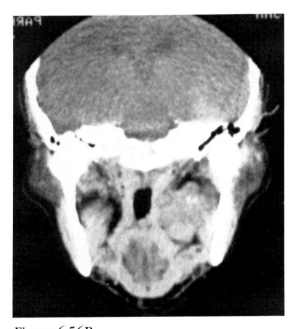

Figure 6.56B

Coronal CT section demonstrates the parapharyngeal mass between the lateral oropharyngeal wall and the medial pterygoid muscle. There is a slight bulge of the oropharyngeal wall medially. The lesion is separated from the deep portion of the parotid gland. Note the calcific densities within the mass.

Right-sided parapharyngeal pleomorphic adenoma arising from minor salivary glands

The patient was a 53-year-old man with swelling in the peritonsillar and soft palate region on the right side.

Figure 6.57

Axial contrast CT reveals a low-density irregular mass in the right parapharyngeal space behind the pterygoid muscle. The mass extends laterally to the deep portion of the parotid, but is separated by a fat plane from the parotid gland. The mass medially abuts the lateral oropharyngeal wall.

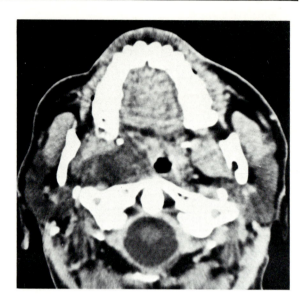

Invasive squamous cell carcinoma in the right side of the parapharyngeal space

This 59-year-old woman had intermittent right-sided frontal and occipital headaches. Physical examination revealed a right-sided serous otitis media. She also developed severe pain on the right side, which required pain medication and an occipital nerve injection. Two months following her initial complaints, she developed some difficulty in swallowing, a right-sided Horner's syndrome, and a non-tender fullness of the right side of the peritonsillar area. Endoscopy with a biopsy of the peritonsillar region revealed a squamous cell carcinoma.

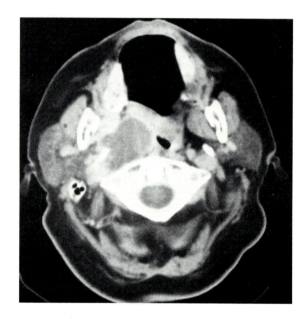

Figure 6.58

Axial contrast CT scan at the angle of the mandible shows a low-density mass in the parapharyngeal space with some rim enhancement. The mass is adjacent to the deep portion of the parotid gland. The soft palate is pushed medially and anteriorly by this parapharyngeal mass.

References

Batsakis, J. G. *Tumors of the head and neck: clinical and pathological considerations.* Baltimore: William & Wilkins, 1979.

Beahrs, O. H. et al. Carcinomatous transformation of mixed tumours of the parotid gland. *Arch. Surg.* 75:605–614, 1957.

Belsky, J. L. et al. Salivary gland tumors in atomic bomb survivors. Hiroshima–Nagasaki, 1959 to 1970. *JAMA* 219:864–868, 1972.

Bergman, F. Tumors of the minor salivary glands. *Cancer* 33:538, 1966.

Blanck, C.; Eneroth, C-M.; and Jakobsson, P. A. Mucoepidermoid adenopapillary (non-epidermoid) carcinomas of the parotid gland. *Cancer* 28:676–685, 1971.

Blanck, C.; Eneroth, C-M.; and Jakobsson, P. A. Oncocytoma of the parotid gland: neoplasm or nodular hyperplasia? *Cancer* 25:919–925, 1970.

Bryan, R. N. et al. Computed tomography of the major salivary glands. *AJR* 139:547–554, 1982.

Carter, B. L. et al. Computed tomography and sialography. Part 2. Pathology. *J. Comput. Assist. Tomogr.* 5:46–53, 1981.

Castro, E. B. et al. Tumors of the major salivary glands in children. *Cancer* 29:312, 1972.

Catlin, D. Surgery for head and neck lymphomas. *Surgery* 60:1160–1166, 1966.

Chaudhry, A. P., and Gorlin, R. J. Papillary cystadenoma lymphomatosum (adenolymphoma). *Am. J. Surg.* 95:923–931, 1958.

Chong, G. C.; Beahrs, O. H.; and Woolner, L. B. Surgical management of acinic cell carcinoma of the parotid gland. *Surg. Gynecol. Obstet.* 138:65–68, 1974.

Christopherson, W. M. Oncocytoma of the parotid gland. *Arch. Pathol.* 68:96–98, 1949.

Clarke, J. S.; Hentz, B. C.; and Mahoney, W. D. Bilateral acinic cell carcinoma of the parotid gland. *Ann. Surg.* 170:866, 1969.

Conley, J. J. *Salivary glands and the facial nerve.* New York: Grune & Stratton, 1975.

Conley, J., and Arena, S. Parotid gland as a focus of metastasis. *Arch. Surg.* 87:757–764, 1963.

Conley, J., and Dingman, D. L. Adenoid cystic carcinoma in the head and neck (cylindroma). *Arch. Otolaryngol.* 100:81–90, 1974.

Crocker, D. J.; Calalaris, C. J.; and Finch, R. Intraoral minor salivary gland tumors: report of 38 cases. *Oral Surg.* 29:60, 1970.

Eneroth, C-M. Histological and clinical aspects of parotid tumors. *Acta Orolaryngol.* (suppl.). 191:1–99, 1964.

Eneroth, C-M. Salivary gland tumors in the parotid gland, submandibular gland and the palate region. *Cancer* 27:1415–1418, 1971.

Eneroth, C-M.; Blanck, C.; and Jakobsson, P. A. Carcinoma in pleomorphic adenoma of the parotid gland. *Acta Otolaryngol.* 66:477–492, 1968.

Eneroth, C-M.; Hjertman, L.; and Moberger, G. Salivary gland adenomas of the palate. *Acta Otolaryngol.* 73:305–315, 1972.

Eneroth, C-M.; Jakobbson, P. A.; and Blanck, C. Acinic cell carcinoma of the parotid gland. *Cancer* 19:1761–1772, 1966.

Ethell, A. T. A rare "parotid tumor." *J. Laryngol. Otol.* 93:741–744, 1979.

Eversole, L. R. Mucoepidermoid carcinoma: review of 815 reported cases. *J. Oral Surg.* 28:490–494, 1970.

Fine, G.; Marshall, R. B.; and Horn, R. C., Jr. Tumors of the major salivary glands. *Cancer* 13:653–659, 1960.

Frazell, E. L. Observations on the management of salivary gland tumors. In *Cancer management.* Philadelphia: J. B. Lippincott, 1968.

Foote, E. W., and Frazell, E. L. Tumors of the major salivary glands. *Cancer* 6:1065–1133, 1953.

Foote, E. W., and Frazell, E. L. *Tumors of the major salivary glands.* U.S. Atlas of tumor pathology, Armed Forces Institute of Pathology, 1954, section 4.

Gerughty, R. M. et al. Malignant mixed tumor of salivary gland origin. *Cancer* 24:471, 1969.

Golding S. Computed tomography in the diagnosis of parotid gland tumors. *Br. J. Radiol.* 55:182–188, 1982.

Goldman, R. L., and Perzik, S. L. Infantile hemangioma of the parotid gland. A clinicopathological study of 15 cases. *Arch. Otolaryngol.* 90:605–608, 1969.

Gore, D.; Rankow, R.; and Hanford, J. Parapharyngeal neurilemmoma. *Surg. Gynecol. Obstet.* 103:193–201, 1956.

Grage, T. B., and Lober, P. H. Malignant tumors of the major salivary glands. *Surgery* 52:284–294, 1962.

Graham, J. W. Metastatic cancer in the parotid lymph nodes. *Med. J. Aust.* 2:8, 1965.

Hales, B., and Hansen, J. E. Bilateral simultaneous Warthin's tumor in a woman. *South. Med. J.* 70:257–258, 1977.

Heydt, S. A ganglion associated with the temporomandibular joint. *J. Oral Surg.* 35:400–401, 1977.

Hornbaker, J. H., Jr. et al. Sjögren's syndrome and nodular reticulum cell sarcoma. *Arch. Intern. Med.* 118:449–452, 1966.

Howard, J. M. et al. Parotid tumors in children. *Surg. Gynecol. Obstet.* 90:307–319, 1950.

Hyman, G. A., and Wolff, M. Lymphomas. In *Diseases of the salivary glands*, eds. R. M. Rankow and I. Polayes. Philadelphia: J. B. Lippincott, 1976, ch. 6.

Janecka, I. P., and Conley, J. J. Synovial cyst of the temporomandibular joint imitating a parotid tumor. *J. Maxillofac. Surg.* 6:154–156, 1978.

Johns, M. E. Parotid cancer: a rational basis for treatment. *Head Neck Surg.* 3(2):132–141, 1980.

Karmody, C. S.; Fortson, J. K.; and Calcaterra, V. E. Lymphangiomas of the head and neck in adults. *Otolaryngol. Head Neck Surg.* 90:283–288, 1982.

Kauffman, S. L., and Stout, A. P. Tumors of the major salivary glands in children. *Cancer* 16:1317–1331, 1963.

Kinkead, L. R.; Bennett, J. E.; and Tomich, E. C. A ganglion of the temporomandibular joint presenting as a parotid tumor. *Head Neck Surg.* 3(5):443–445, 1981.

Krolls, S. O.; Trodahl, J. N.; and Boyers, R. C. Salivary gland lesions in children. *Cancer* 30:459–469, 1972.

Kumar, A. J. et al. Computed tomography of extracranial nerve sheath tumors with pathological correlation. *J. Comput. Assist. Tomogr.* 7(5):857–865, 1983.

Levin, J. M.; Robinson, D. W.; and Lin, F. Acinic cell carcinoma. Collective review including bilateral cases. *Arch. Surg.* 110:64–68, 1975.

Manual for staging of cancer. Chicago: American Joint Committee for Cancer Staging and End Results Reporting, 1978.

Moore, H. D. Parotid cysts. *Br. Med. J.* 1:649, 1950.

Moran, J. J. et al. Adenoid cystic carcinoma: a clinicopathological study. *Cancer* 14:1235–1250, 1961.

Moran, A. G., and Buchanan, D. R. Branchial cysts, sinuses and fistulae. *Clin. Otolaryngol.* 3:77–92, 1978.

Morgan, M. N., and MacKenzie, D. H. Tumors of salivary glands. A review of 204 cases with five year follow-up. *Br. J. Surg.* 55:284–288, 1968.

Patey, D. H.; Thackray, A. C.; and Keeling, D. H. Malignant disease of the parotid. *Br. J. Cancer* 19:712–737, 1965.

Pope, T. H., Jr., and Lehmann, W. B. Parotid metastasis to parotid nodes. *Arch. Otolaryngol.* 86:673, 1967.

Rabinov, K.; Kell, T. J., Jr.; and Gordon, P. H. Computed tomography of the salivary glands. *Radiol. Clin. North Am.,* in press.

Rauch, S. *Die Speicheldrüsen des Menschen.* Stuttgart: Georg Thieme Verlag, 1959.

Reiquam, C. W. Salivary gland tumors in children. *Arch. Surg.* 86:313, 1963.

Rice, D. H.; Mancuso, A. A.; and Hanafee, W. N. Computerized tomography with simultaneous sialography in evaluating parotid tumors. *Arch. Otolaryngol.* 106:472–473, 1980.

Schuller, D. E., and McCabe, B. F. Salivary gland neoplasms in children. *Otolaryngol. Clin. North Am.* 1977.

Seldin, H. M. et al. Lipoma of the oral cavity: report of 26 cases. *J. Oral Surg.* 25:270, 1967.

Silverman, P. M.; Korobkin, M.; and Moore, A. V. Computed tomography of cystic neck masses. *J. Comput. Assist. Tomogr.* 7(3):498–502, 1983.

Simpson, R. A. Lateral cervical cysts and fistulas. *Laryngoscope* 79:30–59, 1967.

Som, P., and Biller, F. The combined computerized tomography-sialogram: a technique to differentiate deep lobe parotid tumors from extra parotid pharyngomaxillary space tumor. *Ann. Otol. Rhinol. Laryngol.* 88:590–595, 1979.

Som, P. M.; Biller, H. G.; and Lawson, W. Tumors of the parapharyngeal space: preoperative evaluation, diagnosis and surgical procedures. *Ann. Otol. Rhinol. Laryngol.* 90 (suppl. 80 1 pt. 4): 1–15, 1981.

Som, P. M., and Sanders, D. E. *The salivary gland.* In *Head and neck imaging excluding the brain.* eds. R. T. Bergeron, A. G. Osborn, and P. M. Som. St. Louis: C. V. Mosby, 1984, ch. 4.

Sone, S. et al. CT of parotid tumors. *AJNR* 3:143–147, 1982.

Spiro, R. H.; Huvos, A. G.; and Strong, E. W. Adenoid cystic carcinoma of salivary origin. A clinicopathologic study of 242 cases. *Cancer* 31:117–129, 1974.

Spiro, R. H.; Huvos, A. G.; and Strong, E. W. Cancer of the parotid gland. *Am. J. Surg.* 130:452–459, 1975.

Spiro, R. H.; Koss, L. G.; and Hajdu, S. I. Tumors of minor salivary origin. A clinicopathologic study of 492 cases. *Cancer* 31:117–129, 1973.

Stebner, F. C. et al. Identification of Warthin's tumors by scanning of salivary glands. *Am. J. Surg.* 116:513–517, 1968.

Stone, D. N. et al. Parotid CT sialography. *Radiology* 138:393–397, 1981.

Talal, N., and Bernim, J. J. The development of malignant lymphomas in the course of Sjögren's syndrome. *Am. J. Med.* 36:529–540, 1964.

Thackray, A. C., and Lucas, R. B. *Tumors of the major salivary glands.* Atlas of tumor pathology, Armed Forces Institute of Pathology, 1974.

Thackray, A. C., and Sobin, L. H. *Histological typing of salivary gland tumors.* International histological classification of tumors, no. 7. Geneva, World Health Organization, 1972.

Wallace, A. C. et al. Salivary gland tumors in Canadian Eskimos. *Cancer* 16:1338–1353, 1963.

Weber, A. L., and Kushner, D. C. Parotid tumor. *Ann. Otol. Rhinol. Laryngol.* 86(2):26, 1977.

Work, W. P., and Hybels, R. L. A study of tumors of the parapharyngeal space. *Laryngoscope* 84:1748–1755, 1974.

Wowro, N. W.; Fredrickson, R. W.; and Tennant, R. Hemangioma of the parotid gland in the newborn and in infancy. *Cancer* 8:595, 1955.

Chapter 7   Hypertrophy of the Masseter Muscles

To some degree this term may be misleading since there may be hypertrophy not only of the masseter muscles but also of the temporalis muscles and the bony areas of attachment of these muscles (Conley 1975).

Masseter muscle hypertrophy has been recognized for more than a century. Legg (1880), in what is believed to be the first recorded instance of this entity, published an apparently complete description of an instance of enlargement of the masseter and temporalis muscles bilaterally in a 10-year-old girl. His observations are still pertinent. He described "tumors at angles of jaw and on temples."

> On each temple there is a tumor of ill-defined outline rising more suddenly in front but gradually subsiding toward the back, the one on the left being rather more marked than the one on the right. It extends upwards as far as the temporal ridge, backwards to the distance of an inch behind the auricle, downwards it would seem to be bounded by the zygoma. To the feel they are both firm, giving no trace of fluctuation; they also move. When she sets her teeth they become hard and rise up.
>
> Both angles of the jaw appear to be especially prominent, there seeming to be a distinct bony enlargement corresponding to the insertion of the masseter. . . . There is also a tumor at each angle of the jaw, that on the left side being, perhaps, slightly more marked. They possess the same characters as those on the temples, giving no sense of fluctuation and becoming hard when she shuts her jaw. They extend upwards to the zygoma, being coterminous with the tumors on the temples; below they are bounded by the jaw-bone. (362–363)

In 1905, Duroux reported bilateral hypertrophy of the masseter muscles in a 22-year-old man. Boldt (1930) reported two cases of bilateral masseter muscle hypertrophy, one in a 16-year-old boy, the other in a 24-year-old woman who also manifested temporalis muscle hypertrophy.

Development

Masseteric hypertrophy of minor degree is common, and the abnormality draws no particular interest until extreme degrees of enlargement are reached (Lash 1963; Trodahl 1970). The enlargement of the muscle may reach such proportions as to become unsightly (Coffey 1942; Guggenheim and Cohen 1959; Conley 1975), constituting a significant cosmetic problem. Such patients may be referred for treatment because of a question of parotid tumor (Maxwell and Waggoner 1951; Guggenheim and Cohen 1959). The muscle may be enlarged as much as three times normal size (Adams 1949). This entity should not be confused with the similar clinical appearance commonly seen in thin patients who have only prominent flaring mandibular angles without abnormal enlargement of the muscles (Maxwell and Waggoner 1951; Barton 1957).

The process of masseteric hypertrophy commonly begins in adolescence or early adulthood (Maxwell 1952; Kern 1954; Masters, Georgiade, and Pickerell 1955; Guggenheim and Cohen 1959). According to Waldhart and Lynch (1971), it rarely occurs in small children or in patients over the age of 30 years. Nevertheless, it is also seen in older patients (Barton 1957) (fig. 7.5). It does occur in children and has been reported in patients 10, 11, and 12 years old (respectively, Legg 1880; Maxwell and Waggoner 1951; Lash 1963). There usually is a history of slow growth of the mass over a period of years (Masters, Georgiade, and Pickerell 1955), but it is not unusual for patients to become suddenly aware of the presence of such enlargement. Gurney (1947) presents a case in which enlargement of the muscles had been present for 20 years.

Sex distribution is about equal (Kern 1954). The process may be unilateral or bilateral (Drummond and McIntosh 1954; Masters, Georgiade, and Pickerell 1955; Barton 1957) and is frequently asymmetrical. The diagnosis of masseter muscle hypertrophy can be suspected clinically because the smooth, nontender swelling is anterior to the usual location of parotid masses and has the consistency of muscle tissue (Drummond and McIntosh 1954). Its outlines correspond with those of the masseter muscle, with indefinite upper border and a lower margin along the inferior portion of the mandible.

The masseter muscle originates on the zygomatic arch and zygomatic process of the maxilla and is inserted upon the lateral aspect of the ramus and angle of the mandible (fig. 7.1). The temporalis muscle originates in the temporal fossa and inserts on the coronoid process of the mandible. With clenching of the teeth, the mass of hypertrophied muscle becomes more prominent, harder, and fixed, and now can be definitely localized anterior to the usual position of the major portion of the parotid gland (fig. 7.6C). The presence of this contractile mass corresponding with the masseter muscle renders the diagnosis all but certain. Simultaneous palpation of the mass externally and intraorally, both at rest and during clenching of the teeth, will confirm that the entire mass consists of the masseter muscle. If the masseter muscle only is enlarged, there is a prominent bulge at the angle of the mandible, producing a squaring of the contour here (figs. 7.3A, 7.6A). If the temporalis muscle also is enlarged, the entire side of the face may attain an outward convexity (Conley 1975) (fig. 7.5A). In addition to these findings, the mandible may be flared and a bony prominence may be palpated deep to the muscle, along the angle of the mandible (Masters, Georgiade, and Pickerell 1955; Barton 1957).

Radiologic Changes

Plain radiographs or panoramic films may show flaring of the angle of the mandible and a bony prominence or external hyperostosis at the lateral aspect and free margin of the angle of the mandible (figs. 7.2A, 7.5B). In advanced cases, this may show irregularity of contour and irregularity of density (Masters, Georgiade, and Pickerell 1955; Guggenheim and Cohen 1959). According to these authors, the lateral cortex at the angle of the mandible may present an irregularly scalloped appearance or may protrude as a more or less rough, spinelike projection and may even assume the appearance of multiple cystic radiolucent areas.

Conventional sialography may show the parotid gland and duct to be displaced laterally from their position (Blatt et al. 1959; O'Hara 1973) (figs. 7.2A,B,C). No intrinsic parotid abnormalities ordinarily accompany masseter muscle hypertrophy.

CT examination, done without contrast material, shows enlargement of the masseter muscle (figs. 7.3C, 7.4, 7.5C,D,E, 7.6B). Coarse, focal bulges in this muscle may correspond with the clinically palpable mass in this region. The temporalis and pterygoid muscles may also be prominent (figs. 7.5E,F).

Histology

Histologic examination of the enlarged muscle has for the most part revealed normal striated muscle or muscle manifesting work hypertrophy (Gurney 1947; Masters, Georgiade, and Pickerell 1955; Batsakis 1979). Guggenheim and Cohen (1960) reviewed the literature in this regard and reported normal muscle in one chronic case of their own, and in one acute case, showed significant hypertrophy of individual masseter muscle fibers together with some small islands of cartilage in the muscle itself, which they interpreted as associated myositis ossificans. Histologic examination of bony prominence at the angle of the mandible has shown only normal cortical bone (Adams 1949; Masters, Georgiade, and Pickerell 1955; Waldhart and Lynch 1971).

Differential Diagnosis

Although the cause of the muscle hypertrophy is unknown in the majority of patients (Maxwell and Waggoner 1951; Soderberg and

Switzer 1954; Masters, Georgiade, and Pickerell 1955; Lash 1963; Waldhart and Lynch 1971), many authors have suggested that the finding may represent physiologic work hypertrophy caused by grinding or clenching of the teeth (Gurney 1947; Kern 1954; Drummond and McIntosh 1954; Barton 1957; Guggenheim and Cohen 1959). Boldt (1930) referred to these patients as "tooth athletes." In the patients reported here, more or less continuous contraction of one or more of the muscles of mastication was found to be present in every instance and throughout all patient examinations. The state of contraction of the muscles is reported to be relieved by general anesthesia (Guggenheim and Cohen 1960).

The significance of the abnormality lies primarily in the possibility of its being mistaken for an inflammatory process or tumor in the parotid gland or nearby tissues (Maxwell and Waggoner 1951; Guggenheim and Cohen 1959; Lash 1963). Surgery has occasionally been performed in such instances (Hersh 1946; Barton 1957), as has irradiation (Lash 1963). It is therefore prudent for all physicians, dentists, and other health care personnel to be aware of this entity.

Treatment

Conservative treatment with reassurance is all that is usually necessary (Coffey 1942; Tempest 1951; Barton 1957; Lash 1963). The patient should be made aware of the nature of the abnormality and advised to try consciously to relax the chewing muscles and to avoid clenching and grinding of the teeth and to avoid any unnecessary exercise of these muscles (such as gum chewing). Any obvious dental or occlusal abnormality or temporomandibular joint abnormality should be corrected. In extreme cases, cosmetic surgery can be done with removal of a portion of the masseter muscle and sometimes removal of the bony angle of the mandible (Gurney 1947; Adams 1949; Masters, Georgiade, and Pickerell 1959; Waldhart and Lynch 1971).

CASES

Diagram of masseter muscle

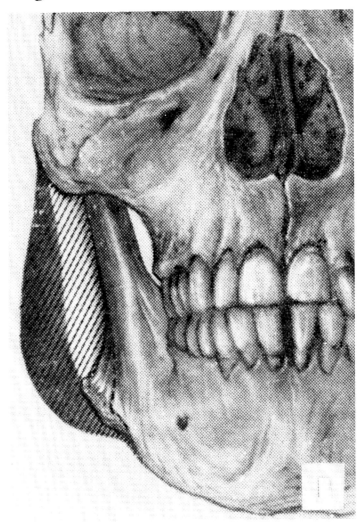

Figure 7.1

Masseter muscle originates on the zygomatic process of the maxilla and zygomatic arch and inserts on the lateral aspect of the ramus and angle of the mandible. The normal muscle is shown in light gray, the hypertrophied muscle in dark gray. (Barton 1954. Reprinted with permission.)

Masseter muscle hypertrophy, right parotid sialogram

C = cannula
Ma = mandible
MM = enlarged masseter muscle
PD = parotid duct
PG = parotid gland
Z = zygomatic arch

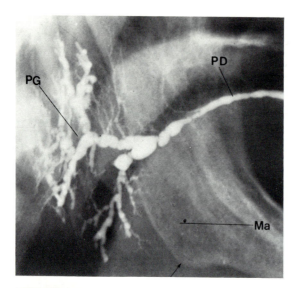

The patient was a 40-year-old man with a history of several episodes of painful swelling in the right parotid area while eating, presumably associated with the sialectasis and stricture formation which are present in the parotid duct system. In addition, however, the masseter muscle was noted clinically to be quite enlarged on each side, in rather symmetrical fashion.

Figure 7.2A

Lateral view, performed with Ethiodol; note the prominent tubercle at the angle of the mandible (*arrow*). There is evidence of moderate sialectasis and stricture formation, presumably unrelated to the muscle hypertrophy (see also fig. 7.2B).

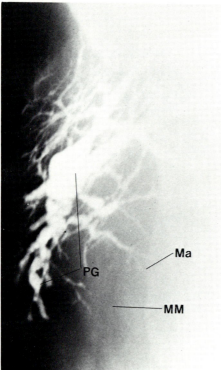

Figure 7.2B

AP view; the lower half of the parotid gland is displaced moderately laterally by the enlarged masseter muscle.

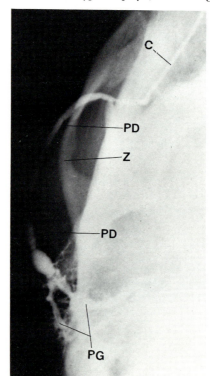

Figure 7.2C

Tilted axial view; the parotid duct is displaced laterally as it passes over the enlarged masseter muscle.

Masseter muscle hypertrophy, mild case

Ma = man-dible
MM = masseter muscle
MPM = medial pterygoid muscle
PG = parotid gland
R = right
L = left

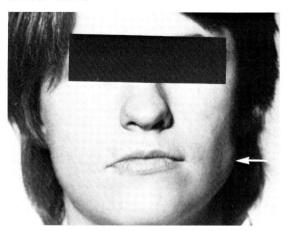

Figure 7.3A

Photograph of the patient; this process is bilateral, but is more evident on the left side than on the right side. The palpable mass is indicated by the arrow.

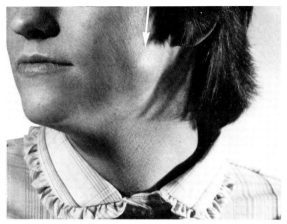

Figure 7.3B

Photograph from slightly different view; arrow indicates palpable mass.

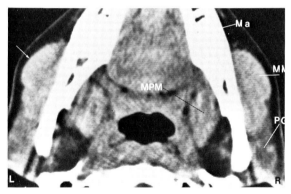

Figure 7.3C

Plain CT performed in the semiaxial position with the chin extended and the gantry angled 20 degrees craniad. The masseter muscles are slightly enlarged bilaterally, that on the left appearing possibly slightly more focally prominent (*arrow*). Their actual measurements are almost the same (compare with figures 2.20, 2.21A, 2.22A,B).

The patient was a 27-year-old woman complaining of a lump in the left jaw area and a feeling of pressure on the left side of the face. There was a history of clicking in the right temporomandibular joint for many years. On clinical examination a hard mass was palpable in the region of the angle of the jaw on the left side, becoming larger with clenching, consistent with enlarged masseter muscle. Minimal similar changes were present on the right. The patient was observed on many occasions, and the jaw was consistently held in a clenched position, especially on the left side. There was no unusual wear of dentition. This case and that in figure 7.4 are examples of slight focal muscle hypertrophy.

Masseter muscle hypertrophy, mild case

Ba = barium marker indicating the palpable mass
Con = condyloid process of mandible
Ma = mandible
Max = maxilla
MM = masseter muscle
MPM = medial pterygoid muscle
PG = parotid gland
SCM = sternocleidomastoid muscle
R = right
L = left

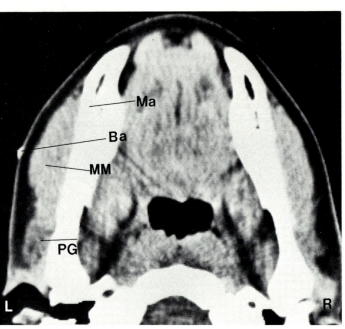

Figure 7.4A

Semiaxial plain CT with the head extended quite high and the gantry angled 11 degrees craniad; near coronal position; low section through the ramus and body of the mandible, with the jaw relaxed. The left masseter muscle is larger than the right one.

The patient was a 20-year-old woman with a three-week history of a mass in the region of the left mandibular angle. The masseter muscle could be seen and palpated to be held in a consistently contracted state by the patient. There was a long history of temporomandibular joint dysfunction on both sides so that the joints opened quite asynchronously with an audible click. There was no unusual wear of dentition. Upon questioning, the patient stated that she realized that she clenched her teeth, especially when she was cold.

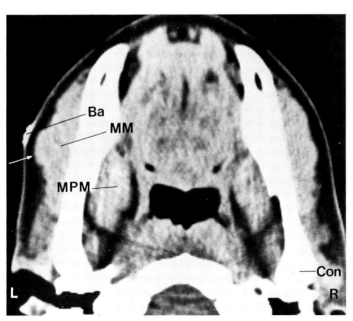

Figure 7.4B

Same position and level as in figure 7.4A, but with
the teeth clenched. Note the prominent muscle
bundle (*arrow*) underlying the barium marker,
which indicates the mass noted in this region by
the patient. Compare with the appearance of
normal masseter muscles in a young man (fig.
2.23A).

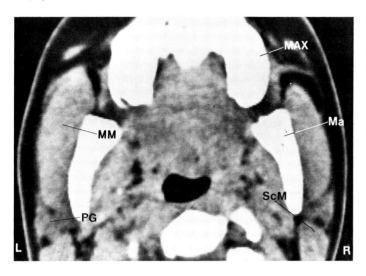

Figure 7.4C

Higher section with the head flexed and the
gantry vertical. The teeth are clenched. The left
masseter muscle is considerably larger than the
right one. Other sections done at a higher level,
not shown, demonstrated the temporalis muscle
to be normal in size. Compare with figures 2.20,
2.22B.

Bilateral hypertrophy of the masseter and temporalis muscles

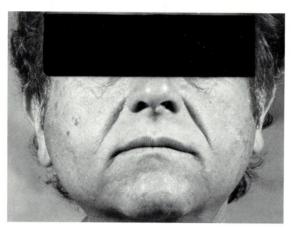

Figure 7.5A

Photograph of the patient showing marked rounded prominence of the facial contour bilaterally.

The patient was a 58-year-old man with a history of episodic pain and swelling and feeling of tension in the side of the face and jaw on each side. Inspection demonstrated marked rounding of the facial contour bilaterally, over the mandibular angles as well as higher. Palpation revealed a hard and large masseter muscle bilaterally, held contracted and tense at all times, and bulging further with voluntary clenching of the teeth. The temporalis muscles were also palpably enlarged.

The patient had first noticed swelling four years earlier and had a long history of temporomandibular joint dysfunction syndrome on the right side, with the jaws locked in partly open position on at least one occasion.

The degree of muscle hypertrophy is much more marked in this patient and in the patient shown in figure 7.6 than in other examples.

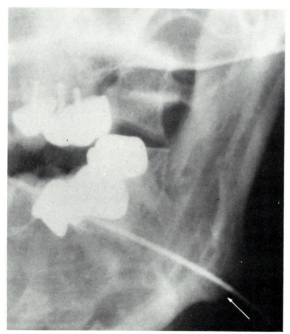

Figure 7.5B

AP radiograph of the mandible; note the prominent tubercle at the angle of the mandible (*arrow*). The catheter overlies this area.

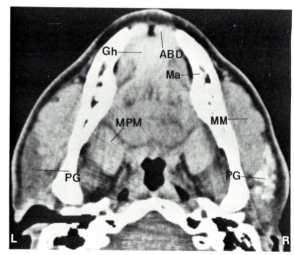

Figure 7.5C

Plain CT through the mandibular ramus and body with the head extended and the gantry angled 20 degrees craniad. Near coronal projection. The masseter muscles are enlarged bilaterally. Note the coarse muscle bundles. The lower pole of the right parotid gland is visible, still containing Ethiodol from sialogram performed five weeks earlier. Compare with figures 2.21A, 2.23A.

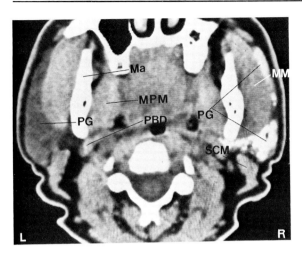
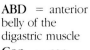

Figure 7.5D

Plain CT through the ramus of the mandible with the head flexed and the gantry vertical. The masseter muscles are markedly enlarged on each side; the parotid gland is compressed by the enlarged masseter muscles. Compare with figures 2.20, 2.22B.

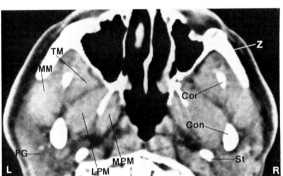

Figure 7.5E

CT section through the lower anterior portion of the zygomatic arch; the head is flexed and the gantry is angled 4 degrees caudad. This section is just below the insertion of the masseter muscles into the zygoma. The enlarged temporal muscles can be seen at their insertions onto the coronoid processes. Compare with figure 2.22A and with normal muscle appearance shown by silver and colleagues (1983).

Figure 7.5F

CT section through the upper part of the temporal fossa. The temporalis muscles are quite large even at this high level.

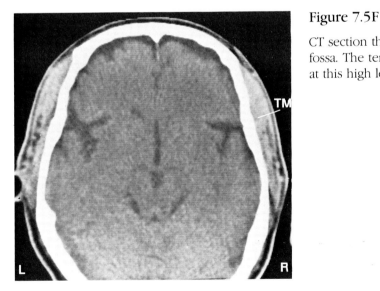

ABD = anterior belly of the digastric muscle

Con = condyloid process

Cor = coronoid process

GH = geniohyoid muscle

LPM = lateral pyterygoid muscle

Ma = mandible

MM = masseter muscle

MPM = medial pterygoid muscle

PBD = posterior belly of the digastric muscle

PG = parotid gland (with retained Ethiodol on right side)

SCM = sternocleidomastoid muscle

St = styloid process

TM = temporalis muscle

Z = anterior portion of the zygomatic arch

Masseter muscle hypertrophy

BB = metal marker on skin indicating palpable mass
Ma = mandible
MM = masseter muscle
MPM = medial pterygoid muscle
PG = parotid gland
St = styloid process

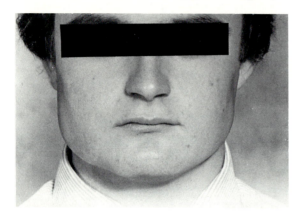

Figure 7.6A

Photograph of the patient; the patient's friends had noted the prominent bulge at the side of the jaw.

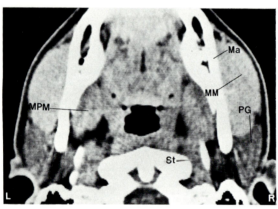

Figure 7.6B

Plain CT of the parotid region with the head extended and the gantry angled 20 degrees craniad; the masseter muscle is enlarged moderately on the right, slightly on the left.

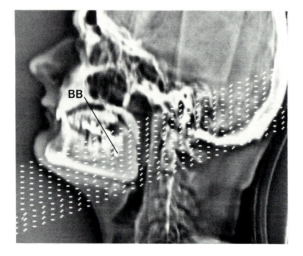

Figure 7.6C

Digital radiograph (topogram) showing the planes imaged. The BB indicates the palpable enlarged masseer muscle, anterior to the usual location of parotid masses.

The patient is a 20-year-old man with a mass first noted at the angle of the right jaw nine months previously. There has been no pain, but there is a possible history of clicking in one of the temporomandibular joints. Physical examination revealed a firm mass anterior to the angle of the jaw and anteriorly to the usual location of parotid masses. Bidigital palpation with the jaw relaxed and clenched demonstrated the mass to be entirely masseter muscle.

References

Adams, W. M. Bilateral hypertrophy of the masseter muscle: an operation for correction. *Br. J. Plast. Surg.* 2:78–82, 1949.

Barton, R. T. Benign masseteric hypertrophy. A syndrome of importance in the differential diagnosis of parotid tumors. *JAMA* 164:1646–1647, 1957.

Batsakis, J. G. *Tumors of the head and neck. Clinical and pathological considerations,* 2nd edition. Baltimore: Williams & Wilkins, 1979.

Blatt, I. M., et al. Secretory sialography in diseases external to the major salivary glands. *Ann. Otol. Rhinol. Laryngol.* 68:175–186, 1959.

Boldt, H. Ein Beitrag zur Kenntnis der einfachen Masseterhypertrophie mit einigen Fällen. Dissertation, Friedrich-Wilhelms-Universität zu Berlin, 1930.

Coffey, R. J. Unilateral hypertrophy of the masseter muscle. *Surgery* 11:815–818, 1942.

Conley, J. *Salivary glands and the facial nerve.* New York: Grune & Stratton, 1975.

Drummond, J. A., and McIntosh, C. A. Unilateral hypertrophy of masseter muscle. *Am. J. Surg.* 87:711–714, 1954.

Duroux, M. Hypertrophie musculaire bilaterale des masseters. *Lyon Med.* 104:1355–1356, 1905.

Guggenheim, P., and Cohen, L. B. External hyperostosis of the mandible angle associated with masseteric hypertrophy. *Arch. Otolaryngol.* 70:674–680, 1959.

Guggenheim, P., and Cohen, L. B. The histopathology of masseteric hypertrophy. *Arch. Otolaryngol.* 71:906–912, 1960.

Gurney, C. E. Chronic bilateral benign hypertrophy of the masseter muscles. *Am. J. Surg.* 73:137–139, 1947.

Hersh, J. H. Hypertrophy of the masseter muscle. *Arch. Otolaryngol.* 43:593–596, 1946.

Kern, A. B. Masseter muscle hypertrophy. *Archives of Dermatology and Syphilology.* 69:558–562, 1954.

Lash, H. Benign masseteric hypertrophy. *Surg. Clin. North Am.* 43:1357–1361, 1963.

Legg, J. W. Enlargement of the temporal and masseter muscles on both sides. *Transactions of the Pathological Society of London* 31:361–366, 1880.

Masters, F.; Georgiade, N.; and Pickrell, K. The surgical treatment of benign masseteric hypertrophy. *Plast. Reconstr. Surg.* 5:215–221, 1955.

Maxwell, J. H. Hypertrophy of the masseter muscle: a clinical entity. *AMA Arch. Otolaryngol.* 55:254–255, 1952.

Maxwell, J. H., and Waggoner, R. W. Hypertrophy of the masseter muscles. *Ann. Otol. Rhinol. Laryngol.* 60:538–548, 1951.

O'Hara, A. E. Sialography: past, present and future. *CRC Critical Reviews in Radiological Sciences* 4:87–139, 1973.

Silver, A. J., et al. Computed tomography of the nasopharynx and related spaces. *Radiology* 147:725–738, 1983.

Soderberg, B. N., and Switzer, W. E. Bilateral hypertrophy of the masseter muscles. *United States Armed Forces Medical Journal* 5:393–396, 1954.

Tempest, M. N. Simple unilateral hypertrophy of the masseter muscle. *Br. J. Plast. Surg.* 4:136–138, 1951.

Trodahl, J. N. Non-neoplastic disorders of muscle. In *Thoma's oral pathology,* ed. R. J. Gorlin and H. M. Goldman. St. Louis: C. V. Mosby Company, 1970, pp. 1071–1090.

Waldhart, E., and Lynch, J. B. Benign hypertrophy of the masseter muscles and mandibular angles. *Arch. Surg.* 102:115–118, 1971.

Index